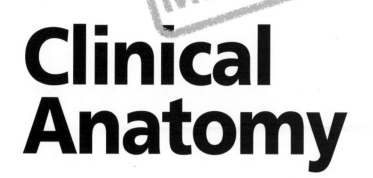

Clinical
Anatomy

Commissioning Editors: Ellen Green
Project Development Manager: Barbara Simmons
Project Controller: Nancy Arnott
Designer: Judith Wright

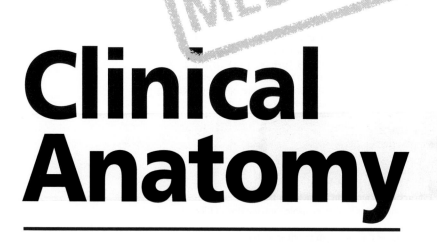

Clinical Anatomy

A core text with self-assessment

STANLEY MONKHOUSE

MA MB BChir PhD
University of Nottingham at Derby,
formerly Professor of Anatomy at the
Royal College of Surgeons in Ireland

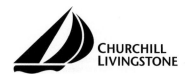

CHURCHILL
LIVINGSTONE

EDINBURGH LONDON NEW YORK OXFORD PHILADELPHIA ST LOUIS SYDNEY TORONTO 2001

CHURCHILL LIVINGSTONE
An imprint of Elsevier Limited

First published 2001
Reprinted 2004 (twice), 2005

ISBN 0 443 063958

British Library Cataloguing in Publication Data
A catalogue record for this book is available from the British Library

Library of Congress Cataloging in Publication Data
A catalog record for this book is available from the Library of Congress

Notice
Medical knowledge is constantly changing. Standard safety precautions must be
followed, but as new research and clinical experience broaden our knowledge,
changes in treatment and drug therapy may become necessary or appropriate.
Readers are advised to check the most current product information provided by
the manufacturer of each drug to be administered to verify the recommended
dose, the method and duration of administration, and contraindications. It is the
responsibility of the practitioner, relying on experience and knowledge of the
patient, to determine dosages and the best treatment for each individual patient.
Neither the Publisher nor the editors/contributor assumes any liability for any
injury and/or damage to persons or property arising from this publication.

The Publisher

ELSEVIER your source for books,
journals and multimedia
in the health sciences
www.elsevierhealth.com

Working together to grow
libraries in developing countries

www.elsevier.com | www.bookaid.org | www.sabre.org

ELSEVIER | BOOK AID International | Sabre Foundation

The
Publisher's
policy is to use
**paper manufactured
from sustainable forests**

Printed in Spain

Acknowledgements

I was introduced to anatomy by Max Bull and Gordon Wright, and I learned the importance of clinical anatomy at the feet of Rex Coupland. Students and patients in Nottingham and Dublin made me reflect on the boundary between 'need to know' and 'nice to know' and provoked me to seek new and better ways to get my message across. I have learned a great deal from my colleagues Andy Sparrow, Norman Thomas, Harold Browne, Clive Lee and, particularly, Tom Farrell, who has read drafts of this book and made a multitude of helpful suggestions. Ellen Green at Churchill Livingstone displayed great faith in me by inviting me to write this text, and I could not have done without Barbara Simmons and Sue Beasley, who helped to keep me on the rails. And finally, I thank Susan, Victoria, Hugh and Edward, with apologies for another summer ruined. To all these people I am indebted, and for them all I am thankful.

Contents

Using this book

This chapter explains how a big subject like anatomy, covered by some other textbooks in over 1000 pages, can be squashed into a small book like this. It also explains how the book is organised, and why, and gives some tips on how to study. In short, this introductory chapter aims:

1. to help you plan your learning
2. to show you how to use the book to increase your understanding as well as your knowledge
3. to show that self-assessment can make learning easier and more enjoyable.

Philosophy of the book

The effective diagnosis and management of disease, whatever the cause, depends upon some knowledge of structures that may be involved. In many disease conditions, symptoms and signs result not only from changes in the affected organ, but also from effects on neighbouring structures and from the spread of disease to them. This is why as a medical professional you need to know something about how the body is put together.

It is possible to learn anatomy in great detail. This has at least two disadvantages. Firstly, it is mind-numbingly boring, and secondly you may be lulled into a false sense of security: there is much variation from person to person, and from birth to death. So a choice has to be made: it has to be recognised that some items of information are important, and some are not; lines have to be drawn between 'need to know' and 'nice to know'. My decisions about where to draw these lines have been based on over 25 years of teaching and reflecting upon clinical anatomy, on over 10 years as a full-time or part-time medical practitioner, and on extensive experience as an examiner in all types of situations (discipline-based exams, integrated exams, postgraduate exams, exams for health care workers other than medical students). The questions I have asked myself when deciding whether or not to include something have generally been 'does it matter to the junior hospital doctor or general practitioner?' and 'does it aid the understanding of an important topic?' If the answer to both these questions is no, then the topic has been omitted. There are plenty more comprehensive books on the market that can be consulted if you want a more in-depth account.

Having said that, there are several topics that are considered in some depth. This is either because they are important and such knowledge is generally clinically useful, or else because a little more detail will, I hope, clarify a complex picture. In such situations I have tried to make it clear that you need not bother with the details. Also, from time to time I stray into physiology and other disciplines if I think it helpful to do so: my experience is that these short digressions are sometimes just the things that help important information to stick. The text, therefore, is more than just lists and bullet points for cramming: it is a mixture of zoological principles, functional and clinical considerations, and opinions. I hope that the inclusion of some explanatory material will stimulate rather than bore you, and that it will not obscure the basics.

Layout of the book

Section 1 (Chs 1–9) includes a consideration of anatomical terminology, followed by a brief survey of the body organised by the main physiological systems – this is systematic anatomy. In Section 2, from Chapter 10 onwards, the body is considered in more depth by region, one chapter for each major region. Within a chapter, each main topic is preceded by an overview and learning objectives. Use these as checklists so that nothing of major importance passes you by. The numerous clinical boxes scattered throughout the text will provide some focus for your study, and I recommend not only that you read these, but also reflect upon them. How are the symptoms produced? What other symptoms could accompany them? Might the manifestation of the disease depend upon anatomical variations? These are some of the questions that you should ask yourself.

Approach to study in general

I am a disorganised and undisciplined student and so I feel unworthy to offer advice to anyone, other than the following:

- Make a plan with realistic targets, but be prepared to adjust it if necessary.
- If a course and guidelines are available, attend and heed them diligently.

- Read about, and reflect upon, all learning material within 1 or 2 days of having considered it, and at most within a week.
- Discuss your studies with friends and colleagues (and I include educators as colleagues). You cannot be certain you have 'got' something until you have successfully explained it to someone else. (The look on the face of a previously perplexed student when the penny drops is one of the things that attracted me to teaching.) It also follows, then, that you can serve others by listening to their explanations. Such two-way sessions will probably be the most productive time you will ever spend educationally.
- If your goal is to pass an examination, find out everything you can about the format of the examination and get hold of as many past papers as possible. Then, when you feel you have done enough work, try to do the papers under exam conditions and discuss your answers with someone else – an examiner if possible, or a colleague if not.
- There is more to life than work: ignore this at your peril.
- Above all, think imaginatively.

Self-assessment

Questions are provided at the end of Section 1, and subsequently after each chapter. Do not be surprised to see that within these questions, the same items of information are tested in more than one question type: this is deliberate.

Multiple choice questions

You are required to mark each statement as true or false. Remember that within a group of five responses, all may be correct, or all may be incorrect. Negative marking is used in some centres, and not in others, so you would do well to find out what you will be confronted by. The combination of negative marking and guessing when you do not know the right answer is not recommended! These questions can easily be adapted to several formats: the simple true/false question; or the more complex, where the answer depends upon which responses are correct from each group of five.

Matching item questions

In these questions you must choose the option from the list provided that best fits the given statement or question. This type of question, not normally associated with negative marking (although there is no reason why it could not be), is used in United States licensing examinations, and similar exams for other bodies, and is used by several undergraduate schools. These questions can easily be adapted to fit multi-disciplinary ('integrated') assessments.

Short answers

Some of these questions require single items of information that may be needed in answering 'filling in the gaps' questions. Others require more extended responses in which there are several different ways of presenting the information, the choice being left up to you. In these, try to limit yourself to no more than one page, and aim to complete these longer questions well within 10 minutes. It is very important that you answer the question that is asked: if specific items of information are requested, you must give them: by all means give additional information if you wish, but not at the expense of what is required. Once again, the topics asked in these short answer questions can easily be adapted to fit multidisciplinary ('integrated') assessments, and you may find it useful to try to construct these questions for yourself.

Essays

I have not provided any titles for essay questions because I can see no purpose served by essays in clinical anatomy that is not better served by short notes, and from the point of view of the marker, short answers are much easier and quicker to deal with. If you are unfortunate enough to be confronted by anatomy essays, many of the short notes topics would serve.

Viva questions

As a visual subject, anatomy has traditionally been associated with visual recognition tests using photographs, living models or displayed specimens. This component of anatomy has traditionally been tested in viva voce (oral) exams. From a clinical point of view, it is essential that you are able to point to where something is: being able to write about it is of minor importance. I base most such assessments in which I am involved on radiographs and surface anatomy live models, using simple clinical skills to test anatomical information. As visual examinations, these assessments can be computer based, and some people, though by no means all, find the impersonal nature of computerised exams less challenging than being forced to indulge in conversation with a real live examiner!

Compose your own questions

You will find it very beneficial to try to construct your own examination questions, and then to produce your own model answers. This will highlight some of the difficulties, and it may give you some sympathy for the poor examiner.

Conclusions

You should amend the framework for using this book according to your own needs and the examinations you are facing. Although rote learning can not entirely be avoided, your aim should always be the acquisition of an understanding of the principles involved, rather than simply the tedious memorisation of a large number of apparently unrelated facts.

SECTION 1
Systematic anatomy

1 Introduction

Studying anatomy

Anatomy is a visual subject: ideally, you need to see, touch and feel to get an idea of three dimensions. When you read a portion of text you should try to picture the structures concerned: dissected parts and a good anatomical atlas, whether on paper or computer, will help.

Different people study differently, and some find an understanding of three dimensions easier to come by than do others. Nevertheless, as a basis for study I recommend that you use the nervous system and the main arteries, together with the following conceptual framework, common to all living things:

- we reproduce
- we seek sustenance
- we absorb and distribute nutrients
- we excrete waste products
- we try to prolong our own existence; and
- we endeavour to control these processes.

Surface markings and vertebral levels

The surface projection of internal organs is important since it forms the basis of the clinical examination of a patient. When you read about any structure, the heart for example, you should try to picture the body and relate the printed word to a precise location. Better still, get a friend to be a surface anatomy model (it is no good looking at yourself in a mirror because right and left are the wrong way round).

The horizontal level of a structure in the body is described by reference to the vertebra(e) at the same level – that is to say in the same transverse plane. This is known as 'the vertebral level'.

Both surface markings and vertebral levels are important and useful in the clinical context.

Study Figure 1.1 and note that:

- the suprasternal notch is at vertebral level T2
- the sternal angle is at vertebral level T4
- the xiphoid process is at vertebral level T9 (about)
- the surface marking of the gall bladder is the tip of the right ninth costal cartilage (at the anterior end of the ninth rib). Its vertebral level is L1.

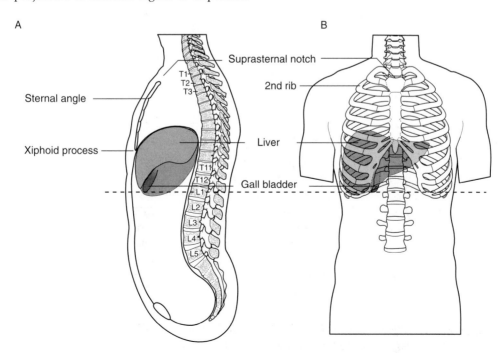

Fig. 1.1 Vertebral levels and surface markings using the gall bladder and liver as examples.
(**A**) Trunk: medial sagittal section. (**B**) Trunk: anterior view.

Regional anatomy and systematic anatomy

The cardiovascular and nervous systems are found in all parts of the body. The respiratory system is in the head, neck and thorax. The alimentary system is in the head, neck, thorax, abdomen and perineum. To study anatomy by systems is relevant to the particular system, but wasteful since it means that, for example, different parts of the thorax must be studied on different occasions for several systems. Study by systems also fails to give an appreciation of the fact that disease knows no boundaries: a bronchial carcinoma may cause symptoms in more than one system because the carcinoma may involve adjacent structures. Both approaches, systematic and regional, are important and after a superficial survey of the anatomically important systems, a regional approach is used in this book.

Prenatal development

Knowledge of prenatal development is necessary to understand how congenital anomalies arise, and it helps in appreciating why the structures of the body are as they are. Development itself is a consequence of history – the succession of living things – and of the demands of the embryo for nutrition and survival. This is not a textbook of embryology, or of anthropology or evolution, but occasional references to these topics will be made where it seems helpful.

Variation

You should bear in mind when you are studying anatomy or examining a patient that variations are found, and in some organs and systems, for example superficial veins, variations are common. Nevertheless, there are 'averages' and it is these, given in this book, that you should be familiar with.

Eponyms

Angle of Louis, foramen of Winslow, Hirschsprung's disease – who are these people? Why do we continue to use their names? Such eponyms are commonly used in medicine despite the best efforts of grey men and women to abolish them. They remind us of history and of personalities and they are sometimes easier to pronounce than the proper names. In this book I use the more commonly occurring eponyms, and give the proper names with them. You will hear eponyms used by others sooner or later, so you might as well start now.

2 Words and the anatomical position

Overview

Studying the medical sciences involves learning a new language, more than half of which is anatomical. A brief excursion into words and grammar is both desirable and necessary, and Table 2.1 gives some of the most commonly occurring words, prefixes and suffixes that you are unlikely to have met before in this context.

Learning Objectives

You should:

- be able to describe and demonstrate the anatomical position

- be able to demonstrate planes: coronal, sagittal, transverse

- have a reasonable working knowledge of the terms in Table 2.1

- try to discern the different components of medical and anatomical terms.

2.1 Anatomical position

Many words and descriptions assume the use of a standard position in relation to which surfaces and movements are defined. This is the anatomical position in which the body is pictured as standing erect with the palms of the hands facing forwards. This reference position is used irrespective of posture: your hand is *always* distal to your elbow, and your head *always* superior to your chest, even if you are upside down.

Relations: caution!

This word is used a great deal. It simply means geographical neighbours and it passes no comment on similarity. Related structures might be similar (e.g. arch of aorta and pulmonary artery), or they might not (arch of aorta and left main bronchus). The oesophagus is related to the left atrium of the heart – they are close neighbours (and this may matter clinically), but they are dissimilar in form and function.

Planes and movements   (Figs 2.1, 2.2)

Study Figures 2.1 and 2.2 and understand the meaning of the terms: you will need them in clinical work.

2.2 Singular and plural

Many anatomical and medical words are from Latin and Greek with plurals that are formed in ways other than by simply adding 's' or 'es'. A few of the more obvious examples are given in Table 2.2. Refer back to this table as necessary: as you become more familiar with its contents, you will be able to predict the meanings of new words when you encounter them for the first time.

2.3 Colloquial or correct?

When you stand in the anatomical position, your head is superior to your chest. In everyday language you say that your head is above your chest. Strict anatomists frown at colloquialisms like this, but they are in common use. In this book I switch between correct and colloquial terms as seems most natural to me. On the whole, I prefer the colloquial in the hope that readability is more important than pedantic fastidiousness. You need to remember, though, that the matter takes on great importance when the patients are lying down, as they so often are.

Table 2.1 Commonly used words, prefixes and suffixes

Term	Meaning and example
ab-	Away from. Abduct: move away from midline
ad-	Towards. Adduct: move towards midline
adeno-	Related to glands
afferent	Travelling towards. Afferent nerve impulse: towards the brain and spinal cord
anastomosis	Network (usually arteries or veins) receiving inputs from more than one source (plural: anastomoses)
anterior	Front (with reference to anatomical position); see ventral
-blast	Primitive cell or structure which gives rise to other cell type or structure. Osteoblast: primitive bone-forming cell. See -cyte
brachial	Pertaining to the arm (shoulder–elbow)
branchial	Associated with the entrance to the digestive system derived from primitive buccopharyngeal structures. Branchial structures are the successors of the gill apparatus in fish
bronchial	Pertaining to the bronchi
cancer	Malignant tumour
carcinoma	Cancer of epithelial (rather than connective tissue) origin
cardiac, -um	Heart
caudal	Nearer the tail (or where it would be). The kidneys are caudal to the diaphragm
cephalic	Nearer to, or pertaining to the head
coronal	Side-to-side plane which divides the structure into a front portion and a rear portion (not necessarily equal)
cranial	Nearer the head
-cyte	Cell. Mature cell type. Osteocyte: cell type found in bone. See -blast
deep	Far, or further, from the surface (see superficial)
distal to	Further away from. The foot is distal to the thigh (see proximal)
dorsal	Towards the back (with reference to anatomical position); similar to posterior in erect humans
-ectomy	Removal. Appendicectomy: removal of the appendix
efferent	Travelling away from. Efferent nerve impulse: away from the central nervous system
endo-	On the inside of. Endocardium: lining of the heart. Endometrium: lining of the uterus. Endoscopy: looking inside
endocrine	Secretion by a cell into its blood vessels (see exocrine)
epi-	On the surface of. Epithelium: all external surfaces. Epidermis: the epithelium of the skin
eversion	Turning the sole of the foot outwards (laterally)
ex-	Out of
exocrine	Secretion by a cell or group of cells into a duct for transport elsewhere (see endocrine)
extend	(Usually) straighten
extra-	Outside. Extracapsular: outside the capsule
fascia	Two meanings: Loose connective and fatty tissue, of variable thickness: superficial fascia, prevertebral fascia Fairly tough sheath or membrane: deep fascia, clavipectoral fascia
fasciculus	Group of axons of nerves all serving similar functions (same as tract)
flex	(Usually) bend
fistula	Artificial connection between two epithelial tubes
foramen	Opening or passage, often through bone
fossa	Depression, hollow, pit
ganglion	A swelling. In the context of the nervous system, its commonest usage, a ganglion is a collection of nerve cell bodies in the peripheral nervous system. It may be a sensory ganglion (without synapses), or an autonomic ganglion (with synapses). See nucleus
gyrus	Eminence of brain tissue between two sulci (see sulcus)
haemo-	Blood. Haemostasis: stagnation or sluggish flow of blood
hiatus	Gap, opening
hilum	Place where vessels and nerves enter
hyper-	Above, increase. Hyperplasia: increased cell division. Hypertrophy: increase in size (see hypo-)
hypo-	Below, decrease. Hypogastric: under the gastric area. Hypoplasia: decrease in cell division (see hyper-)
inferior	Below (with reference to anatomical position)
infundibulum	Funnel, funnel-like part of cavity
inter-	Between
intra-	Inside. Intracapsular: inside the capsule
inversion	Turning the sole of the foot inwards (medially)
-itis	Inflammation. Gastritis: inflammation of the stomach. Arthritis: inflammation of joint
lapar-	Abdomen. Laparoscopy: looking inside the abdomen. Laparotomy: opening the abdomen
lateral	Further from the midline (see medial)
ligament	Connective tissue tying together two or more structures (usually)
limbus	Edge, rim. Limbus of foramen ovale
lumen	Central cavity of a tube (artery, vein, intestine, etc.)
meatus	Pathway or passage

Table 2.1 (*Cont'd*)

Term	Meaning and example
medial	Nearer the midline (see lateral)
median	In the midline
meso-	Between
metrium	Uterus. Myometrium: uterine muscle; endometrium: uterine lining
mucus	Sticky liquid produced by glands. Mucus is a noun (see below)
mucous	Sticky (see serous): this is an adjective (see above)
myo-	Muscle. Myocardium: muscle of the heart
nucleus	In the context of the nervous system, a nucleus is a collection of cell bodies in the central nervous system (brain and spinal cord), all with a similar function. See ganglion
-oma	Swelling (tumour, not necessarily malignant). Lipoma: tumour of fat. Osteoma: bone tumour. Lymphoma: tumour of lymphoid tissues. Melanoma: tumour of cells containing melanin. And so on Malignant tumours. Carcinoma: malignant tumour of epithelial (surface) derivatives. Sarcoma: malignant tumour of connective (non-surface) tissue (bone, muscle, fat)
-ostomy	Making a permanent opening. Colostomy: permanent (or semipermanent) opening of the colon on to the abdominal surface. Tracheostomy: permanent (or semipermanent) opening into the trachea
-otomy	Making a small hole or temporary (e.g. emergency) opening. Laryngotomy: emergency opening into larynx
para-	By the side of, alongside. Paravertebral: by the side of the vertebral column
parietal	Concerning the walls of a cavity
peri-	Around or near. Periosteum: membrane covering the surface of bone
plexus	Network
posterior	Behind or rear (with reference to anatomical position); see dorsal
procto-	From proctodaeum – cloacal origin. Proctoscopy: observation of anal canal and terminal rectum
proximal to	Nearer to. The thigh is proximal to the foot. See distal
raphe	Seam. Line of union of separate parts
sagittal	Front-to-back plane which divides the structure into a right portion and a left portion (not necessarily equal)
sarcoma	Cancer of connective tissue (rather than epithelial) origin
serous	Thin, watery (see mucous)
sinus	Cavity or channel
somatic	Of, or derived from, body wall or somites: skeleton, skeletal (voluntary) muscle and associated connective tissue, and the skin and its appendages (breast, sweat glands, hair, nails, teeth). Nerves that supply these structures tend to be under voluntary control (if motor) and sensation from these structures tends to be immediately and precisely perceptible
sphincter	Muscular valve capable of closing a tube
splanchnic	Much the same as visceral – see later (splanchnic is from the Greek, visceral from the Latin. We do not need two terms, but we have them)
squamous	Flattened, scale-like
stasis	Lack of movement, stagnation. Haemostasis: stagnation of blood
synapse	The site where the terminal of one nerve transmits its electrical impulse to another, separate, nerve
sulcus	Gutter, depression
superficial	Near, or nearer, the surface (see deep)
superior	Above (with reference to anatomical position)
tendon	Attaching muscle to bone
tract	Group of axons of nerves all serving similar functions
ventral	Towards the front (belly) (with reference to anatomical position); similar to anterior in erect humans
visceral	Concerning internal organs (viscus, viscera). Nerves that supply these structures tend to be under involuntary control (if motor) and sensation from these structures tends to be vague and imprecisely perceptible or even imperceptible
viscus	Originally, hollow organ, but now used for any internal organ (liver, spleen, etc.)

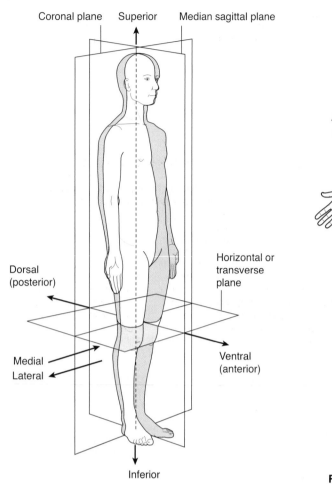

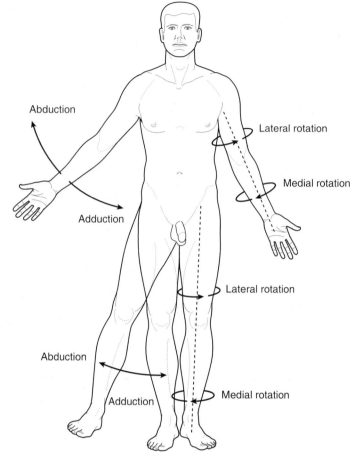

Fig. 2.1 Planes. A plane parallel to the median (sagittal) plane is a parasagittal plane.

Fig. 2.2

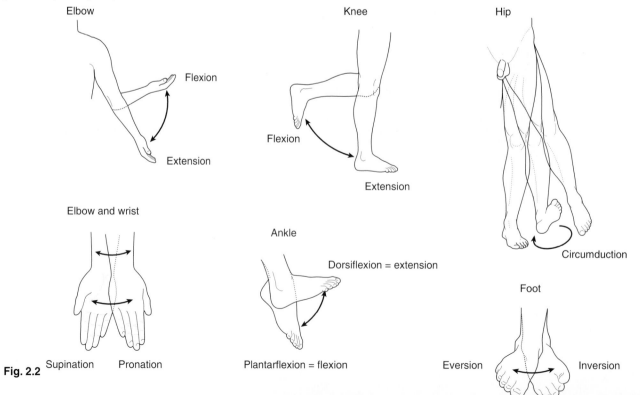

Fig. 2.2

Fig. 2.2 (*Opposite page*) Movements. The terms used in this figure are applicable to most joints, not just those illustrated. The exceptions are pronation and supination (elbow and wrist only), plantarflexion and dorsiflexion (ankle only), and inversion and eversion (foot only). Note that at the knee, flexion is apparently contrary to flexion at the elbow (it is not in fact: there is an embryological explanation for this, as you will see).

Table 2.2 Anatomical words: singular and plural

Change in word ending	Examples	
	Singular	Plural
-um to -a	atrium, diverticulum, epithelium, hilum, etc.	atria, diverticula, epithelia, hila, etc.
-a to -ae	bursa, fossa, placenta	bursae, fossae, placentae (but see below)
-us to -i	gyrus, sulcus	gyri, sulci (see below for meatus, plexus)
-is to -es	metastasis, symphysis, testis	metastases, symphyses, testes
Other	foramen	foramina
	ganglion	ganglia
	meninx (rarely used)	meninges
	phalanx	phalanges
	viscus	viscera

Note. Classical languages should not be used wantonly: these words are now English words and so English plurals can be used, I think, wherever possible. The plurals of meatus and plexus are best rendered as meatuses and plexuses: their Latin plurals are meatus and plexus (spelt the same, pronounced differently). But I am not consistent: I prefer bursas to bursae, fossas to fossae, and placentas to placentae, but would not accept diverticulums!

3 Outline of the body plan

Overview

The human body is built like that of all vertebrates. The trunk consists of a body wall surrounding central cavities that exist in order to allow internal organs to move independently of the wall. These cavities are the pleural (for the lungs), pericardial (for the heart) and peritoneal (for the intestines). Limbs are outgrowths of the body wall. The head houses the brain and main sense organs, and at the other end of the trunk the perineum deals with body effluent and sexual function. The external aspect of the body is covered by skin and skin appendages.

Learning Objectives

You should:

- understand the trunk as a hollow container with walls

- understand that the limbs are outgrowths of the walls of the trunk

- know the names of the body cavities and serous membranes

- understand that the body wall contains skeletal tissue and muscle

- know the difference between superficial and deep fascia.

3.1 A survey of the body

The anatomy of the human body is based upon the plan common to all vertebrates.

- The trunk (thorax, abdomen, pelvis) houses the internal organs (respiratory, digestive, urinary and internal genital).
- Limbs are outgrowths of the wall of the trunk. These are for locomotion, feeding and communicating.
- The head and neck house the brain and the entrance to the digestive and respiratory tracts. Since, in quadrupeds, the head leads the way into new environments, it also houses the special sense organs.
- The perineum, at the other end of the trunk, deals with the effluent from the digestive and urinary systems, and includes the external genitalia (in short, sphincters and sex). Many regard the perineum as part of the trunk.
- The nervous system serves all regions. The functions of the nervous system are control and communication.
- The vascular system serves all regions, delivering nutrients, removing waste products, acting as a transport medium and playing a part in communication (blushing).

3.2 Section through the trunk
(Fig. 3.1)

Body wall

The body wall is composed of muscle and skeletal material (bone, cartilage) covered externally by skin. It encloses the serous cavities that contain the gut tube and its derivatives, and other internal organs.

Serous cavities: pleural, pericardial, peritoneal

Internal organs that require freedom to move are partially enclosed by a potential space, derived from the embryonic coelom, to facilitate this movement. This develops into the serous cavities (serous because they

A

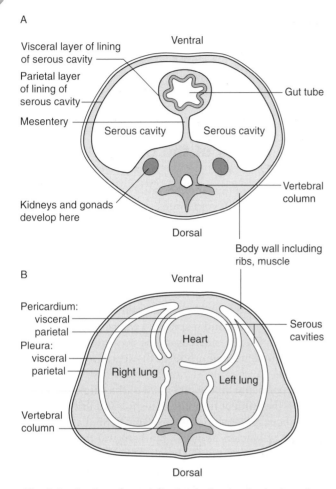

Visceral layer of lining of serous cavity

Parietal layer of lining of serous cavity

Mesentery

Ventral

Gut tube

Serous cavity   Serous cavity

Kidneys and gonads develop here

Vertebral column

Dorsal

Body wall including ribs, muscle

B

Ventral

Pericardium:
  visceral
  parietal
Pleura:
  visceral
  parietal

Heart

Serous cavities

Right lung

Left lung

Vertebral column

Dorsal

Fig. 3.1 Sections through the trunk showing the body wall, internal organs, gut tube and serous cavities. (**A**) Schematic section through the developing abdomen, viewed from below, showing the gut tube free to move within the serous (abdominal) cavity, except for being tethered posteriorly by the mesentery. Note the parietal (body wall) and visceral layers of the lining of the serous cavity. The apparently large extent of the serous cavity is not a true representation since the abdomen becomes filled with coils of intestine. (**B**) A schematic section through the thorax, viewed from below, showing three serous cavities: pericardial and right and left pleural. Note that the cavities, although surrounding most of the heart and lungs, are very narrow. Again, they allow movement as one surface moves on the other.

contain a small amount of lubricating fluid) and the membrane that lines such a cavity is a serous membrane. The serous cavities and membranes in the human are:

- pleural cavities (sometimes called thoracic cavities) permitting movement of lungs during breathing; serous membrane: pleura
- pericardial cavity, permitting movement of the heart as it beats; serous membrane: pericardium
- peritoneal or abdominopelvic cavity, permitting movement of intestines during digestion; serous membrane: peritoneum.

Serous membranes: parietal and visceral layers

The serous membranes secrete lubricating fluid.

- The layer of serous membrane that lines the body wall is the parietal layer.
- The layer of serous membrane that covers the surface of the internal organ is the visceral layer.

Figure 3.1 shows that these two parts are continuous at the point where the internal organ and body wall remain connected by tissue, allowing the passage of nerves, arteries, veins and lymphatics between the internal organ and the body wall. This connection is in some places (e.g. for some of the intestines in the abdomen) elongated to form a mesentery (Fig. 3.1A), a thin sheet covered on both sides by serous membrane, and in other sites the connection remains confined to a small area (e.g. for the lungs), the root or hilum (Fig. 3.1B).

3.3 Fascia and layers

Fascia is a term used in relation to the soft tissues of the body, and most often the body wall where it has two distinct meanings.

- *Superficial fascia.* This is simply loose connective and fatty tissue found immediately beneath the skin. It contains collagen, fat, elastic fibres, and connective tissue. It is variable in thickness: there are regional differences within an individual, and fat people have more than thin people.
- *Deep fascia.* This is a tough fibrous membrane that encircles compartments within the body, particularly in the limbs where it is attached to ridges on the limb bones. It forms partitions which create fascial compartments, sometimes important in limiting the spread of disease.

3.4 Skin

The skin is a barrier, an excretory organ (sodium), a synthetic organ (vitamin D), and a temperature control organ (sweating). The epithelium (external surface) of the skin is the epidermis. It is not necessary to spend much time on the skin except for a few points of clinical importance.

Langer's lines

The orientation of connective and elastic tissue in the skin means that when it is cut in certain planes the edges will lie together, but when it is cut in other planes, the edges will gape. This is important in wound healing: a cut whose edges are gaping will heal less well and with more scarring than a cut whose edges lie together. The (invisible) cleavage lines along which cuts should be made for best healing are Langer's lines and are as shown in Figure 3.2.

Appendages

These are nails, hair, teeth (some people would argue with this), and, in other creatures, horns, hooves and shells. It is worth noting that as you get older your nails become more and more like hooves, and in some cases become long, curved and tough so that they are extremely difficult to trim: onychogryphosis.

Glands

Glands opening onto the surface of the skin are exocrine glands.

- Sweat glands are for temperature control – sweating is a cooling mechanism – and are controlled by the sympathetic nervous system. They also excrete sodium chloride. In the external acoustic meatus (ear canal) these glands are called ceruminous glands because they produce wax (cerumen).
- Sebaceous glands are associated with hair follicles. The sebum they produce is for waterproofing. When their ducts become blocked, sebaceous cysts arise. A boil is an infected sebaceous gland.

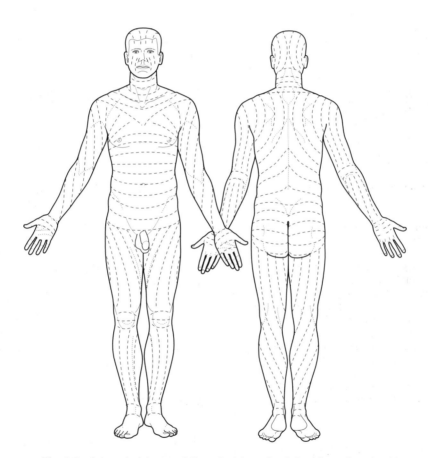

Fig. 3.2 Langer's (cleavage) lines. Incisions that follow these lines heal better than those that do not.

4 Skeleton and muscle

Overview

Skeletal tissue exists for mechanical support. The structure and rigidity of bone reflect its weightbearing function and it is well supplied with blood. Bone formation (ossification) occurs in two ways: direct from membrane, and by means of a cartilaginous precursor. Ossification is not complete until late adolescence, thus allowing bone growth to take place. Joints can be classified as non-synovial (limited movement) and synovial (extensive movement). Another function of bone is the manufacture of blood cells (haemopoiesis). Skeletal muscle (histologically striated) is supplied by voluntary nerve impulses. Smooth muscle is supplied by involuntary nerve impulses. Cardiac muscle, although striated, has intrinsic contractility and is supplied by involuntary nerves.

Learning Objectives

You should:

- understand the role of cartilage and bone

- understand the blood supply of bone and how bone grows

- know the different types of joints and their relative mobility

- know the different characteristics of skeletal, smooth and cardiac muscle

- understand that skeletal muscles work in groups that usually share a common nerve supply.

4.1 Skeleton

Cartilage and bone provide mechanical support. Cartilage is more flexible than bone but confers insufficient rigidity to withstand gravity (large cartilaginous creatures are aquatic, where gravity matters less). Some cartilages remain more or less the same throughout life, while others undergo a gradual conversion to bone – ossification – which takes place before birth or during childhood and adolescence.

Bony skeleton   (Fig. 4.1)

- Axial skeleton: skull, hyoid, vertebral column (including the sacrum), ribs, and sternum.
- Appendicular skeleton: pectoral and pelvic girdles, limb bones:
    - pectoral girdle: clavicle, scapula
    - upper limb: humerus, radius, ulna, carpal bones, metacarpals, phalanges
    - pelvic girdle: hip bone (ilium, ischium, pubis)
    - lower limb: femur, tibia, fibula, tarsal bones, metatarsals, phalanges.

Sesamoid bones are bones that develop in tendons as they cross joints. The patella is an example, and there are others in the wrist and the feet.

Section through bone   (Fig. 4.2)

Important terms are:

- Cortical or compact bone: dense bone around the edges.
- Cancellous, trabecular or spongy bone in which the lines of mechanical stress are evident in the structure of the bone.
- Periosteum: the membranous covering. It has two layers: outer fibrous and inner cellular. The inner layer is vascular and contains stem cells which can when required differentiate into osteoblasts, for example in healing and repair. Damage to periosteum impairs bone healing.
- The medullary (marrow) cavity. This and the spaces in cancellous bone contain haemopoietic (blood-forming) cells; there is therefore a profuse arterial supply.

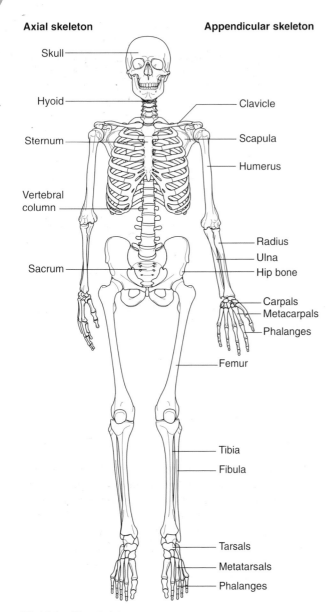

Axial skeleton

Skull

Hyoid

Sternum

Vertebral column

Sacrum

Appendicular skeleton

Clavicle

Scapula

Humerus

Radius

Ulna

Hip bone

Carpals

Metacarpals

Phalanges

Femur

Tibia

Fibula

Tarsals

Metatarsals

Phalanges

Fig. 4.1 The skeleton.

Parts of a long bone

- Head: one end, usually the proximal.
- Neck: the area immediately distal to the head.
- Shaft: the central long portion.
- Condyles: rounded articular surfaces.
- Epicondyles: prominences adjacent to condyles.
- Epiphysis: the name given to the developing ends of a long bone (see later).

Arterial supply of a long bone (Fig. 4.3)

- A large nutrient artery enters through the nutrient foramen (Fig. 4.3 – A). Branches of this reach the ends of a mature long bone, but not of a developing long bone (see below).

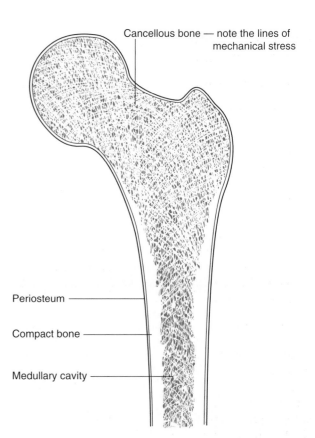

Cancellous bone — note the lines of mechanical stress

Periosteum

Compact bone

Medullary cavity

Fig. 4.2 Longitudinal section through part of a bone. The periosteum is closely applied to the surface of the bone.

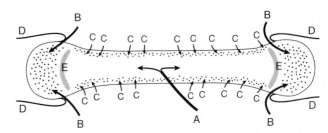

Fig. 4.3 Arterial supply of a long bone: A, nutrient artery; B, retinacular vessels entering at the attachment of the joint capsule; C, numerous small arteries; D, joint capsules; E (shaded area) site of epiphyseal plates of hyaline cartilage in immature bone (absent in mature bones).

- Capsular (retinacular) vessels enter the bone with the attachments of the joint capsule (Fig. 4.3 – B).
- Many small arteries penetrate the periosteum directly, particularly at the site of muscular attachments and near joints (Fig. 4.3 – C).
- Bones have a particularly rich blood supply because haemopoiesis (formation of blood components) takes place in the central marrow cavity.

Ossification and bone growth, the epiphyseal plate

Bone is formed in two principal ways:

- *Membranous (periosteal) ossification.* Osteoblasts from the periosteum invade fetal connective tissue, converting it directly to bone. The clavicle and the flat bones of the skull vault ossify in this manner.
- *Endochondral ossification.* Most bones ossify by passing through an intermediate cartilaginous stage. Fetal connective tissue is converted to cartilage by chondroblasts. This cartilaginous model of the bone may persist for months or years before itself being converted by osteoblasts to bone with the accompanying laying down of minerals, calcium and phosphate. Ossification is not completed until growth has finally ceased.

The ends of bone – the epiphyses – are the last parts of a long bone to ossify, and until then they remain separated from the shaft of the bone by the epiphyseal plate of hyaline cartilage (Fig. 4.3 – E). Since these epiphyseal plates are the sites of growth in length, they are also known as growth plates. Blood vessels never cross epiphyseal plates and so the nutrient artery of the shaft contributes no supply to the ends of a developing long bone until after the epiphyseal plate has disappeared with final fusion of all the components of a bone. This matters: damage to the blood supply can result in death (necrosis) of the bony tissue and if this affects the growing end of a bone in children, normal development may be delayed or prevented. If it affects part of a bone that participates in a joint, movement will be affected.

Bone growth does not stop when ossification is complete: there is a continuous process of bony remodelling in response to altered stress.

Secretion of too much growth hormone before epiphyseal fusion results in gigantism, and after fusion, acromegaly (large extremities). Achondroplasia is a hereditary defect of endochondral ossification in which long bones of the limb fuse early giving short limbs, while the trunk and skull develop normally. Adolescent athletes who use growth hormone will find that it prolongs the life of the epiphyseal plate and delays the fusion of the ends of any long bones not yet united. This can have serious consequences.

4.2 Joints (Fig. 4.4)

Bones confer rigidity; joints permit movement. They may be classified on the basis of structure as fibrous, cartilaginous or synovial. From a clinical point of view, a better classification is simply non-synovial

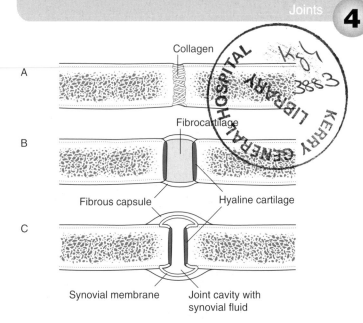

Fig. 4.4 Different types of joints: (**A**) fibrous; (**B**) secondary cartilaginous (symphysis); (**C**) synovial.

and synovial, the former including both fibrous and cartilaginous.

Non-synovial joints

Fibrous joints (Fig. 4.4A)

Two bones are bound together by fibrous tissue. Examples are the inferior tibiofibular joint, part of the ankle, a tooth fitting into the tooth socket (gomphosis), and joints (sutures) between bones of the skull vault. Fibrous joints permit little movement, except that fetal skull bones may move on each other before and during birth, but during early childhood movement becomes increasingly restricted.

Cartilaginous joints

These allow more movement. There are two types:

- *Primary cartilaginous joints* (not illustrated in Fig. 4.4). In these, bony tissue is separated by hyaline cartilage. The junction between the shaft and epiphysis of a long bone constitutes a primary cartilaginous joint. As the constituent parts of a long bone fuse during childhood and adolescence, primary cartilaginous joints gradually disappear, and in an adult there are only a few remaining, most notably the joint between the first rib and the sternum.
- *Secondary cartilaginous joints or symphyses* (Fig. 4.4B). In these, two articular surfaces are each covered by hyaline cartilage and between them is a fibrocartilaginous disc. They are found in the midline of the body and include the joints between

neighbouring vertebral bodies, the joint between the two pubic bones (the pubic symphysis) and the joints between the parts of the sternum.

Age changes in cartilaginous joints. As age advances, cartilaginous joints may ossify, thus limiting movement. This occurs as a matter of course in primary cartilaginous joints (see above) and may occur in secondary cartilaginous joints. The last joint in the body to fuse in this way is that between the sphenoid and occipital bones of the skull in the mid-twenties. This is one reason why the shape of the face and head continues to change until that time.

Synovial joints (Fig. 4.4C)

In a synovial joint, articular surfaces are covered by articular cartilage (usually hyaline, sometimes fibrous) and between them is the synovial cavity limited externally by the joint capsule. Synovial membrane lines the inner aspect of the capsule and any other non-articular surface within the joint. It is important to note that synovial membrane does not cover the articular surfaces themselves. Movement is much freer at these joints, and in some cases extensive. Freedom of movement and stability are mutually incompatible: the more movement, the less stability. Joints at which a wide range of movement is permitted are associated with other means of conferring stability, such as muscles and ligaments.

Why synovial? Synovium is the name given to a specialised connective tissue that produces synovial fluid to lubricate the articular surfaces. Along with peri-cardium, pleura, and peritoneum it is often regarded as one of the serous membranes of the body – all involved in permitting one surface to move on another.

Types of synovial joints

A simple classification, depending upon the number of planes in which movement takes place, is:

- Plane: articular surfaces almost flat for gliding movements, e.g. some carpal joints
- Hinge: movement in one plane, e.g. elbow
- Pivot: movement around a pivot, e.g. atlanto-axial
- Saddle: saddle-shaped articular surfaces, allow movement in two planes, e.g. first carpometacarpal joint
- Ball and socket: relatively unrestricted movement, e.g. shoulder, hip.

Synovial membrane outside joints: bursas, synovial sheaths

Synovial membrane is found outside joints in places where friction resistance is necessary. There are many sites in the body where a muscle tendon or a bulky muscle passes over a bony prominence or beneath a fibrous band, often as a corner is turned. Anatomical arrangements to reduce friction at these sites include isolated synovial cavities between the opposing surfaces: bursas and synovial sheaths.

Bursas. These are bags of synovial membrane and fluid found between tendons or muscles and skin or bone. They may be entirely separate from joints (even if near them), or they may be extensions of the synovial cavity of a joint. Examples of bursas are found in association with the shoulder and knee joints, but they occur elsewhere as well.

Synovial sheaths. These are synovial cavities wrapped around tendons running in confined spaces, notably the wrist, hand and ankle. They will be described in more detail with the limbs.

Nerve supply of joints

Bones and joints are richly supplied with sensory nerve endings: bony and articular trauma and disease are painful. Sensory fibres from joints are found in all nerves supplying muscles that act upon the joint. In general, nerves that supply joints also supply the muscles that act on them, together with the skin over the bony attachments of those muscles: this is Hilton's law, and it is a useful aid to memory.

Diseases of joints and synovium

- Articular surfaces may degenerate, as in osteoarthritis. This may limit movement and eventually such changes may result in two adjacent bones becoming fused.
- Synovium may become inflamed causing pain and limitation of movement. Rheumatoid arthritis is a serious disease in which inflamed and swollen synovium may become trapped between articular surfaces such that it is damaged. This results in more inflammation and swelling, more synovial damage and more limitation of movement … and so on.
  - Inflammation of a bursa: bursitis.
  - Inflammation of a synovial sheath: synovitis.
  - Inflammation of both the synovial sheath and the tendon within it: tenosynovitis.
  - Inflammation of a synovial joint: arthritis.

4.3 Muscle

All cells are potentially capable of movement as a result of contractile proteins within them. Muscle tissue is made up of cells that are specialised for movement, and the more organised the tissue structure is, the quicker and more powerful the movement.

Skeletal muscle: voluntary

Skeletal muscle is supplied by voluntary nerve impulses. Histologically it is striated muscle – that is to say the contractile proteins are so well organised as to give rise to striations visible on microscopy. Skeletal muscle is attached to the skeleton and so causes movements of the trunk or limbs. It is also known as somatic muscle.

Visceral muscle: involuntary

Visceral muscle is supplied by involuntary nerve impulses. It is found in the wall of blood vessels and internal organs (viscera) derived from embryonic cells associated with the wall of the yolk sac or its derivatives.

- Smooth muscle is found in blood vessels and internal organs except the heart.
- Cardiac or heart muscle is striated.

Branchial arch muscle: voluntary

In the head and neck there is a third type of muscle associated with the cranial end of the gut tube (muscles of the mouth, pharynx and larynx). It is therefore visceral, but the muscles are supplied by voluntary nerves and are histologically striated. It is called branchial arch muscle because it is derived embryologically from the branchial (gill) arches.

Muscle attachments

A skeletal muscle is typically attached at both ends to bones. The muscle fibres themselves may be directly attached to an area of bone, or the muscle may form a tendon or aponeurosis (a flattened tendon) which is attached to a small area of the bone. When the muscle contracts, the two bones are approximated, causing movement at the joint between them. It is customary to speak of a muscle as causing a certain movement of a joint: 'biceps flexes the elbow' is preferable to 'biceps flexes the arm'. Some muscles cause movement at more than one joint because they are attached to bones separated by two or more joints. Biceps in the upper limb is such a muscle since it crosses two joints, the elbow and the shoulder. It follows that the action of biceps can be modified by activity of other muscles which stabilise one or other of the joints that biceps crosses.

Some voluntary muscles are attached at one end to the deeper layers of the skin, for example the muscles of facial expression which, when they contract, cause facial movements for expression of emotion, and communication.

Sites of muscle attachments to bone

Muscles are attached to bones either:

- directly, when the muscle fibres themselves are attached to a fairly extensive area of bone
- indirectly, when the muscle fibres converge into a tendon or an aponeurosis (flattened tendon, like a membrane) which attaches to a smaller area of bone.

Wherever a muscle or tendon is attached to a bone, the bony surface will be rough. Such an area is often sufficiently raised above the neighbouring surface to be called a process, a tuberosity, a tubercle, or a trochanter (different words for much the same thing).

It follows that a bony surface that is smooth is free of muscle attachments – indeed, such areas are often directly subcutaneous (e.g. the anteromedial surface of the tibia). You read earlier that arteries enter bones at the site of muscle attachments, and at such bony surfaces that lack muscle attachments the arterial supply is relatively poor. Since the healing process requires a generous blood supply, healing after injury may be impaired. Again, the subcutaneous surface of the tibia is a good example.

Origins, insertion, attachments

The relatively more fixed end of a muscle is known as the origin, and the relatively more mobile end as the insertion. However, there are many cases when one end of a muscle may be more fixed in a certain movement, and the other end more fixed in another movement, depending upon the posture of the body or the action being performed. For example, when you are sitting and you raise your thigh, the proximal end of the thigh muscles is more fixed and the distal end more mobile. But if you then put your feet on the ground and stand up, the distal end of the thigh muscles becomes relatively more fixed since you are raising your vertebral column upon a relatively stable lower limb. For these reasons and others, the term attachments is perfectly satisfactory. The tedious memorising of origins and insertions is quite unnecessary.

Muscle groups

Muscles rarely act in isolation. They are found as part of a group of muscles usually supplied by the same nerve and within one fascial (connective tissue) compartment, and it is the group as a whole that acts. It is more useful clinically to talk of the extensor muscles of the thigh, or the flexor muscles of the arm than to worry about individual muscles within those groups. So not only need you not worry about remembering which end of a muscle is the origin and which the insertion, in many cases you need not worry about individual muscles – only muscle groups. The text will identify those individual muscles that you need to be concerned about.

5 Vertebral column

Overview

The vertebral column provides support. Flexibility is provided by its arrangement into individual vertebrae: 7 cervical, 12 thoracic, 5 lumbar and 5 fused to form the sacrum. Vertebrae are separated by intervertebral discs. Ligaments pass between equivalent parts of adjacent vertebrae to form a ligamentous and bony tube containing the spinal cord. Movements of the column are constrained by the anatomy of individual regions of the column and the rib cage. The venous plexuses around the column and inside the vertebral canal are important in the spread of disease, particularly from the lower abdomen and pelvis.

Learning Objectives

You should:

- know the bones that make up the vertebral column

- understand how the characteristics of vertebrae of the four main regions reflect function

- understand the function and disposition of intervertebral discs

- know the main movements of the column and the muscles that produce them

- understand how the column is supplied with blood, and how its veins are important in the spread of disease.

5.1 Vertebrae

The vertebral column confers rigidity on the trunk: it is an adaptation to deal with gravity. A solid, rigid column would confer maximum rigidity, but then movement would be virtually impossible, so the column is broken up into individual vertebrae as follows:

- 7 cervical
- 12 thoracic (sometimes called dorsal, but this is misleading since they are no more dorsal than the others)
- 5 lumbar
- 5 sacral, fused into one bone, the sacrum
- a few coccygeal which are very small and may be fused; forget about them.

5.2 Intervertebral discs

Intervertebral discs are found between all vertebrae from C2 to S1. They consist of:

- an annulus fibrosus: tough hyaline cartilaginous rim, and
- a nucleus pulposus: fibrocartilaginous core, softer, probably derived from remnants of the notochord.

Rupture of the annulus fibrosus may allow the softer nucleus pulposus to herniate and this may compress the spinal cord or segmental nerve roots in the spinal (vertebral) canal of the vertebral column. This is often somewhat inaccurately referred to as a slipped disc. The symptoms of this condition will depend upon at which level it occurs and which structures are affected.

There is no disc between the base of the skull and vertebra C1 or between vertebrae C1 and C2; this is because of the specialised movements which take place here (see Ch. 14, p. 222).

5.3 Typical vertebra (Fig. 5.1)

Note the following components of vertebrae:

- Body
- Neural arch around the vertebral canal containing the spinal cord:
  - pedicle (joining the body to the transverse process)

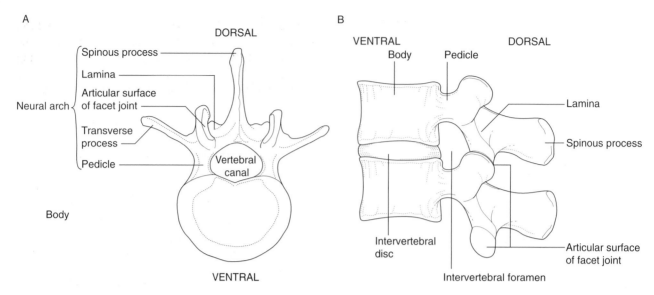

Fig. 5.1 A typical vertebra: (**A**) from above/below; (**B**) from the side. Note the intervertebral foramen through which the spinal nerve passes.

- transverse process
- articular process forming synovial 'facet' joints with the vertebrae above and below
- lamina (joining the transverse process to the spinous process)
- spinous process.

5.4 Regional variations in vertebrae

Cervical vertebrae have:

- a triangular vertebral canal
- a foramen in each transverse process for arteries and veins
- a bifid (two-pronged) spinous process (except C1, C7).

The atlas and axis (C1, C2) are specialised for movement: see Chapter 14.

Thoracic vertebrae have:

- facets for rib articulations
- a spinous process orientated in a marked inferior direction.

Lumbar vertebrae are identifiable by their large size. Sacral vertebrae are fused to form the sacrum.

Junctional zones

Vertebra C7 has some features (for example the non-bifid spinous process) of a thoracic vertebra. Vertebra T12 has some features, notably the bulk, of a lumbar vertebra.

Fusion of vertebra L5 to the sacrum, giving a six-segment sacrum, is known as sacralisation of L5. Separation of vertebra S1 from the sacrum, leaving a four-segment sacrum and six 'lumbar' vertebrae, is lumbarisation of S1. These two conditions will affect strength and mobility and a free S1 vertebra that is out of alignment may compress spinal nerve roots.

Surface anatomy

- *C7.* When you flex your neck and drop your chin onto your chest, the most prominent vertebral spinous process is that of C7 – the vertebra prominens. This is useful clinically should you want to determine a particular vertebral level.
- *L3/4.* A line joining the highest points of the right and left iliac crests intersects the midline at (usually) the L3/L4 junction. This is useful clinically since this level is the usual site for lumbar puncture (see Ch. 6, p. 40).

Spinal curvatures   (Fig. 5.2)

A dorsal convexity is a kyphosis; a dorsal concavity is a lordosis; and a side-to-side bending is a scoliosis.

Before birth the entire vertebral column is kyphotic. After birth, with the demands of weightbearing and the effects of gravity, the cervical and lumbar regions become lordotic. The thoracic and sacral kyphoses are said to be primary curvatures (because they are present at birth); the cervical and lumbar lordoses are secondary curvatures (because they develop subsequently). Age changes in the vertebral bodies and intervertebral discs result in increasing kyphosis as the years advance, more marked in some people than others.

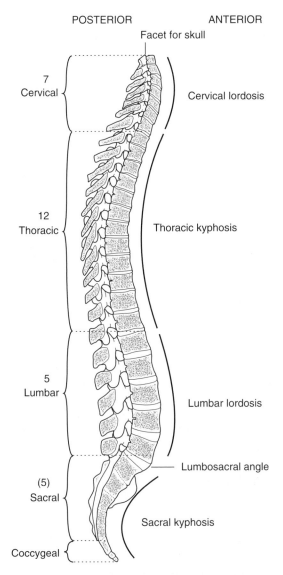

POSTERIOR   ANTERIOR

Facet for skull

7
Cervical — Cervical lordosis

12
Thoracic — Thoracic kyphosis

5
Lumbar — Lumbar lordosis

— Lumbosacral angle

(5)
Sacral — Sacral kyphosis

Coccygeal

Fig. 5.2 Spinal curvatures: median section of vertebral column.

Degrees of scoliosis vary with posture (postural scoliosis), although marked scoliotic deformities, most often developing in adolescent girls, require treatment.

5.5 Joints, ligaments and movements

Each vertebra articulates with the one above and the one below by means of:

- a midline cartilaginous joint – intervertebral disc
- two lateral synovial joints between transverse processes – one on each side. These are often called 'facet' joints.

The movements are flexion, extension and lateral flexion to both sides. All joints are involved in all these movements to some extent, and disease of the facet joints can be particularly troublesome because of the proximity of the joint to the segmental nerves passing through the intervertebral foramina. This can give rise to both back pain at the site of the injury or disease, and pain perceived in the skin and other structures served by the nerve affected (referred pain).

Ligaments of the vertebral column
(Fig. 5.3)

- Anterior longitudinal ligament: connecting the anterior surfaces of the vertebral bodies.
- Posterior longitudinal ligament: on the anterior wall of the vertebral canal, connecting the posterior surfaces of the vertebral bodies. This narrows as it descends and is at its narrowest in the lumbar region, just where the spine bears most weight. In this region, therefore, with a combination of a heavy load and a narrow ligament, herniation of the intervertebral discs is most likely. Such herniations in a posterolateral direction may impinge on the nerve roots or on the spinal cord itself, depending upon the level, causing pain both locally and in the distribution of the nerve concerned.
- Ligamentum flavum: connecting adjacent laminae. This ligament is pierced by a needle (e.g. in lumbar puncture) inserted from behind.
- Articular ligaments. All synovial articulations between the ribs and the vertebral column, and all the synovial facet joints are surrounded by ligaments which may be injured.
- There are also ligaments joining adjacent vertebral spines (interspinous, supraspinous ligaments).

Muscles

Contraction of the muscles of the abdominal wall causes flexion and lateral flexion of the vertebral column. They are assisted by other muscles, depending upon posture, such as lower limb muscles (for example, psoas).

The large muscle bulk posterior and lateral to the vertebral column, between the vertebral spines and the rib cage, is sacrospinalis, sometimes, not strictly accurately, known as erector spinae muscles. They are the postvertebral muscles supplied by the posterior rami of all segmental nerves. You do not need to know the names or attachments of the muscles, but you should realise that they are responsible for maintaining our erect posture and are in constant use during loco-motion and as we shift our weight during postural changes of all descriptions.

At the cranial end immediately below the skull, this group includes the suboccipital muscles supplied by

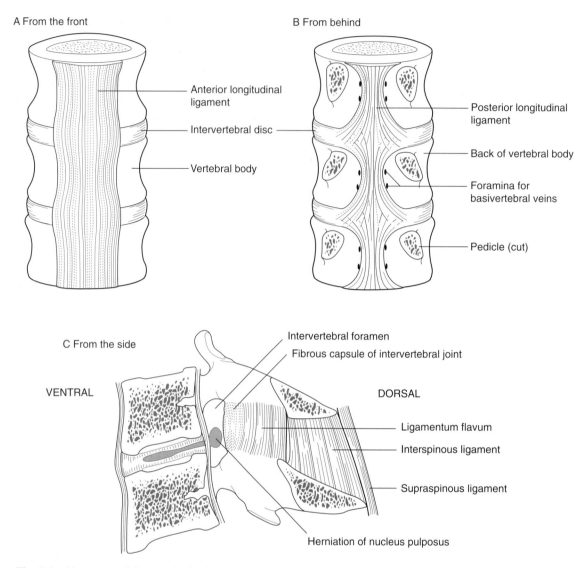

A From the front

Anterior longitudinal ligament

Intervertebral disc

Vertebral body

B From behind

Posterior longitudinal ligament

Back of vertebral body

Foramina for basivertebral veins

Pedicle (cut)

C From the side

Intervertebral foramen

Fibrous capsule of intervertebral joint

VENTRAL

DORSAL

Ligamentum flavum

Interspinous ligament

Supraspinous ligament

Herniation of nucleus pulposus

Fig. 5.3 Ligaments of the vertebral column and disc protrusion (herniation): (**A**) anterior view; (**B**) view of posterior aspect of vertebral bodies and discs, as if from the inside of the vertebral canal; (**C**) lateral view of two adjacent vertebrae with disc protrusion into the vertebral canal.

the dorsal ramus of C1. These are responsible for movements at the atlanto-occipital and atlanto-axial joints. Again, you do not need to memorise them, merely know that they are there.

5.6 Arteries and veins of the vertebral column

Arteries

The vertebral column is surrounded by an arterial network with contributions from the vertebral artery in the neck and the intercostal and lumbar arteries in the trunk. Branches pass through the intervertebral foramina to supply the spinal meninges and cord, and small nutrient arteries supply the bones themselves.

Cartilage is generally held to have no blood vessels, and although a few arteries are found on the surface of intervertebral cartilaginous discs, they do not penetrate far. Since a good blood supply is necessary for the healing process, damaged discs do not heal.

External and internal vertebral venous plexuses

External vertebral venous plexus. This surrounds the vertebral column. It has connections with the pelvic venous plexus, the lumbar veins and the azygos system.

Internal vertebral venous plexus. This is inside the vertebral canal. It anastomoses freely with the external plexus by veins passing through the intervertebral foramina. The internal vertebral venous plexus is in the extradural space and into this plexus drain:

- two or more short veins draining the vertebral body: the basivertebral veins
- veins draining the spinal cord.

These venous connections are important. Since these veins lack valves, blood flow can be in either direction, depending upon intra-abdominal pressure. Pelvic or abdominal malignancy may spread by these venous channels to give secondary deposits (metastases) in the vertebral bodies. These may present as backache, or, if the vertebral body collapses, as nerve entrapments or spinal cord compression. Prostatic malignancy is well known for spreading like this to involve the vertebral column and give rise to vertebral metastases.

Overview

The brain and spinal cord constitute the central nervous system, cranial and spinal nerves the peripheral nervous system. Different descriptive terms are based on direction of impulse (sensory, motor), and nature of sensation or action (somatic, visceral; voluntary, involuntary). Cells of the nervous system are neurons and supporting cells (glial cells, Schwann cells). The central nervous system contains both nerve cell bodies (grey matter) and tracts of axons (white matter), disposed in the spinal cord according to function. Spinal nerves are attached to the spinal cord in such a way that a pair of nerves and the portion of cord to which they are attached constitute a segment. The autonomic (visceral) nervous system controls homeostasis and bodily functions of internal organs, visceral motor impulses forming the sympathetic and parasympathetic nervous systems. Within the vertebral canal the spinal cord is surrounded by spinal meninges. The cord is much shorter than the canal itself, so roots of spinal nerves originating from the low spinal cord must pass within the vertebral canal before they reach the intervertebral foramen through which they pass to the rest of the body.

Learning Objectives

You should:

- know the meaning of central, peripheral, sensory, motor, somatic, visceral, voluntary, involuntary, and the relationships between these terms

- understand the basic organisation of the autonomic nervous system

- know the names and functions of different types of neurons and glial cells

- understand the basic organisation of the brain, spinal cord and spinal nerves

- understand the related concepts of segmentation, dermatomes and myotomes

- know how the spinal cord is surrounded by spinal meninges, and the anatomy of lumbar puncture.

6.1 Parts and definitions

The nervous system consists of the brain, spinal cord and peripheral nerves. It is one of the means by which central control of bodily functions is maintained, and allows the body to respond to stimuli of various sorts. There are several ways of classifying the components of the nervous system (Fig. 6.1).

Geographical: central/peripheral

Central nervous system. This is the brain and spinal cord.

Peripheral nervous system. This is everything else, i.e.:

- cranial nerves arising from the brain: 12 pairs
- spinal nerves arising from the spinal cord: 31 pairs (usually).

Direction of nerve impulse: sensory or afferent/motor or efferent

A nerve impulse in a peripheral nerve may travel:

- towards the central nervous system: a sensory or afferent impulse; or

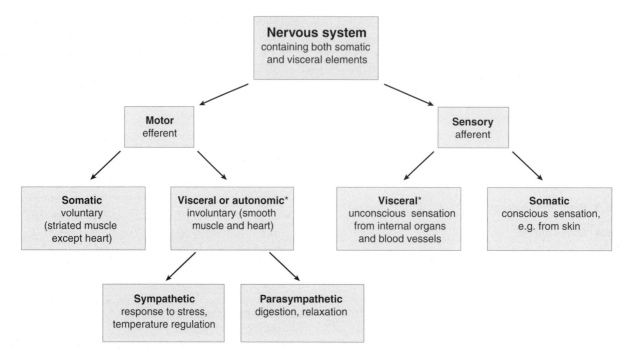

Fig. 6.1 Schematic layout of the nervous system.

- away from the central nervous system: a motor or efferent impulse.

Nature of perception: somatic sensory/visceral sensory

- Somatic sensory impulses are those of which we are acutely aware, and which we are well able to localise (e.g. sharp pain, touch). These generally originate in body wall structures (rather than internal organs). These fibres may run in either cranial or spinal nerves.
- Visceral sensory impulses are either imperceptible, only vaguely localisable, or only become perceptible in disease. They arise from blood vessels or internal organs (viscera), may run in either cranial or spinal nerves and are also found in a network of nerves associated with the internal organs.

Type of action: voluntary motor/visceral (involuntary) motor

Voluntary motor impulses. These control skeletal muscle over which we have voluntary control. From various parts of the brain, nerve impulses pass down in the spinal cord to connect with neurons whose axons pass out of the central nervous system into peripheral nerves.

- The neuron or neurons entirely within the central nervous system are upper motor neurons.
- The neurons with cell bodies in the central nervous system, but whose axons pass into the peripheral

nerves, are lower motor neurons. They are found in both cranial and spinal nerves.

Visceral (involuntary) motor or autonomic. These impulses control muscle over which we do not normally have voluntary control. These fibres may run in either cranial or spinal nerves, and are considered in more detail below and in 6.6.

Autonomic (visceral) nervous system

The visceral components of the nervous system, visceral sensory and visceral motor, supply internal organs and blood vessels. They may be grouped together as the autonomic nervous system, although it is not an anatomically distinct entity. Some components are central, some peripheral: some are in cranial nerves, some in spinal nerves, and some in autonomic plexuses (networks) in and around internal organs.

I recommend that you use the term *autonomic* to include only visceral motor fibres: use the term *visceral sensory* for afferent impulses from internal organs and blood vessels.

6.2 Cells of the nervous system, synapse

Neuron   (Fig. 6.2)

Neurons are nerve cells. They consist of cytoplasm and

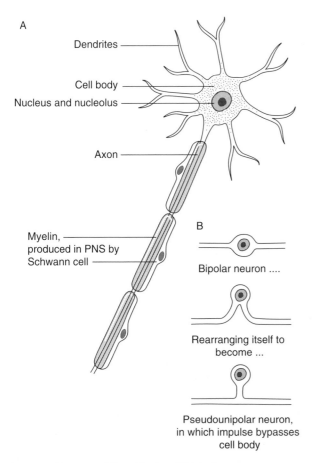

Fig. 6.2 Neurons: (**A**) multipolar; (**B**) bipolar.

a nucleus. The long cytoplasmic process that transmits impulses away from the cell body is the axon. The process that transmits impulses towards the cell body is the dendrite.

- *Multipolar neurons.* These are found throughout the central nervous system. Motor neurons in the spinal cord are multipolar (have more than one cytoplasmic process), one of the poles being the axon (Fig. 6.2A).
- *Bipolar neurons.* Peripheral sensory neurons are originally bipolar with one cytoplasmic process which conducts the nerve impulse from the receptor towards the cell body, and one which conducts the impulse from there to the central nervous system. For spinal nerves, and some cranial nerves, the bipolar cell rearranges its processes during development (Fig. 6.2B) to become pseudounipolar, presumably in the interests of speed of conduction. The sensory neurons which remain truly bipolar are those of olfaction (smell), vision, hearing and balance where the receptors are close to the brain.

The cell bodies of sensory neurons in a peripheral nerve are all collected together in one site, a ganglion (swelling). In a spinal nerve the sensory ganglion is attached to the dorsal (posterior) root of the nerve (see below), and so is known as the dorsal (posterior) root ganglion; it is found in the region of the intervertebral foramen through which the nerve passes out of the vertebral canal. For a cranial nerve it is simply known as the sensory ganglion of that nerve, and is often given another name peculiar to itself.

Synapse

Neural pathways involve a chain of separate neurons. Junctional zones are called synapses: here the impulse at the end of one neuron stimulates the neuron to release chemicals (neurotransmitters) that cause electrical impulses to be generated in the succeeding neuron. Synapses are thus relay stations in the neural pathway.

Supporting cells: glial cells, Schwann cells

Supporting cells provide structural support and myelin. In the brain these are glial cells: oligodendrocytes for myelin production, astrocytes for structural support. In the spinal cord myelin is produced by Schwann cells. Glial cells give rise to the commonest brain tumours: gliomas.

6.3 Brain and spinal cord

Brain

The brain consists of:

- The brain stem: the central, midline portion made up of (from bottom up) medulla oblongata, pons and midbrain. It is continuous below with the spinal cord and above with the forebrain.
- The cerebellum, behind the pons.
- The forebrain: thalamic structures and right and left cerebral hemispheres.

Cranial nerves

There are 12 pairs of cranial nerves arising from the brain. They are usually designated by Roman numerals (I–XII) as in this text, and are concerned mainly with structures in the head and neck.

The cranial nerves and brain are considered in more detail in Chapters 14 and 15.

Spinal cord

The spinal cord is found within the vertebral (spinal) canal. It has a number of functions.

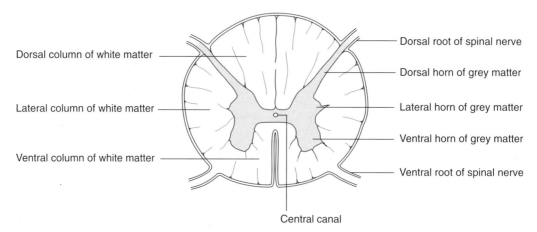

Dorsal column of white matter

Lateral column of white matter

Ventral column of white matter

Dorsal root of spinal nerve

Dorsal horn of grey matter

Lateral horn of grey matter

Ventral horn of grey matter

Ventral root of spinal nerve

Central canal

Fig. 6.3 Spinal cord: grey and white matter. The lateral horn of grey matter is present only in the thoracic and upper lumbar regions of the spinal cord.

- It serves as a coordinating centre for each spinal cord segment, e.g. spinal reflexes.
- It receives sensory information from peripheral nerves and sends it on to the brain and to other places for the purposes of perception and for eliciting appropriate responses.
- It receives commands from the brain, and other centres, which it distributes to appropriate peripheral nerves.

Grey and white matter (Fig. 6.3)

Neural tissue of the entire central nervous system consists of both axons and cell bodies. Axons are surrounded by myelin, a fatty substance which, like most fatty tissues, is almost white in colour. Thus, areas of the central nervous system that are rich in axons surrounded by myelin constitute the white matter. Areas of the central nervous system that largely consist of cell bodies rather than axons do not appear white, and these areas constitute the grey matter. In the spinal cord, grey matter is distributed in a butterfly shape around the central canal.

Regions of grey matter

These are described as horns because of their appearance on cross-section. There are, though, no structural barriers between the different areas.

Ventral (anterior) horn. Cell bodies of lower motor neurons innervating voluntary muscle are found in the ventral grey horn, and so are called ventral (anterior) horn cells, often abbreviated to VHC or AHC. Disease of these cells, for example poliomyelitis, causes paralysis of voluntary muscle. The ventral horns are largest in those parts of the spinal cord that serve regions of the body with many muscles – the limbs: spinal cord segments C5–T1 for the upper limb and L2–S4 for the lower limb.

Lateral horn. Cell bodies of motor neurons of the sympathetic system are found in the lateral horn. The lateral horn is present only in the thoracic and lumbar areas of the spinal cord.

Dorsal (posterior) horn. The dorsal horn handles sensory impulses.

Regions of white matter: tracts

White matter is described as being disposed in columns around the grey matter: anterior, lateral and dorsal columns; again, there are no structural barriers between them. Within white matter, axons are arranged so that those of similar functions are grouped together to form a tract. These tracts are not sharply demarcated from each other: there may be some overlap between them.

Bundles of axons carrying impulses up to the brain form sensory tracts; bundles of axons carrying impulses down from the brain to neurons in the grey matter of the spinal cord form motor tracts. Their names usually reflect the journey of the impulses they carry: a tract beginning with spino- (e.g. spinothalamic, spinotectal) is a sensory tract, and a tract ending with -spinal (e.g. corticospinal, tectospinal) is a motor tract. The largest regions of white matter are the dorsal (posterior) columns: they contain heavily myelinated sensory fibres of large diameter (the degree of myelination and the large diameter giving a fast conduction speed).

6.4 Spinal nerves

Note. In descriptions of the human nervous system, because humans stand erect, the terms dorsal and posterior are interchangeable, as are ventral and anterior. For the nervous system, I prefer dorsal and ventral to anterior and posterior.

Spinal nerves arise in pairs: 8 cervical, 12 thoracic, 5 lumbar and 5 sacral (forget about the coccygeal nerve). Each spinal nerve arises by a series of dorsal rootlets and ventral rootlets. As a general rule, dorsal rootlets convey sensory information into the spinal cord, and ventral rootlets convey motor information away from the spinal cord. These rootlets unite in or near the intervertebral foramen to form the spinal nerve. Nerves C1–7 emerge above the correspondingly numbered vertebrae; C8 nerve arises below vertebra C7 (remember, there are only 7 cervical vertebrae), and thereafter the nerves emerge below the correspondingly numbered vertebra.

Dorsal root ganglion   (Fig. 6.4)

As the dorsal rootlets converge, there is a swelling, the dorsal (posterior) root ganglion, which houses the cell bodies of all the sensory neurons in that particular nerve.

Branches of a typical spinal nerve

(Figs 6.4, 6.5)

Dorsal ramus.   This supplies the dorsal one-third (about) of the body wall; dorsal rami do not contribute to the limbs.

Ventral ramus.   This supplies the ventral two-thirds (about) of the body wall including the limbs.

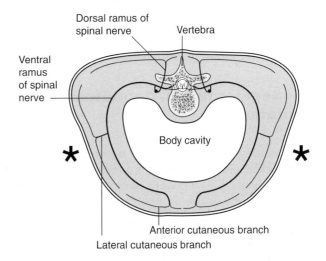

Fig. 6.5   Typical spinal nerve in relation to the trunk. Schematic section through the trunk in the plane of one spinal nerve: * marks the position of the limb bud, in the territory of the ventral ramus of a spinal nerve.

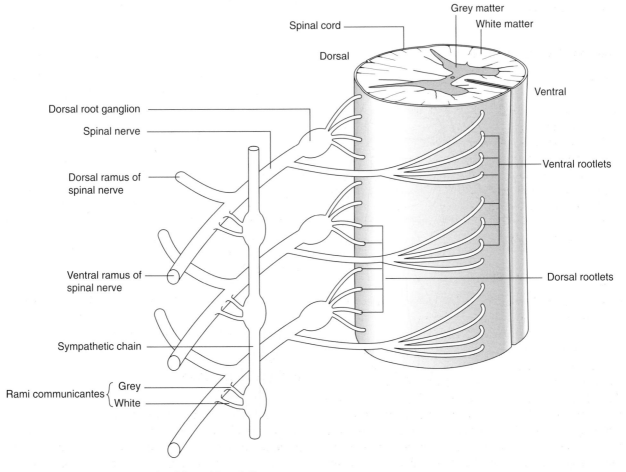

Fig. 6.4   Spinal nerve formation (viewed from left).

Beware of confusion!

Dorsal and ventral roots are not the same as dorsal and ventral rami. Dorsal roots convey sensory impulses; ventral roots convey motor impulses. Once these roots unite to form the nerve, all subsequent branches, including the rami, convey both sensory and motor impulses.

6.5 Segmentation, dermatomes, myotomes

The repeating pattern of spinal nerves reflects the pattern of somites in the embryo. Spinal nerves are called segmental nerves, and the area of the spinal cord from which they arise is known as a spinal cord segment: C5 spinal nerves arise from C5 segment of the spinal cord.

Dermatomes   (Fig. 6.6)

The strip of skin supplied by one spinal nerve is the

dermatome: the dermatome of C5 is supplied by C5 nerve which arises from C5 segment of the spinal cord. Dermatomes are useful clinically. If you find on examination of a patient that there is sensory loss that corresponds to an entire dermatome then you know that something is interfering with either the spinal nerve, the dorsal (sensory) rootlets, the dorsal root ganglion or the spinal cord itself. It is worth noting that there is sufficient overlap between dermatomes for damage to one spinal nerve to cause few if any sensory symptoms. Damage to two adjacent spinal nerves would be more apparent.

Dermatomes bear no relation to Langer's lines (Fig. 3.2, p. 17) despite their apparent similarity at first glance.

Shingles

Shingles illustrates the segmental arrangement of the nervous system and the dermatomes. A viral infection of a dorsal root ganglion causes pain and vesicular eruptions in the strip of skin innervated by the nerve on which the ganglion is situated.

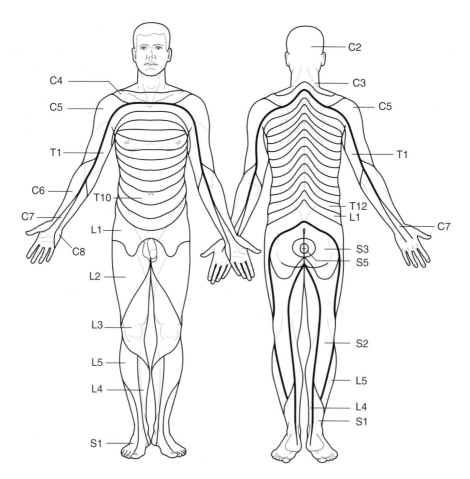

Fig. 6.6   Dermatomes. Note that C1 has no dermatome.

Myotome

Similarly, the skeletal muscle supplied by one spinal cord segment is a myotome. Damage to ventral horn cells of spinal cord segment C5, or damage to the ventral roots of C5 nerve, will cause weakness or paralysis of muscles supplied by that nerve.

6.6 Autonomic nervous system

There are two parts: sympathetic and parasympathetic. The sympathetic system prepares us for action:

- it is active when we are alert, fearful or stressed, dilating the pupil (mydriasis) and speeding the heart
- it is important in temperature regulation, supplying muscles that move cutaneous hair, regulate the calibre of cutaneous blood vessels, and provoke secretion of sweat (for cooling).

The parasympathetic system relaxes us for gut tube activity:

- it provokes salivary secretion, gastric activity and emptying, intestinal peristalsis, anal sphincter relaxation
- it constricts the pupil (miosis)
- it slows the heart
- and it has important reproductive functions.

There are two peripheral motor neurons to smooth muscle

Unlike motor impulses to voluntary muscle, autonomic (visceral motor) impulses to smooth muscle pass in two peripheral motor neurons with an intervening synapse, the two neurons being called presynaptic and post-synaptic. The synapses are found in autonomic ganglia, and the terms preganglionic and postganglionic are also used (more often, in fact).

Layout of the sympathetic nervous system (Fig. 6.7)

Sympathetic impulses arise only from spinal cord segments T1 to L1 or 2, and so the term thoracolumbar is used to describe the sympathetic outflow from the cord. This limited origin demands that, in order for sympathetic impulses to reach all parts of the body, there must be a redistribution system. This is the sympathetic chain which is found on either side of the vertebral column: it certainly extends between T1 and L2, but it also extends higher than T1 so that impulses can pass to cervical spinal nerves and the head, and lower than L2 so that impulses can pass to nerves L3 and below.

In the spinal cord, sympathetic preganglionic impulses arise from the lateral horn cells between T1 and L1 or 2, an impulse passing into the spinal nerve of that segment and thence through a connection, the white ramus communicans, to the sympathetic chain. Once in the chain, several things may happen.

- The preganglionic impulse may synapse on the cell body of a postsynaptic (postganglionic) neuron, the axon of which passes back into the spinal nerve through the grey ramus communicans (grey because less myelinated than the white ramus) to be distributed in the territory of that same spinal nerve in which it emerged from the spinal cord.

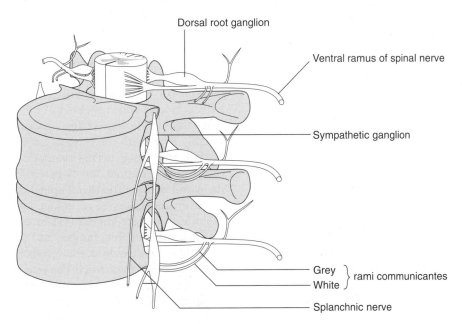

Dorsal root ganglion

Ventral ramus of spinal nerve

Sympathetic ganglion

Grey ⎫ rami communicantes
White ⎭

Splanchnic nerve

Fig. 6.7 Elements of the sympathetic nervous system.

- The preganglionic impulse may synapse on the cell body of a postsynaptic (postganglionic) neuron, the axon of which passes on to an adjacent segmental artery. By this means sympathetic impulses may pass to all branches of that artery.
- Having passed into the sympathetic chain, the preganglionic impulse may ascend or descend in the chain to gain another spinal nerve. This 'new' spinal nerve may be above T1 or below L2 – here is the sympathetic chain acting as the redistribution system referred to earlier. The preganglionic impulse synapses in the ganglion at the 'new' level and proceeds through the grey ramus of the 'new' level into the 'new' spinal nerve for distribution.
- The preganglionic impulse may pass through the ganglion without synapsing, into one of the branches of the sympathetic chain serving the thoracic and abdominal viscera. These are the cardiac and pulmonary branches and the splanchnic nerves. These impulses will synapse in a group of ganglia in plexuses in and around the aorta and its branches (cardiac, pulmonary, coeliac, superior mesenteric, renal, inferior mesenteric, hypogastric).

Layout of the parasympathetic nervous system

As in the sympathetic system, parasympathetic impulses traverse two peripheral motor neurons (pre- and postganglionic). Some arise from the brain stem and pass into cranial nerves III, VII, IX and X, and others arise from cell bodies in the sacral spinal cord and pass into spinal nerves S2, S3 and S4, with none arising between these two regions of the central nervous system. The word craniosacral is used to describe this pattern. The peripheral ganglia are in or on the destination organ, so postganglionic parasympathetic neurons are very short.

Visceral sensation

Sensory (e.g. pain) fibres from internal organs reach the central nervous system using either sympathetic or parasympathetic pathways (or both). But since in the sensory system there is no peripheral synapse, the terms pre- and postganglionic fibres are irrelevant and wrong for visceral sensory nerves. The cell body of a visceral sensory neuron is in the sensory ganglion of whichever nerve delivers the impulse to the central nervous system, so sensory ganglia contain cell bodies of both somatic sensory and visceral sensory neurons.

Referred pain

Disease of internal organs and the gut tube may cause pain which the patient interprets as arising from skin. This is because, to put it simply, the brain is confused into thinking the pain is coming from skin (which is where pain often comes from) rather than from an internal organ supplied by a neuron of the same spinal segment that supplies the skin. The internal pain is said to be 'referred' to a particular dermatome. The physiology of this is not understood.

Ganglion – beware!

You have met two types of ganglion in the preceding sections: a sensory ganglion in 6.2 and an autonomic ganglion in 6.6. Both consist of a collection of cell bodies in the peripheral nervous system, but one has synapses and the other does not.

- A sensory ganglion is simply the site at which the cell bodies of all the bipolar or pseudounipolar sensory neurons in that particular nerve are gathered together.
- An autonomic ganglion is the site of the synapse between preganglionic and postganglionic autonomic neurons.
- Ganglia are either sensory or autonomic: they are never both.

6.7 Spinal cord in the vertebral canal and spinal meninges (Fig. 6.8)

The vertebral (spinal) canal extends throughout the vertebral column, but the spinal cord in the adult is considerably shorter than this. This was not so in fetal life when the cord more nearly filled the canal, but as development proceeds the vertebral column grows more than the spinal cord so that by adulthood there is a considerable discrepancy. In the newborn, the end of the spinal cord is level with vertebra L3, but in the adult it is level with vertebra L2 or even L1. This means that while the origin of the cervical spinal nerves is roughly level with the cervical vertebrae, the thoracic, lumbar and sacral nerves originate higher than their companion vertebrae, the disparity increasing towards the sacral region. The sacral spinal cord (giving origin to sacral spinal nerves) is, in fact, level with the lower thoracic and upper lumbar vertebrae.

As a result of this, lumbar and sacral spinal nerve roots must pass down in the vertebral canal for quite a distance before they reach the intervertebral foramen through which they pass, and after which they are numbered. The collection of these nerve roots that occupy the vertebral canal below the bottom of the spinal cord is the cauda equina.

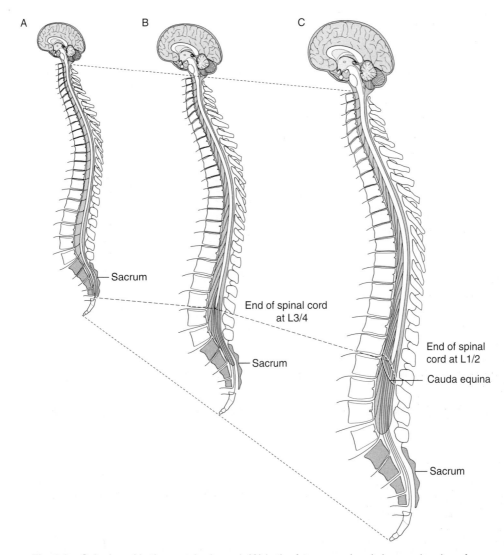

Fig. 6.8 Spinal cord in the vertebral canal: (**A**) in the fetus – cord ends in sacral region of vertebral canal; (**B**) at birth – cord ends about vertebral level L4; (**C**) in the adult – cord ends at vertebral level L1/2.

Meninges (Fig. 6.9)

The spinal cord is surrounded by the meninges (covering membranes) which are continuous with the meninges of the brain (see Ch. 14).

- Pia mater: on the surface of the spinal cord and inseparable from it (Greek: *pia* = tender).
- Arachnoid mater: joined to the pia by thin strands of tissue (Greek: *arakhnes* = spider).
- Dura mater: tough and fibrous (Latin: *dura* = hard), longitudinal fibres. At about the point where the spinal nerve passes through intervertebral foramen, the dura is continued along the nerve as a thick fibrous envelope, the perineurium. Nerve roots in the subarachnoid space lack this covering and so are more fragile than spinal nerves. In traumatic injury to the vertebral column, nerve roots are more often torn than nerves themselves.

The meninges are themselves supplied by sensory nerve fibres which are branches of cranial and spinal nerves, so inflammation of the meninges (meningitis) is painful.

Filum terminale

At the lower margin of the spinal cord, at about vertebral level L2, the pia mater surrounding the cord is prolonged down to attach to the coccyx in the vertebral canal, even though it contains no neural tissue. It is as if this prolongation of pia mater had been occupied by spinal cord in fetal life, but as the spinal cord apparently withdraws upwards during development and maturation, the sleeve of pia mater that contains it becomes empty. This 'envelope' of pia mater is the filum terminale and it is found amidst the nerve roots making up the cauda equina.

POSTERIOR

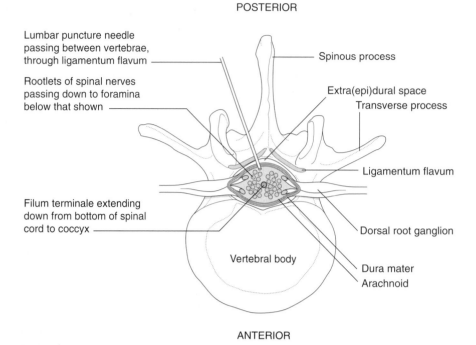

Lumbar puncture needle passing between vertebrae, through ligamentum flavum

Rootlets of spinal nerves passing down to foramina below that shown

Filum terminale extending down from bottom of spinal cord to coccyx

Spinous process

Extra(epi)dural space
Transverse process

Ligamentum flavum

Dorsal root ganglion

Vertebral body

Dura mater
Arachnoid

ANTERIOR

Fig. 6.9   Spinal meninges and lumbar puncture. Section through upper lumbar region.

Subarachnoid space and cerebrospinal fluid

Between the pia and the arachnoid is the subarachnoid space containing cerebrospinal fluid. The pressure of the cerebrospinal fluid in the subarachnoid space keeps the thin arachnoid in contact with the dura such that the space between the arachnoid and dura, the subdural space, is not normally present. The arachnoid and the dura mater normally occupy the vertebral canal well into the sacrum, down to about vertebral level S2.

Denticulate ligament

This is a lateral extension of the pia mater extending from the cord in a coronal plane about midway between the dorsal and ventral nerve roots to meet the internal aspect of the arachnoid in a series of sawtooth-like projections. It helps to tether the spinal cord within the subarachnoid space.

Extradural or epidural space

Outside the dura mater, between it and the walls of the bony canal, is the extradural or epidural space. This contains connective tissue, fat and the internal vertebral venous plexus.

Surface anatomy

- Vertebral level (about) T11–L1/2: sacral region of spinal cord.

- Vertebral level L1/2: end of spinal cord in adult.
- Vertebral level L3/4: end of spinal cord at birth.
- Vertebral level S2: end of dural sac and subarachnoid space.

Lumbar puncture   (Fig. 6.9)

The subarachnoid space below vertebral level L1/2 is occupied by cerebrospinal fluid and the cauda equina, but not by the spinal cord. This is the lumbar cistern of cerebrospinal fluid (a cistern is a region of the subarachnoid space), and into it needles may be inserted to sample the cerebrospinal fluid without risk of damaging the spinal cord itself. This is a lumbar puncture.

A hollow needle is inserted through the skin of the back, usually slightly off centre, and approaches the vertebral column from behind. The needle passes through the ligamentum flavum (a 'give' is felt) between adjacent vertebral laminae. The tip of the needle is now in the extradural space. It should be further advanced until it has pierced the dura and arachnoid together (another 'give'), at which point clear cerebrospinal fluid should pass through the needle and a sample can be taken for analysis.

In the adult this is best done at vertebral level L3/4, the surface marking for which is a line drawn between the highest points of the right and left iliac crests. In the child, where the spinal cord is relatively longer with respect to the vertebral column, lumbar puncture would be performed one or two intervertebral spaces lower.

Epidural anaesthesia and spinal anaesthesia

A liquid anaesthetic agent may be injected into the extra(epi)dural space. This is an epidural anaesthetic and it will anaesthetise the spinal nerve roots it surrounds. It is normally performed as would be a lumbar puncture except that the needle is not advanced after the first 'give' (see above). It is particularly useful for procedures in the pelvis and perineum (supplied by lumbar and sacral nerves) where the patient is unfit for a general anaesthetic.

In spinal anaesthesia, the needle is inserted as in a lumbar puncture and the anaesthetic agent is injected into the subarachnoid space. The specific gravity of these agents is greater than that of the cerebrospinal fluid and so by altering the position of the patient the anaesthetic can be restricted to the lower region of the subarachnoid space. It produces a more profound anaesthesia and lasts longer than an epidural anaesthetic.

7 Cardiovascular system and lymph vessels

Overview

The cardiovascular system consists of a series of closed blood vessels lined by endothelial cells, and a pump: the heart. Arteries may be described as: systemic, taking blood from the left ventricle of the heart to the tissues of the body; and pulmonary, taking blood from the right ventricle to the lungs. Veins may be described as: systemic, conveying blood towards the right atrium of the heart from all tissues of the body except the intestines; pulmonary, conveying blood from the lungs to the left atrium of the heart; and hepatic portal, conveying blood from the intestinal bed to the liver. The lymphatic system conveys tissue fluid back to the venous system: it is important in the spread of disease.

Learning Objectives

You should:

- understand the basic structure of the arterial system

- understand the basic structure of the venous system.

- know the names of the most commonly palpated arterial pulses

- know the meaning of: systemic, pulmonary, portal

- understand the clinical importance of the lymphatic system and the positions of the most commonly palpated groups of lymph nodes.

7.1 Heart

The heart is in the thorax and consists of two pumps, right and left, lying side by side in one organ. The left heart (left atrium and left ventricle) receives oxygenated blood from the lungs and pumps it around the body, and the right heart (right atrium and right ventricle) receives deoxygenated blood from the body and pumps it to the lungs for oxygenation. It is described in Chapter 10.

7.2 Arteries   (Fig. 7.1)

Arteries convey blood from the heart to the tissues. There are two arterial systems:

- the aorta and its branches – systemic arteries – which convey blood from the left ventricle to the capillary beds; and
- pulmonary arteries, which convey deoxygenated blood from the right ventricle to the lungs.

The pulsations of the heartbeat are strongest in large arteries, and palpation of arterial pulses is one of the components of clinical examination of the body. The most commonly palpated pulses are: carotid, radial, aortic, femoral, popliteal, posterior tibial, dorsalis pedis. Other pulses are also used occasionally: brachial, ulnar and anterior tibial. Pulses are marked with an asterisk on Figure 7.1. More precise details of their surface markings are given later in the text.

7.3 Veins   (Fig. 7.2)

Veins convey blood from the tissues back to the heart. The arrangement of veins is much more variable than that of arteries and knowledge of only the principal veins is necessary.

Systemic veins

These convey blood towards the two vena cavas and the heart.

- The superior vena cava receives blood from the upper limbs, head and neck, chest wall and part of the upper abdominal wall.

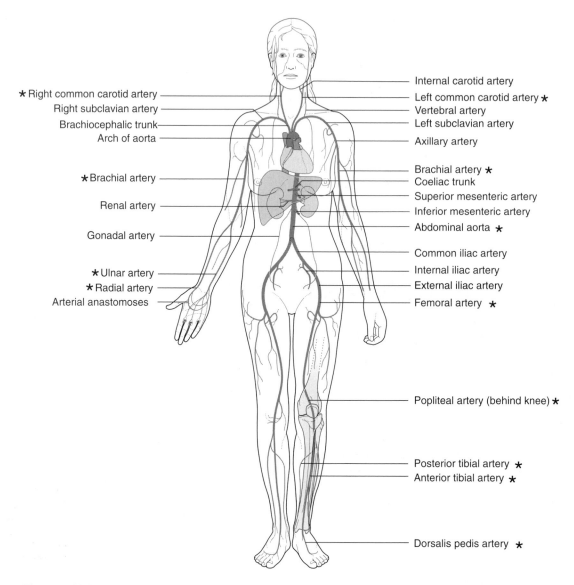

★Right common carotid artery

Right subclavian artery

Brachiocephalic trunk

Arch of aorta

★Brachial artery

Renal artery

Gonadal artery

★Ulnar artery

★Radial artery

Arterial anastomoses

Internal carotid artery

Left common carotid artery ★

Vertebral artery

Left subclavian artery

Axillary artery

Brachial artery ★

Coeliac trunk

Superior mesenteric artery

Inferior mesenteric artery

Abdominal aorta ★

Common iliac artery

Internal iliac artery

External iliac artery

Femoral artery ★

Popliteal artery (behind knee) ★

Posterior tibial artery ★

Anterior tibial artery ★

Dorsalis pedis artery ★

Fig. 7.1   Main arteries and palpable pulses: * indicates the most commonly palpated pulses.

- The inferior vena cava receives blood from the lower limbs, pelvis, abdominal organs, most of the abdominal wall, and the liver (see below).

Pulmonary veins

The right and left pulmonary veins convey oxygenated blood from the lungs to the left atrium of the heart.

Portal venous system   (Fig. 7.3)

Portal veins are veins that connect two capillary beds. All venous blood from the alimentary canal between the lower oesophagus and the anal canal reaches the liver in the hepatic portal vein, usually referred to as simply the portal vein. This with its tributaries (splenic, superior mesenteric, inferior mesenteric veins) constitute

the portal system, blockage of which, for example in liver disease, has serious consequences (see later). From the liver, short veins convey blood to the inferior vena cava – the hepatic veins. In certain forms of liver disease in which blood from the intestines is unable to pass through the liver, anastomoses between portal and systemic veins develop or enlarge to allow blood from the intestines to bypass the liver (see portosystemic anastomoses, p. 124).

Superficial and deep veins

Veins that are easily visible under the skin are superficial veins in the superficial tissues of the body: these may be used clinically as access points for injections or for the insertion of catheters etc. Their anatomy is particularly variable. There is also a venous network alongside the

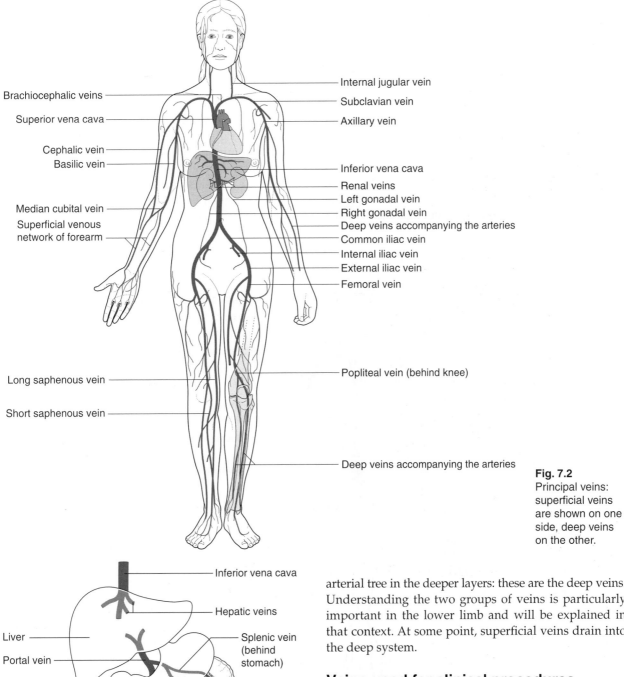

Brachiocephalic veins

Superior vena cava

Cephalic vein

Basilic vein

Median cubital vein

Superficial venous
network of forearm

Long saphenous vein

Short saphenous vein

Internal jugular vein

Subclavian vein

Axillary vein

Inferior vena cava

Renal veins

Left gonadal vein

Right gonadal vein

Deep veins accompanying the arteries

Common iliac vein

Internal iliac vein

External iliac vein

Femoral vein

Popliteal vein (behind knee)

Deep veins accompanying the arteries

Fig. 7.2
Principal veins:
superficial veins
are shown on one
side, deep veins
on the other.

Inferior vena cava

Hepatic veins

Liver

Portal vein

Splenic vein
(behind
stomach)

Superior
mesenteric
vein

Inferior
mesenteric
vein

Fig. 7.3   The portal venous system.

arterial tree in the deeper layers: these are the deep veins. Understanding the two groups of veins is particularly important in the lower limb and will be explained in that context. At some point, superficial veins drain into the deep system.

Veins used for clinical procedures

Veins used most frequently for the insertion of catheters and cannulas are: great saphenous vein at the ankle, femoral vein, antecubital veins, cephalic vein, subclavian vein, brachiocephalic vein, scalp veins (particularly in babies).

7.4 Lymph vessels (lymphatics)

These small, thin-walled vessels convey 'used' extracellular fluid back to the venous system though various groups of lymph nodes. The clinical importance of lymph nodes and lymphatics is out of all proportion to their insignificant size, since it is by the lymphatics that disease, especially malignant disease, often spreads. The lymphatic drainage of one organ to another may result in disease of the first organ becoming apparent as disease of the second. You therefore need to know the main lymphatic channels and lymph node groups.

From the interstitial spaces of the tissues, lymph passes into small lymphatic channels which join to form progressively larger vessels. They are lined by endothelial cells and, like veins, many lymph vessels contain valves. In general, lymph vessels accompany arteries, and arterial pulsations provide the force, squeezing the lymphatics so that lymph flows through them in the direction permitted by the valves. As with veins, there are superficial and deep lymphatics that eventually unite.

The main lymph channels are shown in Figure 7.4, and details of the lymph drainage of specific organs are presented in the text as the organs and regions are considered.

● Lymph from the entire body, *except* the right upper limb and right side of the head, neck and upper thorax, drains to the cisterna chyli in the upper abdomen, then onwards through the thoracic duct to enter the venous system at the junction of the left internal jugular and left subclavian veins as they unite to form the left brachiocephalic vein.

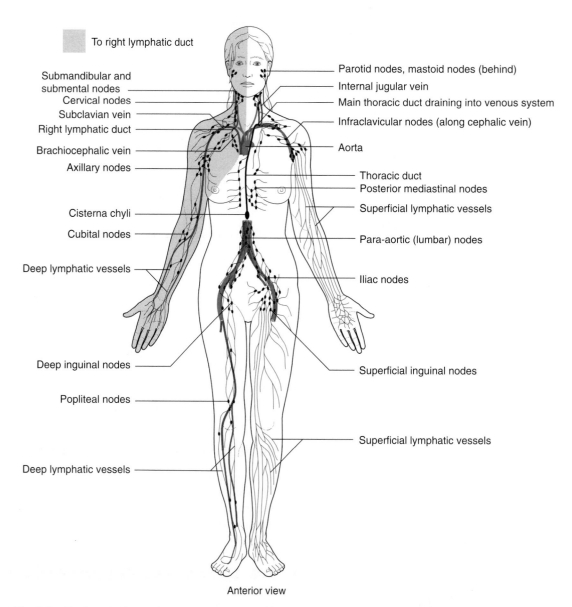

To right lymphatic duct

Submandibular and submental nodes
Cervical nodes
Subclavian vein
Right lymphatic duct
Brachiocephalic vein
Axillary nodes
Cisterna chyli
Cubital nodes
Deep lymphatic vessels
Deep inguinal nodes
Popliteal nodes
Deep lymphatic vessels

Parotid nodes, mastoid nodes (behind)
Internal jugular vein
Main thoracic duct draining into venous system
Infraclavicular nodes (along cephalic vein)
Aorta
Thoracic duct
Posterior mediastinal nodes
Superficial lymphatic vessels
Para-aortic (lumbar) nodes
Iliac nodes
Superficial inguinal nodes
Superficial lymphatic vessels

Anterior view

Fig. 7.4 The lymphatic system. The right side of the head and neck and the right upper limb drain to the right lymphatic duct. The remainder of the body drains to the (main) thoracic duct. Superficial lymphatics are shown on one side, deep lymphatics on the other.

- Lymph from the right upper limb and right side of the head, neck and upper thorax drains to the right lymph duct which enters the venous system at the junction of the right internal jugular and right subclavian veins, which unite to form the right brachiocephalic vein.

Most commonly palpated lymph node groups

These are: parotid, mastoid, submandibular, deep cervical, supraclavicular, axillary, para-aortic, inguinal.

8 Alimentary and respiratory systems

Overview

The alimentary and respiratory systems develop from the embryonic gut tube. Their common origin is reflected in both anatomy – they share a common upper portion (the pharynx) – and function, absorption of material from the external environment and excretion of waste products. They are associated with glands that secrete substances into the lumen of the tube for digestion or lubrication, and with numerous aggregations of lymphoid tissue in the walls that help repel foreign organisms.

Learning Objectives

You should:

- know in the correct order the components of the alimentary canal from mouth to anus

- understand the function of glands, and the definitions of exocrine and endocrine

- know the main features of the respiratory system.

8.1 Alimentary system (Fig. 8.1)

The alimentary system consists of everything between the mouth and the anus together with all the tubes and secretory units (exocrine glands) that open into it.

Exocrine glands

The glands which secrete substances into the lumen of the gut tube (exocrine glands) include:

- submandibular, sublingual, parotid and minor salivary glands secreting substances that begin the digestive process

- mucous glands secreting mucus for lubrication (particularly in the colon where the contents become progressively more solid)
- acid-secreting glands in the stomach for digestion
- glands secreting enzymes for digestion. These include exocrine pancreatic tissue and the bile-secreting cells of the liver. It is important to understand that these are both part of the alimentary system, as are all the smaller glands opening into the gut tube lumen.

Endocrine tissue

Endocrine cells secrete a variety of substances:

- insulin, glucagon and other digestive hormones
- amines such as catecholamines.

In some places endocrine cells are aggregated to form distinct endocrine organs, while in other places they remain isolated as single endocrine secretory units scattered throughout the epithelium.

Lymphoid tissue

The lumen of the gut tube is part of the external environment and gut epithelium is therefore a potential site of entry of foreign matter. Lymphoid material, which is concerned with the recognition of self/non-self and the defence of the organism from foreign invasion, is present in the wall of the gut tube to monitor potential trouble arising from this part of the outside world. It is particularly obvious in the mouth and pharynx where a 'ring' of lymphoid tissue (Waldeyer's ring: tonsils, adenoids) encircles the oropharynx, the ileum (Peyer's patches) and the appendix. From the lymph plexuses in the walls of the gut tube, lymph passes to nodes that drain, as for the rest of the body, to the thoracic duct.

Muscular coat of the gut tube

This involuntary muscle allows propulsion of contents through the gut tube and in the stomach is especially important for the churning movements of digestion. For the most part there are two muscular layers – inner circular and outer longitudinal – although there is an extra partial coat in the stomach. These muscles are

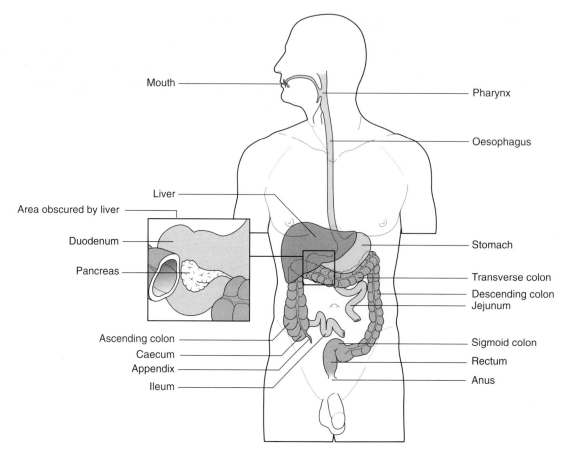

Fig. 8.1 The alimentary system.

supplied by the myenteric plexuses in and around the muscle coats of the gut tube.

Mobility of the gut tube: mesenteries

Those parts of the gut tube that are most mobile are in the abdomen and are surrounded by a serous membrane, the peritoneum, to allow friction-free movement. Figure 3.1A (p. 16) shows the original primitive state of the arrangement of the peritoneum with the mesentery of the gut tube connecting the gut tube to the body wall and allowing vessels and nerves access. For some parts of the intestines this persists (stomach, jejunum, ileum, transverse colon, sigmoid colon), even if somewhat modified, but for other parts of the gut tube, there is no apparent mesentery, it having been incorporated into the dorsal body wall, as described in Chapter 11.

8.2 Respiratory system (Fig. 8.2)

The respiratory system consists of:

- The upper respiratory tract: nasal passages, Eustachian tubes, middle ear and mastoid cavities, pharynx, larynx. A common cold is an upper

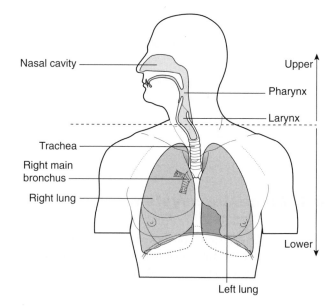

Fig. 8.2 The respiratory system.

respiratory tract infection: sore throat, nasal congestion, earache.
- The lower respiratory tract: trachea, bronchi, lungs.

They are separated by the vocal cords.

Walls of the respiratory passages

The respiratory tubes must remain patent for the passage of air. They are held open by skeletal elements, notably the hyoid bone and laryngeal cartilages in the neck, and hyaline cartilage in the walls of the trachea and bronchi. Apart from the numerous small mucous glands, there are no important associated exocrine glands. As in the alimentary canal, endocrine cells are found in the walls and may (rarely) give rise to tumours. There is no significant lymphoid tissue in the walls of the respiratory system except for lymphatics and Waldeyer's ring referred to earlier.

9 Urogenital system

Overview

The urinary and genital components of the urogenital system are derived from common embryological sources. Their functions are at first sight dissimilar: the urinary system is mainly for excretion of waste products from the blood stream, and the genital system for reproduction. In mammals, organs of both systems are confined to the lower abdomen, pelvis and perineum.

Learning Objectives

You should:

- know the main organs making up both systems

- understand the common origin and shared anatomy.

9.1 Disposition and origin

The urogenital system is confined in mammals to the abdomen, pelvis and perineum. The two components, urinary and genital, have a common embryological origin.

- The gonads and kidneys (and adrenal cortex) are from embryonic tissue on the posterior coelomic wall. This common origin is reflected, despite subsequent movements during development, in the blood supply, lymph drainage and, for the adrenal cortex and the gonads, the secretion of steroid hormones.

- Much of the duct systems of the urogenital organs originate with the terminal portion of the gut: they are either cloacal derivatives, or they open into the cloaca (Latin: sewer). These structures include:
  - in both sexes, the urethra, bladder, ureters, collecting ducts of the kidney
  - in the female, the vagina, uterus and Fallopian tube
  - in the male, the ductus (vas) deferens and seminal vesicles.

9.2 Urinary tract (Fig. 9.1)

Urine is produced in the right and left kidneys and passes through the right and left ureters to the bladder. It is expelled from the bladder through the (midline) urethra. This is short in the female and longer in the male, traversing the penis.

9.3 Reproductive tract

Male reproductive organs (Fig. 9.2)

The paired testes develop high on the posterior body wall and before birth descend to the scrotum. Spermatozoa are produced in the testis and at ejaculation are propelled along the ductus (vas) deferens on each side to join the (midline) urethra in the substance of the prostate gland. They travel to the tip of the penis in the urethra.

Female reproductive organs (Fig. 9.3)

The ovaries also develop high on the posterior body wall but do not descend as far as the testis so that the ovaries remain in the lower abdominal cavity. The uterus and Fallopian (uterine) tubes develop from a paired tubular system that partially unites. Those parts which remain paired are the Fallopian tubes; those that unite form the uterus in which the fetus develops, and the vagina which receives the penis at copulation and through which the baby is born.

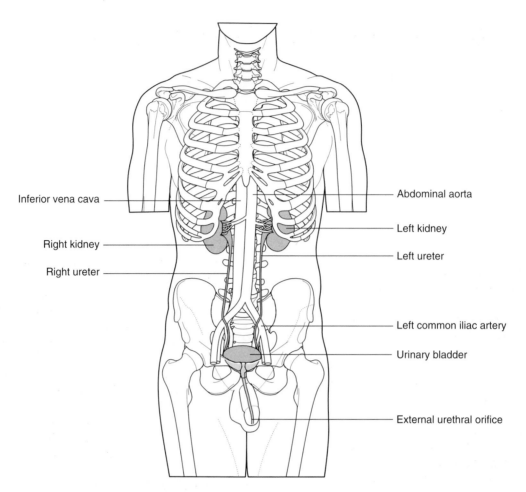

Inferior vena cava

Right kidney

Right ureter

Abdominal aorta

Left kidney

Left ureter

Left common iliac artery

Urinary bladder

External urethral orifice

Fig. 9.1 The urinary tract.

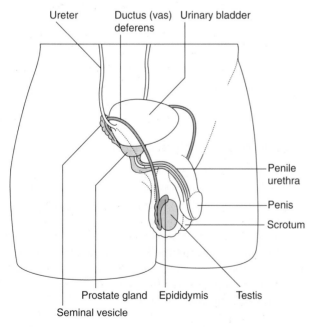

Ureter

Ductus (vas) deferens

Urinary bladder

Penile urethra

Penis

Scrotum

Prostate gland Epididymis Testis

Seminal vesicle

Fig. 9.2 Male reproductive organs: viewed obliquely from the front.

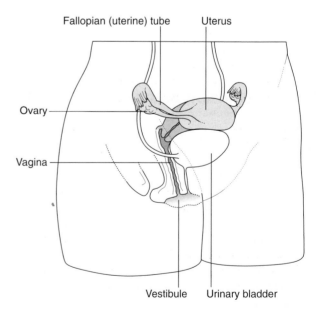

Fallopian (uterine) tube

Uterus

Ovary

Vagina

Vestibule Urinary bladder

Fig. 9.3 Female reproductive organs: viewed obliquely from the front.

Self-assessment on Section 1: questions

Multiple choice questions

1. Concerning anatomical nomenclature:
   a. Medial means in the midline of the body.
   b. Inferior means smaller than superior.
   c. A coronal section divides a structure into a right portion and a left portion.
   d. Sensory nerve impulses pass towards the central nervous system.
   e. The autonomic nervous system supplies smooth muscle.

2. Concerning ribs and sternum:
   a. Typical ribs articulate with vertebrae at the head and at the tubercle.
   b. The first costosternal joint is synovial.
   c. Hyaline cartilage is found between the anterior end of a typical rib and the sternum.
   d. The upper part of the sternum is the manubrium.
   e. The fourth rib articulates with the sternum at the sternal angle of Louis.

3. Synovial joints are present:
   a. Between costal cartilages and the sternum.
   b. Between articular processes of vertebrae.
   c. Between adjacent vertebral bodies.
   d. Between the two pubic bones.
   e. Between the head of a rib and the vertebral column.

4. The epiphyseal plate:
   a. Is at the junction of the head and the shaft of a developing long bone.
   b. Is the site of growth in length.
   c. Is present in a mature bone.
   d. Is composed of hyaline cartilage.
   e. Prevents arteries passing from the shaft to the head of the bone.

5. Concerning the meninges and meningeal spaces:
   a. The pia mater is prolonged below the spinal cord as the cauda equina.
   b. The dural sac ends below at vertebral level S2.
   c. The spinal extradural space contains adipose tissue and a plexus of veins.
   d. The pia mater is firmly adherent to the spinal cord.
   e. The arachnoid mater is outside the dura mater.

6. Blood from the following veins reaches the heart in the superior vena cava:
   a. Subclavian veins.
   b. Internal jugular veins.
   c. Hepatic veins.
   d. Veins of the upper thoracic wall.
   e. Femoral veins.

7. Upper limb arteries include:
   a. Axillary.
   b. Brachial.
   c. Popliteal.
   d. Radial.
   e. Dorsalis pedis.

8. Concerning lumbar puncture and the vertebral column:
   a. At lumbar puncture, a needle inserted between the laminae of adjacent vertebrae will penetrate the ligamentum flavum.
   b. Lumbar puncture is normally performed between vertebrae L1/2 in an adult.
   c. During lumbar puncture, cerebrospinal fluid is taken from the subdural space.
   d. The posterior longitudinal ligament forms part of the anterior wall of the vertebral canal.
   e. Venous blood from a vertebral body drains to the internal vertebral venous plexus.

9. In the spinal cord:
   a. Grey matter consists of collections of myelinated axons.
   b. Myelin is manufactured in peripheral nerves by Schwann cells.
   c. Disease of the ventral horn cells would result in paralysis or weakness of skeletal muscle.
   d. The lateral horn of grey matter is concerned with the innervation of smooth muscle.
   e. The dorsal column of white matter is concerned with sensory perception.

Matching item questions

Questions 1–5

Match the numbered item to the lettered response. Each lettered response may be used once, more than once, or not at all.
   a. Ventral horn cells
   b. Lateral horn cells
   c. Dorsal columns
   d. Schwann cells
   e. Oligodendrocytes

1. Smooth muscle
2. Skeletal muscle
3. Preganglionic sympathetic neurons
4. Sensation
5. Myelin production in peripheral nerves

Questions 6–10

Match the numbered item to the lettered response. Each lettered response may be used once, more than once, or not at all.

   a. Extradural space
   b. Subdural space
   c. Subarachnoid space
   d. Cauda equina
   e. Filum terminale

6. Contains a venous plexus
7. Contains cerebrospinal fluid
8. Consists of rootlets of spinal nerves
9. Ends at vertebral level S2
10. Begins at vertebral level L3/4 in the newborn child

Questions requiring short answers

1. Name the serous cavities of the body. What are the serous membranes, and how are they arranged? What is their function?

2. What are: (a) dermatomes, (b) myotomes, (c) Langer's lines, (d) superficial fascia, (e) deep fascia?

3. What do the following terms mean in respect of veins: (a) superficial, (b) pulmonary, (c) portal, (d) systemic?

4. List the components of the alimentary system in the correct order from mouth to anus.

5. Draw a diagram of a typical vertebra naming the following parts: lamina, pedicle, transverse process, spinous process, body, vertebral canal. How do two typical vertebrae articulate with each other?

6. Describe or draw a cross-section through the mid-thoracic spinal cord labelling grey and white matter, central canal, and spinal nerve attachments. Indicate the position of cell bodies of motor neurons supplying voluntary muscle, cell bodies of motor neurons supplying involuntary muscle, and the dorsal white column. Which cells are attacked in poliomyelitis, and with what result?

7. Describe or draw a cross-section through the vertebral column at vertebral level L3/4 showing the relationship of bone, meninges and the contents of the vertebral canal. Label the meningeal layers indicating the area(s) in which anaesthetic agents may be injected.

8. List the structures that would be penetrated by a lumbar puncture needle. Where would you perform this, and why?

9. What is a dorsal root ganglion? Is it part of the peripheral or the central nervous system? What is its function? What disease may affect it?

Self-assessment on Section 1: answers

Multiple choice answers

1. a. **False**. Medial means nearer the midline than …, but a structure in the midline itself is described as median.
   b. **False**. Inferior means below (when standing in the anatomical position). Inferior is a term of position, not size or quality.
   c. **False**. The division is into anterior and posterior portions, not right and left.
   d. **True**.
   e. **True**. Skeletal muscle is supplied by the somatic nervous system.

2. a. **True**. These are synovial articulations. The head of a typical rib articulates with two vertebrae: that corresponding in number to the rib, and that above. The tubercle of a typical rib articulates with the transverse process of the corresponding vertebra.
   b. **False**. The first costosternal is a primary cartilaginous joint.
   c. **True**. There is also a small synovial cavity between the cartilage and the sternum.
   d. **True**.
   e. **False**. The second rib articulates at the sternal angle.

3. a. **True**.
   b. **False**. These are synovial.
   c. **False**. These are symphyses (secondary cartilaginous).
   d. **False**. This is also a symphysis.
   e. **True**.

4. a. **True**.
   b. **True**.
   c. **False**. It is only present in immature bone.
   d. **True**.
   e. **True**. This may have important consequences in the supply to the head of a bone in a child.

5. a. **False**. This is the filum terminale, not cauda equina. The cauda equina is the name given to the collection of nerve rootlets.
   b. **True**.
   c. **True**. These veins are important in the spread of disease to the vertebral column.
   d. **True**.
   e. **False**. It is inside the dura mater.

6. a. **True**.
   b. **True**.
   c. **False**. Hepatic veins drain blood from the liver to the inferior vena cava. Do not confuse the hepatic veins (liver–IVC) with the (hepatic) portal vein (intestines–liver).
   d. **True**. These empty into the azygos vein which is a tributary of the superior vena cava.
   e. **False**. Blood from the femoral veins reaches the heart in the IVC.

7. a. **True**.
   b. **True**.
   c. **False**. It is a lower limb artery, at the back of the knee.
   d. **True**.
   e. **False**. It is an artery of the foot.

8. a. **True**.
   b. **False**. It is between L3/4 in an adult and lower in the newborn child.
   c. **False**. It is taken from the subarachnoid space.
   d. **True**.
   e. **True**. Two or more basivertebral veins emerge from the posterior aspect of the vertebral body and drain into the plexus.

9. a. **False**. This is white matter. Grey matter is predominantly made up of cell bodies.
   b. **True**. It is made by oligodendrocytes in the central nervous system.
   c. **True**. These cells are affected in poliomyelitis.
   d. **True**. Cell bodies of preganglionic sympathetic neurons are here.
   e. **True**.

Matching item answers

1. b.
   Lateral horn cells give rise to autonomic neurons supplying visceral smooth muscle.

2. a.
   Ventral horn cells give rise to somatic neurons supplying voluntary skeletal muscle.

3. b.
   See 1 above.

4. c.
   The dorsal columns are large tracts of white matter conveying sensory information up towards the brain.

5. d.
   Oligodendrocytes produce myelin in the central nervous system.

6. a.
   The extradural (epidural) space contains the internal vertebral venous plexus.

7. c.

8. d.
   The rootlets are present because the spinal cord is so much shorter than the vertebral column, so rootlets for the lumbar and sacral nerves have to pass for some distance in the subarachnoid space and vertebral canal before they reach the appropriate intervertebral foramen.

9. c.

10. e.
    See Figure 6.8 (p. 39).

Short answers

1. The serous cavities are the pleural (right and left), the pericardial and the peritoneal. They are lined by serous membranes: pleura, pericardium and peritoneum. These are arranged such that one layer – the parietal layer – is on the internal aspect of the body wall and one layer – the visceral layer – almost completely surrounds the internal organ (lungs, heart, guts). The parietal and visceral layers are continuous at the site where the internal organ is connected to the body wall (e.g. the hilum of the lung). See Figure 3.1 (p. 16).

2. a. A dermatome is the area of skin supplied by one spinal nerve. See Figure 6.6 (p. 36).
   b. A myotome is the group of skeletal muscle fibres supplied by one spinal nerve.
   c. Langer's lines are invisible cleavage lines along which cuts should be made for good healing; they arise from the orientation of connective and elastic tissue in the skin (see Fig. 3.2, p. 17).
   d. Superficial fascia is subcutaneous tissue of varying thickness; it includes fat, connective tissue, blood vessels and nerves.
   e. Deep fascia is the fibrous layer, almost a membrane, which limits the superficial fascia; deep fascia often forms the sheath of a muscle.

3. a. Superficial veins are those that run in the superficial fascia (see above) and are, if there is not too much fat, visible under the skin.
   b. Deep veins accompany the principal arteries deep to the deep fascia. Deep and superficial veins communicate.
   c. Portal veins are those which begin and end in capillary beds. The term portal veins usually means the hepatic portal vein conveying blood rich in nutrients to the liver from the alimentary canal between the lower oesophagus and anal canal. Its tributaries are the splenic, superior and inferior mesenteric veins (Fig. 7.3, p. 45).
   d. Systemic veins are all other veins that convey blood from the body back to the heart through the superior and inferior vena cava. The term does not usually include the pulmonary veins conveying blood from the lungs to the heart.

4. Components of the alimentary system in order from mouth to anus are: mouth, pharynx, oesophagus, stomach, duodenum, jejunum, ileum, caecum, ascending colon, transverse colon, descending colon, sigmoid colon, rectum, anal canal.

5. See Figure 5.1. (p. 26).

6. See Figure 6.3 (p. 34). Cell bodies of motor neurons supplying voluntary muscle are in the ventral horn of grey matter. Cell bodies of motor neurons supplying involuntary muscle of the trunk are mostly in the lateral horn of grey matter. Ventral horn cells are attacked in poliomyelitis, leading to weakness or paralysis of the muscles supplied.

7. See Figure 6.9 (p. 40). The needle in Figure 6.9 is in the subarachnoid space containing cerebrospinal fluid. Anaesthetic agents injected here would give spinal anaesthesia. Anaesthetic agents injected into the extra(epi)dural space would give an epidural anaesthesia. When drawing the diagram, it would not be necessary to include the rootlets of spinal nerves, although it may be helpful if you let the examiner know that you knew they were there.

8. Assuming that the needle were inserted just to one side of the midline, it would pass through: skin, subcutaneous tissue (superficial fascia), postvertebral muscle, ligamentum flavum, extradural space (fat and vessels), dura mater, arachnoid mater. In an adult you would perform this between vertebrae L3 and L4, well below the termination of the spinal cord at L1/2. In a newborn child you would insert the needle between L4 and L5.

9. A dorsal root ganglion is a swelling on the dorsal root of a spinal nerve as it passes through the intervertebral foramen. It houses the cell bodies of all sensory (pseudounipolar) neurons within that nerve and so destruction of if would result in sensory changes in the dermatome concerned. These ganglia may be infected by microorganisms: the herpes zoster virus is an example. This may give rise to shingles in which there is a vesicular eruption in the skin over the affected dermatome, and dermatome pain.

2 SECTION 2
Regional anatomy

10 Thorax

Introduction

The thorax consists of:

- the chest wall
- the two pleural cavities surrounding the lungs
- the area between these cavities, the mediastinum, in which are found the heart, great vessels, trachea and oesophagus, vagus and phrenic nerves, thymus gland and the thoracic duct.

On the external surface of the anterolateral chest wall are the breasts (mammary glands), also considered in this chapter.

Below, the thorax is separated from the abdomen by the diaphragm; above, it is continuous with the neck at the thoracic inlet (between sternum and vertebra T1) through which structures pass between thorax and neck (Fig. 10.1).

10.1 Chest wall

Overview

The chest wall consists of the ribs and sternum laterally and anteriorly, and the vertebral column posteriorly, which provides most of the structural support. Ribs articulate with the vertebral column behind and the sternum in front, these articulations permitting the movements of breathing. Intercostal (between the ribs) spaces are occupied by muscle and a neurovascular bundle that supplies the muscles, the skin over them and the lining of the pleural cavity deep to them. The repeating pattern of vertebrae, ribs and the intercostal neurovascular bundle is an illustration of segmentation.

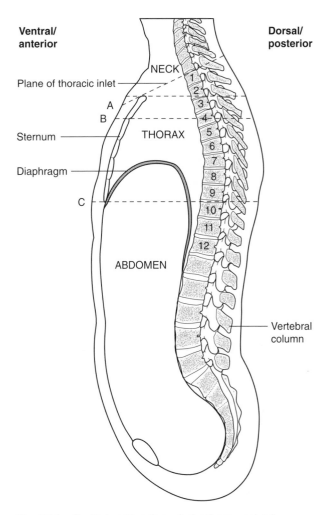

Fig. 10.1 Sagittal section through the thorax: point A (suprasternal border) is at vertebral level T2; point B (sternal angle of Louis) is at vertebral level T4; point C (xiphoid process) is at about vertebral level T9.

Learning Objectives

You should:

- appreciate the orientation of the ribs

- know the vertebral levels of the suprasternal notch, angle of Louis, and xiphisternum

- understand how ribs articulate with vertebrae and sternum

- appreciate the structure and contents of an intercostal space
- know the formation and function of intercostal nerves and the dermatomes of the chest wall
- know where and how to insert a chest drain.

Vertebral levels and surface markings

(Fig. 10.1)

Remind yourself of the significance of vertebral levels and surface markings.

- The suprasternal notch (in which you can palpate the trachea) is at vertebral level T2.
- The sternal angle (of Louis) is at vertebral level T4.
- The xiphisternum (xiphoid process) is at vertebral level T9 (about).
- Note the downwards orientation of the ribs when you consider an anterior view of the rib cage: the second rib articulates with vertebra T2 posteriorly, but with the sternal angle at vertebral level T4 anteriorly. Therefore, a transverse (horizontal) section of the thorax, such as a scan, intersects several ribs.

Bones and joints of the chest wall

(Fig. 10.2)

The chest wall is made up of the 12 pairs of ribs, the sternum and the intercostal muscles. Ribs are numbered 1–12 from above down and articulate with the vertebral column posteriorly and (mostly) the sternum anteriorly. The ribs are angled with respect to the horizontal plane – the sternal end is lower than the vertebral – and so in horizontal section, or a transverse CT or MRI scan, several ribs will be seen sectioned obliquely. Ribs are united at their anterior end to cartilage: the costal cartilages.

Vertebrae

The main features of a typical vertebra are described in Chapter 5. A thoracic vertebra is identifiable because of its facets for articulation with the ribs. Vertebrae T2–T9 have two demifacets on each side, other vertebrae having only one.

Ribs

Each rib has a head, neck, tubercle and shaft. Figure 10.3 shows the main features of a typical rib (ribs 2–10). Of the atypical ribs (1, 11, 12), you need only bother with the first.

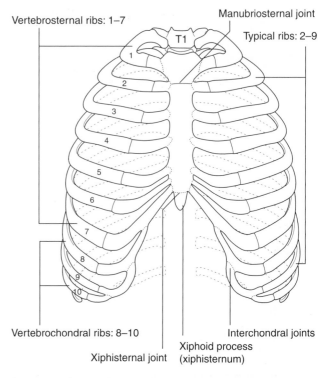

Vertebrosternal ribs: 1–7

Manubriosternal joint

Typical ribs: 2–9

T1

Vertebrochondral ribs: 8–10

Xiphisternal joint

Xiphoid process (xiphisternum)

Interchondral joints

Fig. 10.2 Thorax from the front. Note the orientation of the ribs: a horizontal section through the thorax (e.g. a CT scan) intersects several ribs.

First rib

- Scalene tubercle on the upper surface, to which is attached scalenus anterior muscle.
- Groove for subclavian vein, anterior to the tubercle.
- Groove for subclavian artery, posterior to the tubercle.

Sternum

There are three parts, from superior to inferior: manubrium, body and xiphoid process (or xiphisternum). There may be a hole in the centre of the body, since it is formed by a number of individual sternebrae that should fuse together, but may fail to do so.

Joints between vertebrae and ribs

Typical ribs have three synovial articulations with the vertebrae.

- The head has upper and lower articular facets set almost at a right angle to one another, the lower articulating with the vertebra corresponding in number to the rib, and the upper with the vertebra above. Ribs 1, 10, 11 and 12 have only one facet and articulate only with the numerically corresponding vertebra.

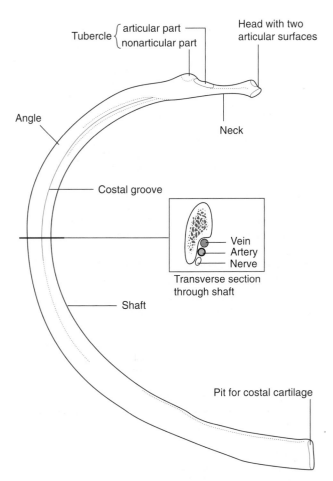

Tubercle { articular part / nonarticular part

Head with two articular surfaces

Angle

Neck

Costal groove

Vein
Artery
Nerve

Transverse section through shaft

Shaft

Pit for costal cartilage

Fig. 10.3 A typical rib, inferior aspect. The head articulates with two vertebrae, those corresponding in number to the rib, and the rib above. The costal groove on the internal aspect of the rib is shown with the neurovascular bundle.

- The tubercle of most ribs (not 11 or 12) articulates with the transverse process of the numerically corresponding vertebra.

These joints allow the ribs to move in breathing.

Ligaments

These ligaments are not of great importance. They include:

- triradiate ligament: from the head of the rib to the vertebra above, the intervertebral disc, and the vertebra below
- costotransverse ligaments between the vertebral transverse process and the tubercle of the rib.

Joints between ribs, sternum and vertebral column

- The first costal cartilage is continuous with the manubrium (primary cartilaginous joint) and

Table 10.1 Articulation of ribs with vertebral column and sternum

Rib	Posterior articulation	Anterior articulation
1	Vertebra T1 only	Sternum (primary cartilaginous joint, so first rib and sternum move as one)
2–7	Vertebra of same number and one above	Small synovial cavity between sternum and costal cartilage
8–9	As above	Costal cartilage articulates with cartilage immediately above
10	Vertebra of same number only	Costal cartilage articulates with cartilage immediately above
11, 12	Vertebra of same number only	None

remains so throughout life, unless it ossifies completely.

- Costal cartilages 2–7 have synovial articulations with the sternum. The second costal cartilage articulates at the sternal angle with the manubrium and the body of the sternum. The sternal angle (of Louis) is easily palpable and when you are counting ribs as part of a physical examination, it is best to start at the sternal angle with the second rib. In any case, the first rib is difficult to find because it is underneath the clavicle.
- Costal cartilages 8–10 have synovial articulations with the costal cartilage immediately above.
- Costal cartilages 11 and 12 are free of any anterior articulations, but provide attachments for muscles.

Articulations are summarised in Table 10.1.

- Ribs 1–7 are vertebrosternal, or true ribs.
- Ribs 8–10 are vertebrochondral or false ribs.
- Ribs 11 and 12 are floating ribs.

Muscles of chest wall

Intercostal muscles and spaces (Fig. 10.4)

There are three layers of tissue between ribs, partly muscle and partly membrane: external, internal and innermost intercostals, with the intercostal neuro-vascular bundle running between the internal and innermost. The area between ribs, occupied by these intercostal muscles, is the intercostal space.

- External intercostal muscle. Muscle at the back and sides, membrane anteriorly. Fibres pass from the upper rib downwards and forwards to the upper border of the rib below.

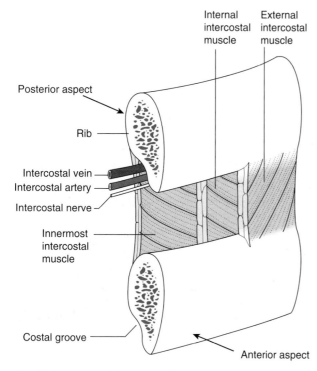

Internal intercostal muscle · External intercostal muscle

Posterior aspect

Rib

Intercostal vein

Intercostal artery

Intercostal nerve

Innermost intercostal muscle

Costal groove

Anterior aspect

Fig. 10.4 Intercostal space and muscles.

- Internal intercostal muscle. Muscle at the front and sides, membrane posteriorly. Fibres pass upwards and forwards, more or less at right angles to those of the external intercostal.
- Innermost intercostal muscle: as internal intercostal.
- Inside the chest wall there are (usually) muscle fibres that fan out from the sternum to the internal aspect of ribs 3–6. This is transversus thoracis, and it is equivalent to the transversus abdominis in the abdomen. It is not important.

Neurovascular bundle, costal groove

These muscles are supplied by the segmental intercostal nerve corresponding in number to the intercostal space. The rib has a groove underneath most of its length on the internal aspect. This costal groove provides some shelter for the intercostal neurovascular bundle. Within the groove the neurovascular bundle is arranged, from top to bottom, vein, artery, nerve (VAN). In each intercostal space, there are also smaller branches of the intercostal nerve and artery (collateral branches) which run on top of the rib below.

Muscles of the pectoral girdle

Overlying the ribs and intercostal muscles externally are muscles which attach the upper limb (humerus, clavicle and scapula) to the trunk: pectoralis major, pectoralis minor, latissimus dorsi, levator scapulae,

rhomboids, and trapezius. These are considered in Chapter 12.

> **Clinical box**
>
> **Insertion of chest drains** (Fig. 10.5)
> It is occasionally necessary to insert a chest drain (a hollow tube) through the chest wall into the pleural cavity. This procedure, properly termed thoracocentesis (also thoracentesis, pleurocentesis), is performed to remove either fluid (excess pleural fluid, blood) or air that had collected in the pleural cavity (see Pneumothorax, p. 70). The position of various structures which should be avoided (heart, liver, spleen, etc.) means that there are two places on either side where this may most safely be done:
> - second intercostal space in the midclavicular line
> - fourth or fifth space in the midaxillary line.
>
> To avoid any risk of damage to the main intercostal neurovascular bundle, it is better to insert the chest drain in the lower half of an intercostal space.

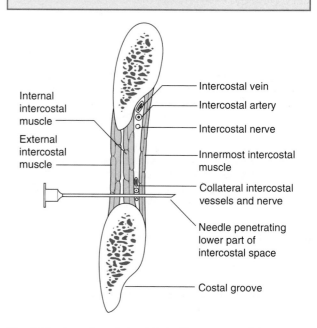

Internal intercostal muscle

External intercostal muscle

Intercostal vein

Intercostal artery

Intercostal nerve

Innermost intercostal muscle

Collateral intercostal vessels and nerve

Needle penetrating lower part of intercostal space

Costal groove

Fig. 10.5 Insertion of chest drain (thoracocentesis).

Blood supply of chest wall

Arteries: branches of the aorta and the subclavian/axillary artery

- Posterior intercostal arteries (Fig. 10.6). These are branches of the aorta (so-called segmental arteries), except for the first and second which come from the costocervical trunk, a branch of the subclavian artery (not from the aorta because it does not pass high enough in the thorax).
- Anterior intercostal arteries (Fig. 10.7). These arise from the right and left internal thoracic arteries,

A

B

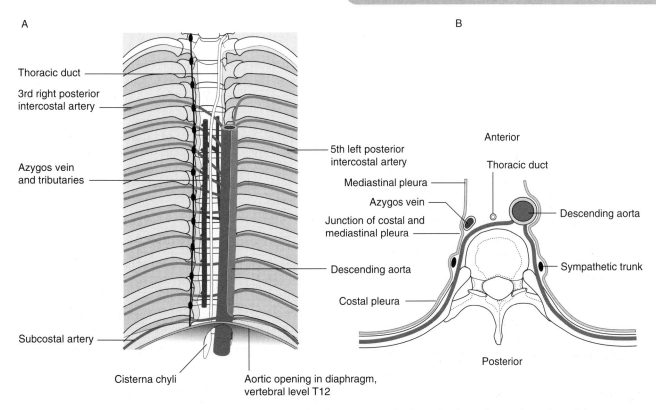

Thoracic duct

3rd right posterior intercostal artery

Azygos vein and tributaries

Subcostal artery

Cisterna chyli

Aortic opening in diaphragm, vertebral level T12

5th left posterior intercostal artery

Mediastinal pleura

Azygos vein

Junction of costal and mediastinal pleura

Descending aorta

Costal pleura

Anterior

Thoracic duct

Descending aorta

Sympathetic trunk

Posterior

Fig. 10.6 Posterior intercostal arteries. (**A**) Anterior view. The first two posterior intercostal arteries are branches of the subclavian artery and approach the spaces from above. They are of no great clinical significance. (**B**) Schematic cross-section showing the origin of posterior intercostal vessels from the aorta.

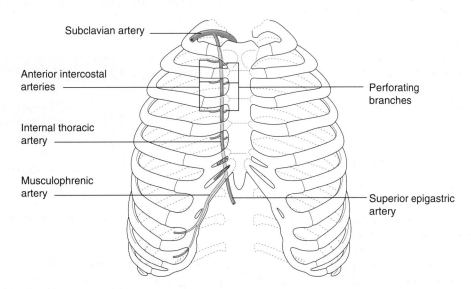

Subclavian artery

Anterior intercostal arteries

Internal thoracic artery

Musculophrenic artery

Perforating branches

Superior epigastric artery

Fig. 10.7 Right internal thoracic artery. Note the anterior intercostal arteries.

branches of the subclavian which run internally down the chest wall 1 or 2 cm lateral to the sternal border. They are important in supplying the breast. Anterior and posterior intercostal arteries anastomose with each other in the intercostal space, and this potential route between the internal thoracic artery and the aorta is important in

congenital aortic coarctation (narrowing) as a bypass for the narrowing (see later and Fig. 10.25, p. 86).

- Lateral thoracic artery. Again, this is important for the breast.
- Other branches of the subclavian/axillary arteries: thoracoacromial (acromiothoracic), superior (or supreme or highest) thoracic (don't bother with these).

Veins

- Anterior intercostal veins drain to the internal thoracic veins, thence to the subclavian – brachiocephalic – superior vena cava (SVC).
- Posterior intercostal veins drain to the azygos system and the SVC. As the first one or two posterior intercostal arteries arise differently from the rest, so the posterior intercostal veins of the first few spaces drain differently: to the brachiocephalic veins (see later).

Intercostal nerves (Fig. 10.8)

Intercostal nerves are ventral rami of the thoracic segmental nerves (see Ch. 6). Having been formed in the region of the intervertebral foramen, they run in the costal groove of each rib and supply the intercostal muscles, a strip of skin overlying the intercostal muscles and a similar strip of parietal pleura on the internal aspect of the chest wall. Anteriorly, when the ribs turn upwards, the neurovascular bundle parts company with the ribs and continues in the direction already established. Lower intercostal nerves therefore also supply skin of most of the anterior abdominal wall and the parietal peritoneum deep to it (the abdominal equivalent of parietal pleura).

Intercostal nerves contain both motor and sensory fibres

- Cell bodies of motor fibres to skeletal muscle (voluntary motor fibres) are in the ventral horn of grey matter of the correspondingly numbered spinal cord segment.
- Cell bodies of sensory fibres in an intercostal nerve are in the dorsal root ganglion of the parent segmental nerve.

This arrangement gives rise to the concept of segmental innervation, and allows automatic reflex action within one segment – a physiological pheno-menon particularly important clinically in the limbs.

Intercostal nerves also convey sympathetic fibres (see later).

Segmentation, dermatomes

Segmentation is most obvious in the thorax: segmental bones (ribs), segmental nerves, dermatomes, segmental vessels, and, in a way, the vertebrae. Study again Figure 6.6 (p. 36), the dermatome pattern for the whole body, and in the chest memorise these dermatomes:

- skin over the second intercostal space (landmark: sternal angle of Louis): spinal nerve T2; and similarly down the chest to
- skin over the xiphoid process: T7 or 8.

10.2 Pleural cavities, tracheobronchial tree, lungs
(Figs 10.9, 10.10)

Overview

The pleural cavities surround the lungs. Air is conducted to and from the alveoli by, in order, the trachea, right and left main bronchi, lobar bronchi, segmental bronchi, and finally bronchioles. The right lung has three lobes, the left two, and within these the functional units of the lung are bronchopulmonary segments. The lungs are invaginated into the pleura such that the pleura is disposed as a visceral layer on the lung surface and a parietal layer on the inside of the chest wall, visceral and parietal being continuous at the pulmonary hilum. The pleural cavities and lungs extend beyond the rib cage and are intimately related inferiorly to the liver, spleen and kidneys, and superiorly to the root of the neck.

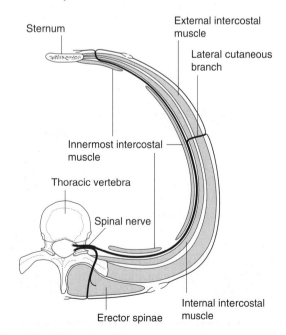

Fig. 10.8   Thoracic wall: oblique section showing one intercostal nerve.

Learning Objectives

You should:

- know the structure of the tracheobronchial tree and its surface landmarks

- know the extent of the pleural cavities and the lungs within them in relation to surface landmarks

- know where major abdominal organs are most closely related to the lungs

- know the pattern of lobes and bronchopulmonary segments for each lung

- understand the movements of breathing and how disease can modify the pattern

- know what you are listening to when you place your stethoscope over different areas of the lungs.

Pleural cavities, mediastinum

The right and left pleural cavities surround the right and left lungs. The tissue between them that contains heart and great vessels etc. is the mediastinum.

The pleural cavities are, like the pericardial and peritoneal cavities, serous cavities derived from the embryonic coelom. Serous cavities, which also include synovial cavities, are lined by mesothelium, a simple squamous lining which, with associated connective tissue and basement membrane, makes up the serous membranes (pleura, pericardium, peritoneum, synovium).

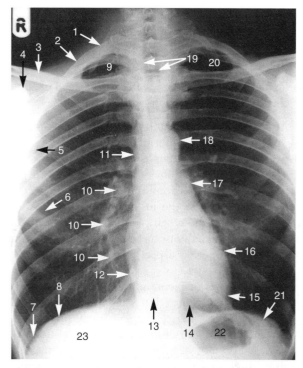

Fig. 10.10 Radiograph of chest: 1, cervical rib (rare); it may compress the lower trunk of the brachial plexus; 2, first rib; 3, clavicle; 4, coracoid process of scapula; 5, medial border of scapula; 6, anterior portion of fifth rib; 7, right costodiaphragmatic recess; 8, right dome of diaphragm; 9, apex of lung; 10, pulmonary vessels and bronchi at hilum of lung; 11, right border of superior vena cava; 12, right heart border – right atrium; 13, position of inferior vena cava entering right atrium; 14, inferior heart border – right ventricle; 15, apex of heart; 16, left heart border – left ventricle; 17, pulmonary artery (left atrial appendage may be apparent here); 18, arch ('knuckle') of aorta; 19, margins of trachea (dark area between); 20, apex of lung; 21, left dome of diaphragm; 22, air in stomach; 23, liver.

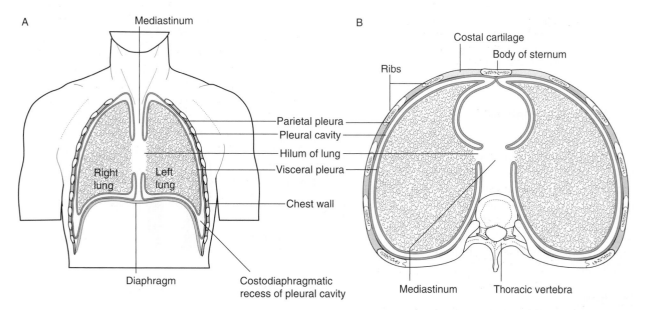

Fig. 10.9 The lungs and pleura: (**A**) coronal section of trunk; (**B**) transverse section of thorax. Note that the visceral and parietal layers of pleura are continuous at the hilum (root) of the lung.

They are, strictly speaking, only potential cavities. Each lung invaginates each pleural cavity as it forms in such a way that the serous lining of the cavities, the pleura, is found:

- on the inside of the chest wall – the parietal pleura
- covering the lung – the visceral pleura.

At the place where the bronchial tree passes from the mediastinum into the lung, parietal and visceral pleura are continuous: this is the *root* or *hilum* of the lung and it should be obvious that nothing can pass into or out of the lung except through the hilum.

Parietal pleura on the inside of the chest wall is sometimes called the costal pleura, that on the medial side of the pleural cavity the mediastinal pleura, and that on the superior aspect of the diaphragm the diaphragmatic pleura.

The two layers of pleura glide on one another (for movement in breathing), but since there is normally nothing between the visceral and parietal pleura other than a minute amount of lubricating pleural fluid, the two layers do not separate. The surface tension of pleural fluid ensures that the two layers remain adherent. A simple analogy is two sheets of glass with water between them: the two sheets may move on one another but can not easily be separated because of the film of fluid between them.

Clinical box

Pneumothorax, haemothorax

If air finds its way between the visceral and parietal pleura (e.g. a lung alveolus bursts, or a person is stabbed), then the two 'plates of glass' separate, the lung does not move with the chest wall and the elastic tissue in the lungs causes them to collapse, thus preventing normal breathing. This is a pneumothorax (Fig. 10.11). If a blood vessel bleeds into the pleural cavity, a haemothorax develops. These conditions are treated by the insertion of a chest drain (Fig. 10.5, see p. 66).

Tracheobronchial tree (Fig. 10.12)

The respiratory system consists of all the air-conducting passages from the nose to the alveoli of the lungs. The respiratory system clinically is divided into upper and lower, separated by the vocal cords. An upper respiratory tract infection (URTI, or head cold) leads to symptoms we have all experienced: nasal, throat, and ear discomfort, which reminds us that the upper respiratory tract also includes an extension to the middle ear.

Trachea

The trachea begins at the level of the cricoid cartilage

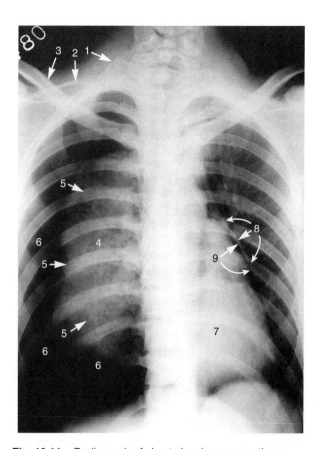

Fig. 10.11 Radiograph of chest showing pneumothorax, pneumopericardium: 1, first rib; 2, superior border of scapula; 3, clavicle; 4, collapsed lung; 5, margin of collapsed lung; 6, the areas between the ribs are completely black (an absence of normal lung radiographic appearance), signifying the presence of air in the pleural cavity on this side; 7, heart; 8, the fibrous and parietal pericardial layers are visible because 9, air is also present in the pericardial cavity – pneumopericardium.

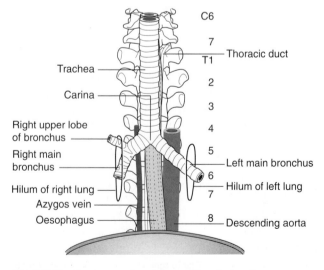

Fig. 10.12 Trachea and main bronchi; anterior view.

(vertebral level C6) and descends to its bifurcation (vertebral level about T4 in the supine position and T5 or 6 in the erect position). Its walls are made up of incomplete rings of hyaline cartilage closed posteriorly by connective tissue and trachealis muscle (involuntary muscle). Behind it is the oesophagus and between the two in the neck are the recurrent laryngeal nerves (see later).

Clinical box

Palpating the trachea
The trachea should be central in the suprasternal notch (vertebral level T2), and palpation of this is a routine part of a thorough clinical examination. If the trachea is deviated to one side or the other, this implies that it has been displaced by disease (e.g. a tumour or a pneumothorax pushing it to the other side).

Tracheal bifurcation and main bronchi

At the bifurcation of the trachea, the two main bronchi arise and these pass into the lungs at the hila with the pulmonary (Latin: *pulmo* = lung) arteries and veins. At the bifurcation, the internal ridge that separates the two main bronchi is the carina (Latin: keel) and this should be fairly sharp. The area immediately beneath the bifurcation is occupied by tracheobronchial lymph nodes, which are often involved in malignant disease. If, at bronchoscopy, the carina is less than sharp, it is likely that tracheobronchial lymph nodes are enlarged.

The right main bronchus is slightly larger in calibre than the left, and this is one reason why inhaled foreign bodies more often pass into the right main bronchus. Both bronchi pass inferolaterally from the tracheal bifurcation, but the angulation of the bronchi is by no means constant. In some people the arrangement is more or less symmetrical, whereas in others the right main bronchus is more in line with the trachea than the left. The right main bronchus passes directly to the hilum of the right lung. The left main bronchus passes anterior to the oesophagus, which it indents (vertebral level T4/5, see later) and thence to the hilum of the left lung.

Lobar bronchi

The right and left main bronchi each give lobar bronchi to the lobes of the lungs, and these divide into segmental bronchi, each serving its own bronchopulmonary segment (see later). The incomplete cartilaginous rings, like those in the trachea, persist into the lobar bronchi. Structural support to smaller bronchi is provided by randomly arranged plates of cartilage in the wall.

Lungs

Lobes and fissures

The lungs are divided by fissures into lobes. The right lung has three lobes: upper, middle and lower; the left lung has two: upper and lower. The left-sided equivalent of the right middle lobe is the lingula – part of the left upper lobe. The lobes are demarcated by fissures: oblique and horizontal on the right, and oblique only on the left. The horizontal fissure is sometimes incomplete.

Occasionally on the right, the developing azygos vein may invaginate its way into the apical portion of the right upper lobe, thus creating a 'peninsula' of lung tissue. This azygos fissure and lobe may be mistaken on a chest radiograph for a pathological condition.

Bronchopulmonary segments   (Fig. 10.13)

Each lung is made up of a number of broncho-pulmonary segments, each with its own bronchus, its own branch of the pulmonary artery, and its own tributary of the pulmonary vein. These discrete units enable surgeons to excise one or more broncho-pulmonary segments when disease is confined to them without compromising the function of other segments. You need to know them.

Right lung
- Upper lobe: apical, posterior and anterior bronchopulmonary segments.
- Middle lobe: lateral and medial bronchopulmonary segments.
- Lower lobe: apical, medial, anterior, lateral and posterior bronchopulmonary segments.

Conventionally, the segments are numbered 1–10 in the order given. To avoid confusion between upper and lower lobes, the lower lobe segments are often called apical basal, medial basal, and so on.

Left lung
The pattern is modified somewhat:
- The middle lobe is replaced by the superior and inferior segments of the lingula (parts of the upper lobe).
- There is no medial basal segmental bronchus and the left medial basal segment may be much reduced in size or even absent as a result of the presence of the heart.
- There may be a common origin from the left upper lobe bronchus for the left upper lobe apical and posterior segmental bronchi, although the segments themselves are separate, as on the right.

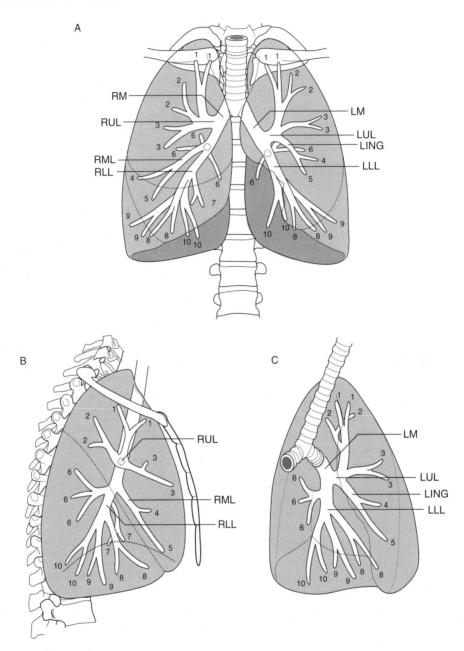

Fig. 10.13 Bronchi and bronchopulmonary segments: (**A**) anterior view; (**B**) lateral view of right lung showing right bronchi; (**C**) oblique view of left lung showing left bronchi. RM, right main bronchus; RUL, right upper lobe bronchus; RML, right middle lobe bronchus; RLL, right lower lobe bronchus; LM, left main bronchus; LUL, left upper lobe bronchus; LING, lingular bronchus; LLL, left lower lobe bronchus.

Right segmental bronchi:

- Upper lobe: 1, apical; 2, posterior; 3, anterior
- Middle lobe: 4, lateral; 5, medial
- Lower lobe: 6, apical basal; 7, medial basal; 8, anterior basal; 9, lateral basal; 10, posterior basal.

Left segmental bronchi:

- Upper lobe: 1, apical; 2, posterior; 3, anterior; 4, superior lingular; 5, inferior lingular
- Lower lobe: 6, apical basal; 8, anterior basal; 9, lateral basal, 10, posterior basal.

Note: There is no medial basal bronchus (7) on the left.

You should bear in mind that there is, as usual, some variation in this pattern from person to person. It is interesting, but of no relevance, to know that in pigs, sheep, llamas and tigers one of the right lobar bronchi arises from the trachea itself.

Pulmonary hila

These are the regions where arteries, veins, the bronchial tree, nerves and lymphatics pass between mediastinum and lungs. You need not bother with the precise arrangement of structures at the hilum except to know that the bronchi are posterior and the pulmonary arteries superior. The pulmonary ligament is the narrow inferior extension of the hilum, containing nothing of importance.

Relations of lungs to other organs

A number of important mediastinal structures are intimately related to the lungs and create impressions on the medial aspect of both lungs. On the right lung, those formed by the superior vena cava, the azygos vein and the oesophagus are noteworthy. On the left side, the impressions of the heart, the aortic arch and descending aorta are obvious.

Sensory nerve supply of pleura and lungs

Parietal pleura

- Costal: local intercostal nerves.
- Diaphragmatic: local intercostal nerves (peripherally), phrenic nerve (centrally).
- Mediastinal: phrenic (mainly).

Parietal pleural sensation is somatic sensation, and pain from irritation of parietal pleura will be sharp and well localised by the patient.

Lungs and visceral pleura

The lungs and visceral pleura, like all internal organs, are supplied by visceral sensory nerves that travel back to the central nervous system in nerves also conveying sympathetic and/or parasympathetic fibres. Visceral pain is much more vague and poorly localised by the patient. Inflammation of the pleura is called pleurisy and the sharp pain commonly associated with it arises not from irritation of the visceral pleura but from irritation of parietal pleura to which the disease has spread.

Clinical box

Movements of breathing

Normal breathing is the result of movement of the diaphragm. The diaphragm descends, the diaphragmatic parietal pleura descends and, since the two layers of pleura can not separate, this pulls the visceral pleura down so that the lung alveoli and airways expand and air is sucked in. In expiration, the diaphragm relaxes and the elastic tissue in the lung recoils, thus expelling air in the airways. In forced inspiration other muscles are used and these include any muscles that will enlarge the rib cage in any way. Neck muscles (sternocleidomastoid) will pull it up, abdominal muscles (quadratus lumborum) will pull it down, and by fixing the upper limbs, pectoral girdle muscles (pectoralis major, latissimus dorsi) will pull it out. These are *accessory muscles of respiration* and you will see them in action in any patient suffering a bronchitic or asthmatic attack. The function of the intercostal muscles is not fully understood, despite what anyone may tell you, but obviously they afford a degree of flexibility between the more rigid ribs.

The shape of the costotransverse joints allows the lateral aspect of the lower ribs to swivel up and out, thus increasing the lateral diameter of the chest. The anterior ends of all ribs can swing up and out, thereby increasing the anteroposterior diameter of the chest. Disease resulting in limitation of movement at these joints can be a cause of respiratory distress.

Lymphatics of the thorax

Chest wall

Lymph vessels pass:

- posteriorly with the main intercostal neurovascular bundle to reach paravertebral nodes and drain into the main thoracic duct (except for the upper few spaces on the right, which drain into the right lymphatic duct)
- anteriorly with the internal thoracic vessels to parasternal nodes and thence to the thoracic duct.

Both these lymphatic channels communicate with those of the breast and may be involved in the spread of breast disease.

Lungs and trachea

There are communicating lymph plexuses immediately under the visceral pleura and around the bronchial tree. From here lymph passes to the hilum where hilar nodes are found and thence to the mediastinal nodes and the thoracic duct.

Tracheobronchial nodes

These are the mediastinal lymph nodes immediately beneath the carina. They constitute the largest collection of lymph nodes in the body and receive lymph from heart, lungs and mediastinal structures such as the oesophagus. Enlargement of these nodes will cause a widening of the carina when viewed at bronchoscopy (see above).

Surface markings of lungs (Fig. 10.14)

Pleural cavities and reflections

These are important. The pleura extends above the clavicle into the neck where it is vulnerable to stab wounds, so do not be surprised if a patient who has been stabbed above the clavicle is breathless: there may be a pneumothorax. In this region the superior limit of the pleural cavity is formed by the suprapleural membrane, a half-tent of membrane suspended from the transverse process of vertebra C7 to attach to the inner aspect of the first rib.

Remember 2, 4, 6, 8, 10, 12. From about 2 cm above the clavicle, the line of pleural reflection passes behind the sternoclavicular joint and almost meets its fellow of the other side behind the sternal angle (level of second costal cartilage), then down to the level of the fourth costal cartilage where the left line passes laterally but the right continues down to the sixth. The lines then pass obliquely laterally across the sixth cartilage, crossing the eighth rib in the midclavicular line, the tenth rib in the midaxillary line and the twelfth rib (behind now) in the midscapular line, or even lower.

Costodiaphragmatic recess

The inferior recess of the pleural cavity, between the ribs and the diaphragm, is the costodiaphragmatic recess. Its lower extremities are not normally occupied by lung tissue except possibly during extreme deep inspiration. In normal circumstances the costal pleura and the diaphragmatic pleura here are in contact.

Note that at the back the costodiaphragmatic recesses of the pleural cavities are behind the upper poles of the kidneys.

Pleura below the ribs

The three sites where the pleural reflection is below the costal margin are:

- right costosternal region (not the left, because of the heart)
- between the twelfth rib and the vertebral column on the right
- between the twelfth rib and the vertebral column on the left.

In these places abdominal incisions may enter the pleural cavity.

Lungs

These are similar to the pleura except that lung tissue does not normally extend much below vertebral level T10, and of course the extent of the lungs varies during breathing with inspiration and expiration.

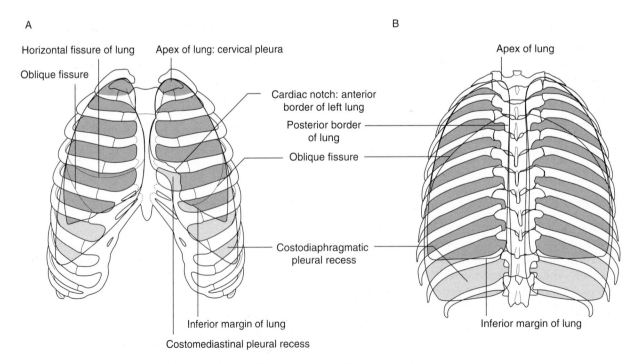

A

Horizontal fissure of lung — Apex of lung: cervical pleura

Oblique fissure

Cardiac notch: anterior border of left lung

Posterior border of lung

Oblique fissure

Costodiaphragmatic pleural recess

Inferior margin of lung

Costomediastinal pleural recess

B

Apex of lung

Inferior margin of lung

Fig. 10.14 Surface anatomy of pleura and lungs: (**A**) anterior view; (**B**) posterior view.

Table 10.2 Effect of breathing on position of lung structures

Structure	In forced expiration	In forced inspiration
Bifurcation of trachea	T4	T5/6 or lower
Hilum of lung	T5	T6 or lower
Lower border of lung	T8 (med.) to T9 (lat.)	T9 (med.) to T12 (lat.)

- Oblique fissure (both sides): spine of vertebra T2 or T3 – sixth costal cartilage.
- Horizontal fissure (right lung only): level of fourth costal cartilage, sternal edge – line of oblique fissure.

Variations in position depending upon posture and breathing

You should bear in mind that structures move during breathing. Vertebral levels are given in Table 10.2.

Finally, it should be obvious that everything will be lower when you are standing erect than when you are lying down. For these reasons, surface markings and vertebral levels are only approximate.

Clinical box

Listening to (auscultating) the lungs
From a clinical point of view you should note the following:

- When you place your stethoscope on a patient's back, you are listening mainly to the lower lobe. There is a small area of upper lobe, but no middle lobe at all.
- When you place your stethoscope on a patient's anterior chest wall, you are listening mainly to the upper and middle lobes.
- You will listen to the middle lobe best by placing the stethoscope at the side and in the axilla.
- You can not listen to individual bronchopulmonary segments, or even to individual lobes.
- When a patient is lying in bed on his back, the most dependent bronchopulmonary segments are the apical and posterior segments of the lower lobe. These segments are most often affected by lung infections in ill, bedridden patients.
- In normal breathing, lung tissue does not occupy the lower extremities of the costodiaphragmatic recesses, but it may in deep inspiration. This means that in this region the surface markings of the extent of the lungs is different from the surface markings for the extent of the pleural cavities.

10.3 Heart and pericardial cavity

Overview

The heart is surrounded by visceral and parietal layers of serous pericardium (equivalent to the pleura), and external to these the fibrous pericardium. The heart and pericardial cavity are in the anterior mediastinum, behind the sternum slightly to the left of the midline. The heart is orientated such that the right chambers of the heart are more anterior, and the left chambers more posterior. The outflow from each chamber is guarded by a valve: right atrium – tricuspid; right ventricle – pulmonary; left atrium – mitral; left ventricle – aortic. The cardiac conducting system is the means by which contraction is coordinated. Right and left coronary arteries from the ascending aorta supply heart muscle with freshly oxygenated blood. The inherent rhythmicity of cardiac muscle is modulated by the autonomic innervation of the heart, amongst other things.

Learning Objectives

You should:

- understand the arrangement of the pericardium around the heart, and the importance of cardiac tamponade
- know the surface markings of the heart and its borders as seen on a PA chest radiograph
- know the route taken by blood as it passes through the chambers and valves of the heart, and know how to perform external cardiac massage
- know the position, surface anatomy and importance of the cardiac valves
- understand the disposition and importance of the conducting system
- know the anatomy of the right, left, circumflex, anterior interventricular and posterior interventricular coronary arteries
- know where to place your stethoscope in order to listen to the various elements of cardiac function.

Pericardium

Serous pericardium (Fig. 10.15)

The heart is surrounded by the serous pericardium,

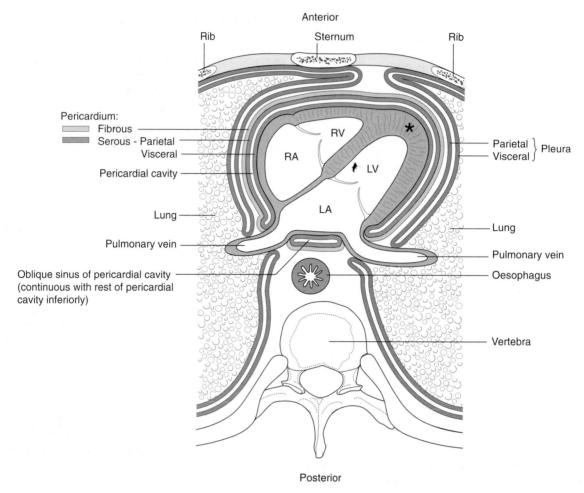

Fig. 10.15 Schematic cross-section through the chest (from below) showing the heart: RA, right atrium; RV, right ventricle; LA, left atrium; LV, left ventricle; *, apex.

equivalent in all respects to the pleura and peritoneum, with a visceral layer immediately covering the heart, and a parietal layer.

Fibrous pericardium (Fig. 10.15)

The serous pericardium, and the heart inside it, are then enclosed in a sac of tough fibrous tissue, the fibrous pericardium. It is simply like a plastic bag closed round the 'neck' of the heart (the great vessels) and is firmly attached to the underlying parietal layer of serous pericardium.

So, there are two types of pericardium, fibrous and serous, and there are two layers of serous pericardium. Note that it is the serous pericardium that is equivalent to the pleura. As in the pleural cavity, the pericardial cavity is only a potential cavity: it contains a minute amount of pericardial fluid and is there to facilitate gliding movements such as occur during the beating of the heart, but it does not allow separation of the two layers of serous pericardium.

Pericardial cavity and sinuses

The cardiac equivalent of the hilum of the lung, that is the place where structures pass between the heart and the rest of the mediastinum, is not as 'tidy' as the pulmonary hilum. The embryology of the great arteries (aorta, pulmonary) and veins (inferior vena cava, superior vena cava and pulmonary veins) results in the area posterior to the heart being complex.

- That part of the pericardial cavity behind the heart is the oblique sinus separating the left atrium (the original left side of the heart is now at the back) from the oesophagus.
- The transverse sinus is the potential communication between the right and left sides of the pericardial cavity found behind the great arteries (ascending aorta, pulmonary artery) and in front of the superior vena cava.

Borders of the heart   (Fig. 10.16)

Clinical box

Cardiac tamponade
It is important to realise that the fibrous pericardium is indeed fibrous and not elastic. If fluid were to collect in the pericardial cavity, the pericardial covering would not be able to expand to accommodate it and the beating of the heart would become increasingly compromised. This is cardiac tamponade – a potentially fatal emergency. It may arise from pericarditis (inflammatory fluid in the pericardial cavity) or from rupture of one of the coronary vessels or even of the heart wall itself, resulting in blood in the pericardial cavity (haemopericardium).

Heart

Surfaces and borders

The heart develops as a midline structure. It subsequently shifts so that the left side becomes posterior and the right side anterior. Despite this, the terms left and right are used and you might bear in mind that right can often, but not always, be translated as anterior, and left as posterior.

Surfaces of the heart

- Anterior or sternocostal (Fig. 10.16).
- Inferior or diaphragmatic.
- Posterior surface.

The most superior aspect of the heart is the area of origin of the great vessels. The term 'base' of the heart is used differently by different groups of people – there are three usages – and so is best avoided altogether.

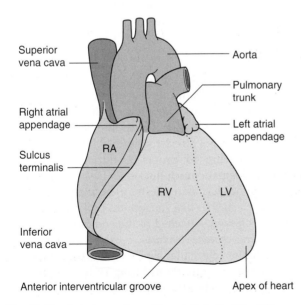

Superior vena cava

Aorta

Pulmonary trunk

Right atrial appendage

Left atrial appendage

Sulcus terminalis

RA

Inferior vena cava

RV   LV

Anterior interventricular groove   Apex of heart

Fig. 10.16   Anterior surface of heart. Note that the left atrium, at the back of the heart, is not evident on this view except (sometimes) for its appendage, as shown: RA, right atrium; RV, right ventricle; LV, left ventricle.

Borders of the heart   (Fig. 10.16)

- Right.
- Inferior or diaphragmatic, at the left extremity of which is the apex, so called for obvious reasons.
- Left, which slopes upwards and medially from apex towards root of great vessels.

Chambers of the heart, septum, conducting system

The heart has four chambers: right and left atria and right and left ventricles. The atria receive blood from veins and have little work to do, so their walls are thin. The right ventricle must contract with sufficient force to propel blood through the lungs and back to the heart, and its walls are significantly thicker than atrial walls. The left ventricle must propel blood throughout the body, and so its walls are much thicker again. The tissue separating the two atria is the atrial (or interatrial) septum, and that separating the two ventricles is the ventricular (or interventricular) septum.

Atria and ventricles are separated by a fibrous skeleton that provides a structural framework for the atrioventricular valves and an anchoring apparatus for contracting ventricular muscle. It is important in the electrical isolation of the ventricles from the atria and it is marked on the external aspect of the heart by the atrioventricular sulcus.

Atria

The left atrium receives blood from the lungs and the right from the rest of the body. Part of each atrial wall is rough owing to the pectinate muscles, and part is smooth. The rough-walled part includes the atrial appendage. Other terms that you may hear used are:

- atrium = auricle
- atrial appendage = auricle = auricular appendage.

The term auricle is ambiguous: do not use it.

Right atrium, fossa ovalis   (Fig. 10.17)
This forms the right heart border. It receives blood from the superior vena cava (SVC) and inferior vena cava (IVC) and may be thought of as being stretched vertically between the two venae cavae. It also receives most of the venous blood from the heart muscle itself through the coronary sinus, the opening of which is adjacent to that of the IVC. The smooth-walled part, which receives the venae cavae, and the rough-walled part are separated by the sulcus terminalis externally (crista terminalis internally).

At the lower end of the crista (internally) are two folds: the 'valves' (non-functional) of the IVC and the

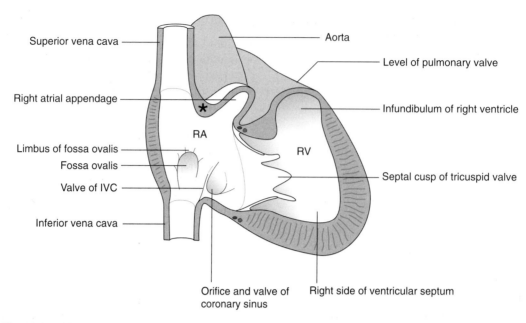

Superior vena cava

Aorta

Level of pulmonary valve

Right atrial appendage

Infundibulum of right ventricle

RA

RV

Limbus of fossa ovalis

Fossa ovalis

Valve of IVC

Septal cusp of tricuspid valve

Inferior vena cava

Orifice and valve of coronary sinus

Right side of ventricular septum

Fig. 10.17 Vertical oblique section through right atrium and ventricle. Papillary muscles and chordae tendineae not shown. RA, right atrium; RV, right ventricle; *, position of sinuatrial node.

coronary sinus which guard the orifices of these vessels. The valve of the IVC is continuous superiorly with the limbus (edge) of the fossa ovalis, a crescentic ridge on the atrial septum marking the site of the prenatal foramen ovale by which means blood passed from right to left atria, bypassing the non-functional lungs. The thicker part of the atrial septum, which ends inferiorly in the limbus of the fossa ovalis, is formed from embryological septum secundum; the thinner part in the floor of the fossa is from septum primum. The two septa normally unite, but they may remain separate forming a probe-patent (that is, a probe may be inserted) foramen ovale. This is not normally a problem because the higher venous pressure in the left atrium normally pushes over the thinner septum primum on the left so that it remains in contact with the thicker septum secundum.

The crista terminalis marks the junction between the two embryological parts of the right atrium. Since the smooth-walled portion is from the sinus venosus (receiving SVC, IVC, coronary sinus) and the rough-walled part is from the primitive atrium, the crista marks the sinuatrial (or sinoatrial) junction. At its upper end, just to the left of the entry of the SVC, is the sinuatrial (SA) node or cardiac pacemaker. Despite the importance of the SA node, there is nothing to see with the naked eye.

The outflow valve of the right atrium is the tricuspid (see later).

Left atrium   (Fig. 10.15)
This is at the back of the heart and receives blood from the pulmonary veins (usually two right, two left). It

may be thought of as being stretched from side to side between the right and left pulmonary veins. Behind the left atrium is the oesophagus, and an enlarged left atrium may result in a narrowing of the lower part of the thoracic oesophagus visible on a barium swallow investigation. The left atrial appendage may be apparent on the left heart border between the left ventricle (below) and the pulmonary artery (above). The smooth-walled part of the atrium is derived from incorporation of pulmonary veins and the rough-walled part from the primitive cardiac atrium. The outflow valve of the left atrium is the mitral (see later).

Ventricles

These are the chambers that do the work: they have thick muscular walls. In the fetus both ventricles share the work more or less equally and their walls are of equal thickness, but after birth the left ventricular walls, which propel blood round the body (as opposed to simply having to propel it through the lungs) become and remain much thicker. In both ventricles the internal surface has many fleshy trabeculations (ridges) and *papillary muscles* like stalagmites projecting into the ventricular lumen. Attached to the end of the papillary muscles are *chordae tendineae* – thin fibrous cords attached to the ventricular aspect of the atrioventricular valves. These are important during systole in preventing 'blowback' of the atrioventricular valves.

Right ventricle
The only noteworthy feature is the septomarginal (moderator) band that contains the right bundle of the

conducting system. The outflow valve is the pulmonary valve, and the part of the ventricle immediately beneath it is the conus arteriosus or infundibulum.

Left ventricle

There is nothing noteworthy about the interior of this chamber. The outflow valve is the aortic.

Ventricular septum

Most of this is thick and highly muscular as befits part of the wall of the left ventricle, but near the atrioventricular junction, part is membranous (pars membranacea), in effect a continuation of the atrial septum. If during development the membranous portion and the muscular portion fail to fuse, a ventricular septal defect results. Neural crest cells contribute to the membranous portion of the septum, and ventricular septal defects may be associated with other anomalies of neural crest origin.

Valves

In the order in which blood flows through the heart, the valves are: tricuspid, pulmonary (lungs), mitral, aortic. The positions of the valves in diastole and systole are shown in Figure 10.18. The mitral valve has two large cusps and the other valves each have three (Fig. 10.19). You should know the cusps of the aortic valve because of their relationship to the origin of the coronary arteries.

Cusps of the aortic valve and the coronary arteries (Figs 10.18, 10.19)

- The right coronary artery arises from the dilatation of the aorta immediately above the anterior cusp of the aortic valve. This dilatation is the anterior aortic sinus. The anterior cusp and anterior sinus are sometimes known as the right cusp and sinus because of the origin of the right coronary artery, but this ignores their actual position in the chest.
- The left coronary artery arises from the left posterior aortic sinus immediately above the left posterior cusp of the aortic valve. Both cusp and sinus are sometimes known as left cusp and left sinus because of the origin of the left coronary artery, but again this ignores their actual position.
- The right posterior aortic cusp and sinus are not associated with a coronary artery, and so may be referred to as the non-coronary cusp and sinus.

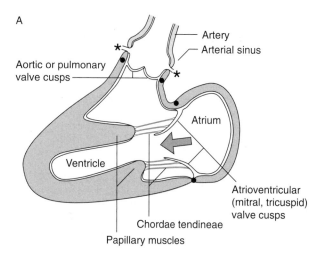

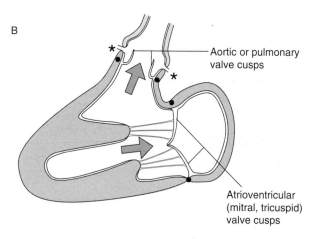

Fig. 10.18 Heart valves: (**A**) in diastole and (**B**) in systole. Arrows indicate direction in which blood is propelled; *, openings of coronary arteries.

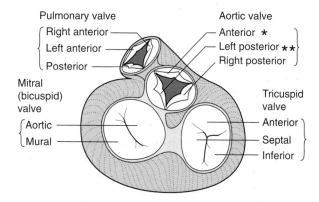

Fig. 10.19 Cusps of heart valves from above with atria and great arteries removed. Dark stippled area is fibrous skeleton: *, right coronary artery arises above this cusp; **, left coronary artery arises above this cusp.

Valve disease

Valve disease is generally of two types: stenosis and incompetence. In stenosis the valves do not open fully, and in incompetence they do not shut properly. One cause of incompetence of the atrioventricular valves you have already met is rupture of the chordae tendineae. Symptoms and signs will vary depending upon which valve is involved.

In stenosis there will be turbulent flow as blood is squeezed as if through a nozzle. This will lead to an audible murmur which will occur in systole if the aortic or pulmonary valve is involved (since blood flows through these during systole) or in diastole if the mitral or tricuspid is involved.

In mitral or tricuspid incompetence, blood will flow back into the atria, leading to a systolic murmur. In mitral incompetence the volume of blood gushing back into the left atrium with each left ventricular contraction will cause significant dilatation of the atrium. This may lead to a sensation of discomfort from pressure on the oesophagus. In aortic or pulmonary incompetence, blood will flow back into the ventricles during diastole, leading to a diastolic murmur. Combinations of sounds and symptoms can be used to diagnose the problem although, in truth, modern diagnostic methods involving ultrasound and pressure transducers are (regrettably) rendering this kind of intellectual detective work redundant.

Why do ventricles have bundles when atria do not?

Simply because ventricular contraction needs to be coordinated in a specific manner to give rise to the 'wringing' action of ventricular contraction. Should the right and left bundles function imperfectly (e.g. in right and/or left bundle branch block), then ventricular function is impaired. The action of the ventricular muscle requires that some structure in the heart will provide a measure of rigidity that is lacking in the atria. This is the fibrous skeleton referred to earlier in which are embedded the atrioventricular valves. It has another very important function. Being fibrous, it is impervious to the electrical impulse and so isolates electrically the atria from the ventricles, *except* where the bundle of His penetrates it. This isolation is very important: were it not so, and electrical impulses could spread unchecked from atria to ventricles, ventricular contraction would be entirely uncoordinated. This may in fact happen if the fibrous skeleton is damaged in disease. In this circumstance, the electrical impulse may pass as normal from atria to ventricles in the bundle of His but then return to the atria through the 'electrical opening' in the fibrous skeleton produced by disease, thus setting up extrasystoles in the atria. These may then travel back into the ventricles, completely disrupting the normal rhythm. These, for obvious reasons, are called *re-entry phenomena*.

Coronary arteries (Fig. 10.20)

Heart muscle requires an extensive supply of freshly oxygenated blood. This is provided by the right and

Conducting system and fibrous skeleton

The pacemaker is the sinuatrial (SA) node in the wall of the right atrium at the top of the crista terminalis. From the SA node the impulse passes to the atrioventricular (AV) node in the lower end of the atrial septum beside the coronary sinus opening. There are probably several distinct routes along which impulses pass in the atrial wall, although they are not histologically distinct. From the AV node specialised cardiac muscle fibres, Purkinje fibres, form the bundle of His. This penetrates the fibrous skeleton that separates the atria from the ventricles, and it passes into the ventricular septum (ventricular septal defects may interfere with it, leading to cardiac dysrhythmias). About half way down the septum it divides into right and left branches. The left bundle passes to the apex and up the left side of the heart. The right bundle crosses to the inferior (embryonic right) side of the ventricle in the septomarginal (moderator) band, an identifiable ridge in the wall of the right ventricle.

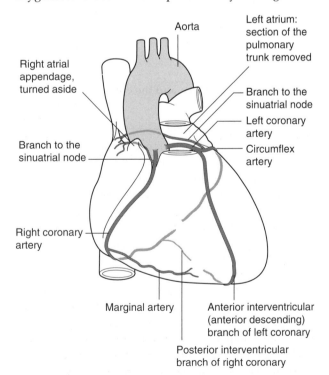

Fig. 10.20 Coronary arteries: anterior view (pulmonary trunk removed).

left coronary arteries arising from the aorta immediately above the aortic valve.

- The right coronary artery arises from the anterior aortic sinus (slight dilatation) above the anterior cusp of the aortic valve. It passes inferiorly in the anterior atrioventricular groove and gives off the marginal branch as it approaches the diaphragmatic (inferior) surface of the heart. The main trunk passes under the heart on the diaphragmatic surface and then turns to the left, running in the posterior interventricular groove towards the apex as the posterior interventricular artery. Branches of the right coronary artery supply both atria, most of the right ventricle, the posterior part of the ventricular septum and the posterior part of the left ventricle, and usually there is a branch to the sinuatrial (pacemaker) node.
- The left coronary artery arises from the left posterior aortic sinus above the left posterior cusp of the aortic valve. It passes forwards behind the origin of the pulmonary trunk for about 2 cm and then divides into the circumflex and anterior interventricular arteries. The circumflex passes posteriorly in the atrioventricular groove behind the heart to anastomose with branches of the right coronary artery. The anterior interventricular artery passes down on the anterior aspect of the heart to the apex. Its alternative name, therefore, much used by clinicians, is the left anterior descending artery. Branches of the left coronary supply both atria, the anterior part of the left ventricle, the anterior ventricular septum and some adjacent right ventricle.

There are extensive anastomoses between the territories of the two arteries and variations are common. For example, the posterior interventricular artery may be a continuation of the circumflex (thus from the left coronary) rather than of the right coronary artery.

Coronary vessels fill during diastole. A little thought will confirm that when the cusps of the aortic valve are open during systole, blood can not enter the coronary vessels, and it is propelled quickly past their openings by the force of ventricular contraction. During diastole with the cusps of the aortic valve in the closed position, the elastic recoil of the aortic wall provides helpful propulsion forcing blood from the aortic sinuses into the coronary vessels. Blood flow through coronary vessels is maximal during diastole: obviously, when heart muscle is contracting, coronary vessels are narrowed and blood flow impeded. Here is another good reason why the openings of the coronary vessels should be outside, rather than in, the myocardium.

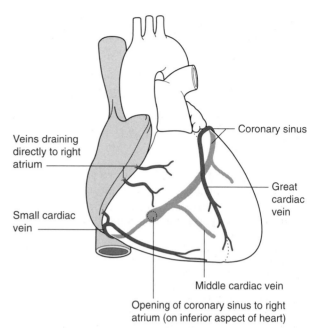

Fig. 10.21 Cardiac veins: anterior view.

Cardiac veins (Fig. 10.21)

A knowledge of these is less important. Most veins are tributaries of the coronary sinus so most venous blood drains into the right atrium through the coronary sinus, but veins from the anterior wall of the heart drain directly into the right atrium. Many small veins in the myocardium open directly into all chambers of the heart (Thebesian veins).

Cardiac autonomic innervation

- Parasympathetic: from the vagus (tenth cranial) nerve. Cardiac branches arise from both right and left vagus nerves in the neck and thorax, and from the recurrent laryngeal branch of the vagus. They cause a bradycardia (a slowing of the heart rate).
- Sympathetic: cardiac branches of the sympathetic chain arise from the cervical and thoracic regions of the sympathetic chain on both sides. Sympathetic stimulation results in tachycardia (increase in heart rate) and increased contractility.

What does the autonomic supply to the heart actually do?

At heart transplant operations, you can be sure that the surgeon makes no effort to reconnect sympathetic or parasympathetic connections. And yet the heart usually works well enough (given that it is not rejected). You might then wonder about the importance of what physiology textbooks tell you. Heart muscle possesses inherent rhythmicity: its innervation merely modulates this.

Surface markings of the heart (Fig. 10.22)

These are very important: they form the basis of the clinical examination of the heart. Here is a fairly reliable scheme: $2 \times 3 = 6$:

(a) second intercostal space near the left sternal edge
(b) third intercostal space near the right sternal edge
(c) sixth intercostal space at the right sternal edge
(d) fifth intercostal space in the midclavicular line (the apex).

Back to (a).

Position of the heart valves (Fig. 10.22)

All the heart valves are retrosternal. The highest is the pulmonary at about the level of the third costal cartilage, then the aortic at the third space, then the mitral at the fourth costal cartilage, and finally the tricuspid at the fourth space. This may be conveniently remembered as PAMT 3344 – but remember, all retrosternal, close to the midline.

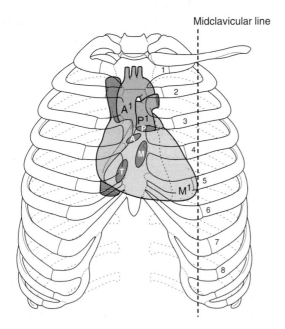

Midclavicular line

Fig. 10.22 Surface markings of heart and auscultation of heart valves: A, position of aortic valve; A¹ aortic valve best heard here; M, position of mitral valve; M¹, mitral valve best heard here; P, position of pulmonary valve; P¹, pulmonary valve best heard here; T, position of tricuspid valve.

Clinical box

Coronary artery bypass graft (CABG)
Heart disease is sometimes caused by narrowing or blockage of coronary arteries. Once located, the areas of narrowing can be bypassed by grafting material from elsewhere to form a replacement segment of artery. A section of great saphenous vein from the lower limb is sometimes used (but remember to orientate it so that the valves in the vein allow blood to flow in the required direction). There is another option for the anterior interventricular (anterior descending) artery. This vessel runs more or less parallel to, and not far distant from, the left internal thoracic artery, which may be anastomosed to it.

Cardiac pain
Visceral sensory fibres pass back to the central nervous system in sympathetic nerves. They enter the spinal cord in lower cervical and upper thoracic spinal nerves and so (see Referred pain, p. 38) it is not surprising that cardiac pain is felt in the dermatomes of these segments: upper chest, upper limb, possibly neck. But it is not easy to explain why, given that the heart is a midline structure and (presumably) innervated equally by nerves from both sides, cardiac pain should be predominantly left sided.

Apex beat (Fig. 10.22)
The apex beat is the most inferolateral point on the chest wall at which the heartbeat may be palpated. Should it be found other than in the normal position of the apex (see above), then you may assume that the heart is either enlarged or displaced. This may not necessarily indicate disease: for example, an athlete may have an enlarged heart.

Listening to (auscultating) the heart valves
(Fig. 10.22)
Blood passing through the valves transmits the sounds away from the valves themselves, and this means that the valves are best heard at places other than their surface markings (Table 10.3).

External cardiac massage
The object of external cardiac massage as used in cardiopulmonary resuscitation is to empty the blood from the ventricles by compressing the heart between the sternum and the spinal column (see Fig. 10.15). The compression of the chest also forces blood from the lung capillaries through the heart into the aorta. It is attempted by laying the patient on his back on a hard surface, and vigorously compressing the lower sternum at the rate of 80–100 per minute with sufficient force to produce pulsations in the carotid and femoral arteries. This force may fracture ribs, but being alive with fractured ribs is probably better than being dead with intact ones.

Radiology of the heart (Fig. 10.10)

PA view, inspection of the cardiac outline

Right border, from above down:

● right brachiocephalic vein

Table 10.3 Surface markings and auscultation of the heart valves

Valve	Position	Best heard
Pulmonary	Retrosternal, level of 3rd rib	2nd space just to left of sternal edge
Aortic	Retrosternal, level of 3rd space	2nd space just to right of sternal edge
Mitral	Retrosternal, level of 4th rib	Apex (5th space, midclavicular line)
Tricuspid	Retrosternal, level of 4th space	Lower sternal edge, side depending upon the condition

- SVC
- right atrium.

Diaphragmatic surface, right to left:

- right ventricle
- very small portion of left ventricle
- apex.

Left border, from apex up:

- left ventricle
- (left atrial appendage, sometimes)
- pulmonary artery
- aortic knuckle (junction of aortic arch with descending aorta).

10.4 Mediastinum

Overview

The mediastinum is the area between the two pleural cavities. It is divided into the superior mediastinum above vertebral level T4 and, below this, the anterior mediastinum (in front of the pericardial cavity), middle mediastinum (pericardial cavity and contents) and posterior mediastinum (behind the pericardial cavity). The organs of significance are the oesophagus, trachea, great arteries and veins, thoracic duct, vagus nerve, phrenic nerve and sympathetic chain. The arch of the aorta gives rise to the great arteries supplying the head, neck and upper limbs. The tributaries of the superior vena cava are important clinical access routes. The trachea, oesophagus and vagus and phrenic nerves are closely interrelated and may be affected in malignant tumours of the lung. The sympathetic chains are found in the superior and posterior divisions of the mediastinum, and give rise to the cardiac branches and splanchnic nerves supplying thoracoabdominal viscera.

Learning Objectives

You should:

- know the subdivisions and contents of the mediastinum
- know the disposition of the great arteries and veins and their principal branches and tributaries
- know the anatomy of insertion of catheters etc. into the right brachiocephalic vein
- know the formation, course and functions of the phrenic nerves
- know the formation, course and functions of the vagus nerves and branches
- understand how thoracic disease may give rise to signs and symptoms in the head, neck and upper limb
- know the basic anatomy of the sympathetic nervous system in the thorax.

Parts of the mediastinum

The mediastinum is divided horizontally by the plane from the sternal angle (of Louis) to vertebra T4 into:

- the superior mediastinum, above this plane
- the inferior mediastinum below this plane, which is itself divided into:
  - anterior mediastinum: anterior to the heart and pericardium
  - middle mediastinum: the heart and pericardium
  - posterior mediastinum: behind the heart and pericardium, containing the oesophagus, trachea, vagus and phrenic nerves, thoracic duct, and sympathetic chain.

There is nothing in the anterior mediastinum worthy of attention other than the thymus gland extending down from the superior mediastinum, and the internal thoracic vessels. Having considered the heart, only the superior and posterior compartments remain to be considered in any detail.

Thymus gland

This is found in children anterior to the trachea, extending from the level of the cricoid cartilage (vertebral level C6) down to the retrosternal area. Thymic tumours may compress the tributaries of the superior vena cava leading to venous engorgement in the neck. During childhood the thymus gradually regresses so that in the adult thymic tissue is more or less confined to the retrosternal connective tissue.

Great arteries

Ascending aorta, pulmonary trunk, arch of the aorta   (Figs 10.23, 10.24)

The aorta is divided into three parts: ascending, arch, and descending. At its origin the aorta is behind the pulmonary trunk, but as they ascend they spiral round each other: the pulmonary trunk passes to the left of the aorta, bifurcating behind it into the right and left pulmonary arteries which pass to the pulmonary hila. The ascending aorta and the pulmonary trunk arise from a single embryonic artery, the truncus arteriosus, which is divided into two vessels by the growth of a spiral septum. This accounts both for the spiral arrangement and the fact that they are inseparable.

The aorta then arches posteriorly and to the left, over the bifurcation of the pulmonary trunk and the left main bronchus, to the posterior mediastinum where it descends on the left of the midline towards the diaphragm. It leaves the thorax, passing behind the diaphragm, at vertebral level T12.

Branches of the ascending aorta and aortic arch are, in order:

- coronary vessels
- brachiocephalic artery, which gives rise to the right common carotid and right subclavian
- left common carotid
- left subclavian.

As the aorta descends posterior to the bifurcation of the pulmonary trunk, there is a fibrous connection between them. This is the ligamentum arteriosum, a remnant of the ductus arteriosus, which in fetal life conveyed blood from the pulmonary trunk to the descending aorta, thus bypassing the lungs.

Branches of the descending aorta are the posterior intercostal arteries from the third onwards (the first two are branches of the costocervical trunk).

Brachiocephalic and subclavian arteries

The asymmetric origins of these arteries is readily explained embryologically and you should bear in

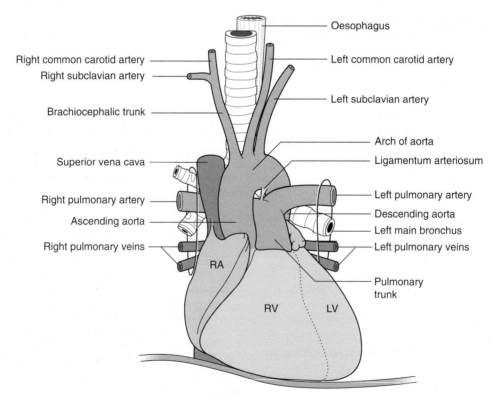

Fig. 10.23   The great vessels and relations (anterior view): LV, left ventricle; RA, right atrium; RV, right ventricle.

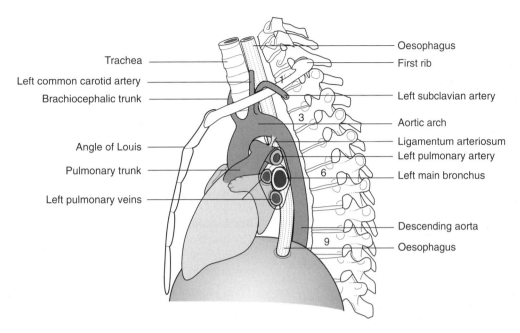

Fig. 10.24   Mediastinum from left side: LA, left atrium; LV, left ventricle.

mind that anomalies in these arrangements may arise. For example, the right subclavian artery may arise independently from the aorta on the left of the midline, and as it passes to the right it may compress the oesophagus, passing either in front of or behind it, causing dysphagia (discomfort on swallowing or an uncomfortable feeling of oesophageal obstruction).

From its origin on each side, the subclavian artery passes laterally, grooving the superior surface of the first rib behind the scalene tubercle (the attachment of scalenus anterior muscle), to reach the lateral border of the first rib where it becomes the axillary artery.

The subclavian artery is divided into three parts for descriptive purposes: first part medial to the scalenus anterior, second part behind the muscle, and third part between the muscle and the first rib.

Branches of the first part are important:

- the vertebral artery
- the internal thoracic artery
- the thyrocervical trunk.

Branches of the second and third parts are unimportant: they supply the top of the rib cage and scapular region, and one of them, the costocervical trunk, gives rise to the first one or two posterior intercostal arteries.

Internal thoracic artery

From its origin from the first part of the subclavian artery, this descends on the internal aspect of the rib cage, just lateral to the sternal edge.

- It gives rise to the anterior intercostal arteries, branches to the medial portion of the breast, and the

pericardiophrenic artery that accompanies the phrenic nerve as it runs on the pericardium.
- It terminates by dividing into:
  - superior epigastric artery: continues down to the anterior abdominal wall and anastomoses with the inferior epigastric artery
  - musculophrenic artery: runs laterally in the angle formed between the trunk wall and the diaphragm, giving branches to both.

These arteries are accompanied by veins draining into the brachiocephalic veins.

Clinical box

Bypassing a blocked aorta   (Fig. 10.25)
In a blockage of the descending aorta, such as a coarctation (narrowing), blood may bypass the blockage as follows:

- Ascending aorta – subclavian arteries – internal thoracic arteries – superior epigastric arteries – inferior epigastric arteries (retrograde flow) – femoral arteries, thence down to the lower limb and up (retrograde) to the iliac arteries and abdominal aorta. In this case the internal thoracic arteries will be much enlarged.
- Ascending aorta – subclavian arteries – scapular anastomosis – posterior intercostal arteries (retrograde flow) – descending aorta. In this case the intercostal arteries will be much enlarged leading to deepening of the costal grooves in which the arteries run. This may be evident on a chest radiograph as 'notching of the ribs'.

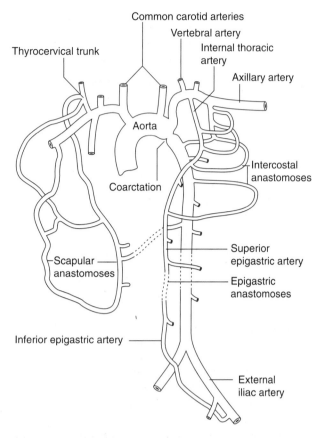

Common carotid arteries
Vertebral artery
Internal thoracic artery
Axillary artery
Thyrocervical trunk
Aorta
Intercostal anastomoses
Coarctation
Superior epigastric artery
Scapular anastomoses
Epigastric anastomoses
Inferior epigastric artery
External iliac artery

Fig. 10.25 Bypassing an aortic coarctation (anterior view). Scapular anastomosis shown on right side, internal thoracic/superior epigastric anastomosis on the left side.

Great veins (Figs 10.26–10.28)

Superior vena cava (SVC)

The SVC lies immediately to the right of the ascending aorta. However, the aorta and the SVC are not adherent and it is possible to pass a finger between them: this is the transverse sinus of the pericardial cavity – a feature of embryological interest and practical utility if you wish to clamp either vessel.

The SVC has three tributaries: the right and left brachiocephalic veins and the azygos vein.

Brachiocephalic veins

The brachiocephalic veins are formed by the junction of the internal jugular and subclavian veins immediately posterior to the sternoclavicular joints (vertebral level

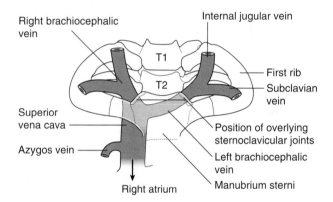

Right brachiocephalic vein
Internal jugular vein
T1
First rib
T2
Subclavian vein
Superior vena cava
Position of overlying sternoclavicular joints
Azygos vein
Left brachiocephalic vein
Manubrium sterni
Right atrium

Fig. 10.26 Great veins (anterior view).

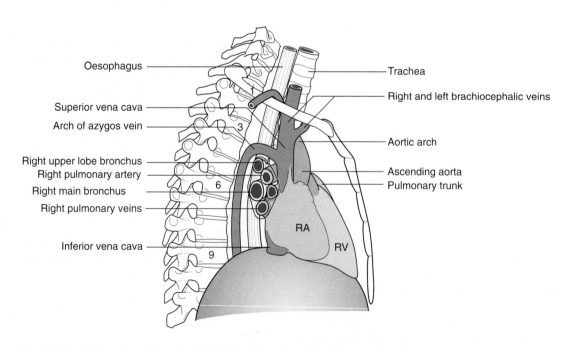

Oesophagus
Trachea
Superior vena cava
Right and left brachiocephalic veins
Arch of azygos vein
Aortic arch
Right upper lobe bronchus
Right pulmonary artery
Ascending aorta
Right main bronchus
Pulmonary trunk
Right pulmonary veins
Inferior vena cava
RA
RV

Fig. 10.27 Mediastinum (from the right): RA, right atrium; RV, right ventricle.

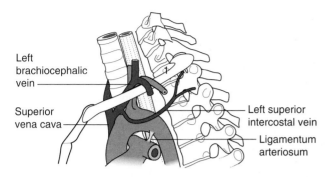

Left
brachiocephalic
vein

Superior
vena cava

Left superior
intercostal vein

Ligamentum
arteriosum

Fig. 10.28 Superior mediastinum (from the left).

about T2): this is an important surface marking. The left brachiocephalic vein crosses the midline to join the right, forming the superior vena cava (SVC) just behind the right sternal edge at the angle of Louis (vertebral level T4). The SVC receives the azygos vein and drains into the smooth-walled part of the right atrium deep to the right third costal cartilage.

Clinical box

Insertion of catheters and central lines, mediastinoscopy
There is almost a straight line from the formation of the right brachiocephalic vein behind the right sternoclavicular joint to the right atrium and beyond into the inferior vena cava (IVC). Catheters and central lines can be inserted into the venous system either directly into the formation of the right brachiocephalic vein from above (between the two heads of sternocleidomastoid) or through the right subclavian vein, a little more laterally.

The subclavian and brachiocephalic veins are anterior to the arteries. To all intents and purposes they are directly behind the sternum and are therefore in danger in mediastinoscopy when a scope is inserted in the suprasternal notch.

Azygos venous system and intercostal veins
The azygos vein receives blood from the posterior intercostal veins and from the segmental veins of the abdomen (connecting veins from the abdomen ascend behind the diaphragm). Veins on the right drain directly into the azygos vein but on the left side the pattern is variable: all you need to know is that segmental veins in the thorax and upper abdomen drain into the azygos system of veins, which ultimately empty into the SVC.

The termination of the azygos vein arches over the hilum of the right lung, on which there is an azygos impression, and the azygos vein enters the SVC about 2 cm above the right atrium.

Superior intercostal veins. Since the azygos vein is found no higher than about vertebral level T4, the first one or two posterior intercostal veins on each side

unite to form a superior intercostal vein that drains into the brachiocephalic veins. The left superior intercostal vein is important to thoracic surgeons since it is vulnerable as it crosses the arch of the aorta between the phrenic and vagus nerves (Fig. 10.28).

Nerves in the mediastinum (Fig. 10.29)

The phrenic and vagus nerves pass down from the neck. The phrenic descends on the pericardium to the diaphragm, so remaining anterior in the chest, and the vagus descends to form a plexus around the oesophagus, so being closer to the vertebral column. The sympathetic chain is found on the internal aspect of the ribs close to the vertebral column. It is intimately related to the intercostal neurovascular bundle and has connections (rami communicantes) with intercostal nerves. Also in this region are branches of the sympathetic chain, the splanchnic nerves, which pass medially and descend towards the diaphragm on their way to the abdomen. For more detailed consideration of the autonomic nervous system in the thorax, see later (p. 91).

Phrenic nerve

This arises from the ventral rami of segmental nerves C3, 4 and 5 and passes down the neck on the anterior aspect of scalenus anterior muscle. At the first rib, the nerve passes medially, between the subclavian vein (anterior) and the subclavian artery (posterior), just lateral to the origin of the thyrocervical trunk. The asymmetrical arrangement of the great vessels in this region means that from this point, the right and left sides must be considered separately.

- The right phrenic runs on the right wall of the SVC and directly to the right side of the fibrous pericardium. It passes directly down on the pericardium over the right atrium to the diaphragm near the orifice for the IVC.
- The left phrenic, having passed deep to the formation of the left brachiocephalic vein, passes over the left side of the arch of the aorta and the pulmonary trunk before descending on the pericardium over the left ventricle to the diaphragm near the cardiac apex.

The phrenic nerves innervate mediastinal pleura (sensory), pericardium (sensory) and diaphragm (motor to the entire diaphragm, sensory from the central tendon region).

Vagus and recurrent laryngeal nerves in the thorax

The vagus on each side enters the thorax from the

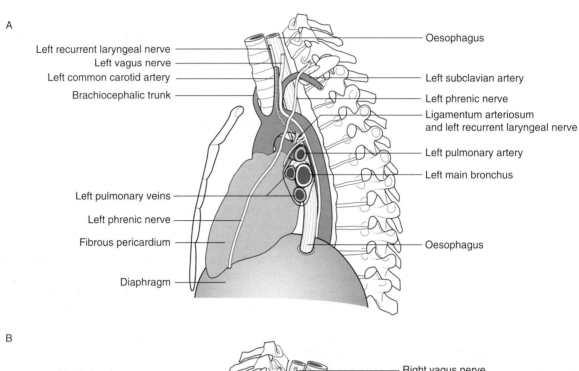

A

Left recurrent laryngeal nerve
Left vagus nerve
Left common carotid artery
Brachiocephalic trunk

Oesophagus

Left subclavian artery
Left phrenic nerve
Ligamentum arteriosum and left recurrent laryngeal nerve
Left pulmonary artery
Left main bronchus

Left pulmonary veins
Left phrenic nerve
Fibrous pericardium

Oesophagus

Diaphragm

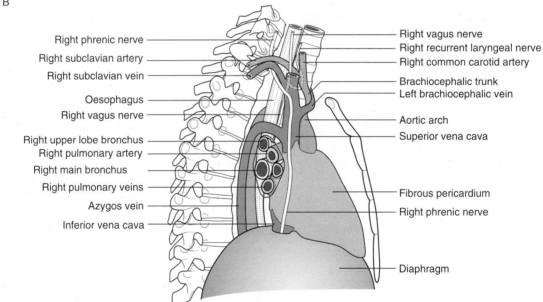

B

Right phrenic nerve
Right subclavian artery
Right subclavian vein
Oesophagus
Right vagus nerve
Right upper lobe bronchus
Right pulmonary artery
Right main bronchus
Right pulmonary veins
Azygos vein
Inferior vena cava

Right vagus nerve
Right recurrent laryngeal nerve
Right common carotid artery
Brachiocephalic trunk
Left brachiocephalic vein
Aortic arch
Superior vena cava

Fibrous pericardium
Right phrenic nerve

Diaphragm

Fig. 10.29 Mediastinum showing vagus and phrenic nerves: (**A**) from the left; (**B**) from the right.

carotid sheath in the neck, between the common carotid artery (medially) and the internal jugular vein (laterally). Again, the asymmetry of the great vessels requires that the two sides be considered separately.

● The right vagus passes anterior to the origin of the right subclavian artery and then forms a plexus on the oesophageal wall. At the right subclavian, it gives off the right recurrent laryngeal nerve which turns upwards again (thus *recurrent*) behind the origin of the subclavian artery, aiming for the larynx in a groove between the trachea and the oesophagus.

● The left vagus remains on the lateral wall of the common carotid artery all the way to the aortic arch. It passes between the descending aorta and the left pulmonary artery and then forms the oesophageal plexus with its fellow of the other side. As it crosses the arch of the aorta it gives the left recurrent laryngeal nerve which passes medially, below the ligamentum arteriosum, before going back up (recurring) to the larynx.

The origin of the left recurrent laryngeal nerve is thus about two vertebral levels lower than the origin of the right. The reasons for this are easily understood.

The recurrent laryngeal nerves innervate muscles of the sixth branchial arch (laryngeal muscles). They are intimately related to the sixth branchial arch arteries and when both of these arteries are present in the embryo, the arrangement of the recurrent laryngeal nerves is symmetrical. However, during subsequent development, the right sixth arch artery degenerates, thus allowing the right sixth arch nerve to take a shorter course to its destination, so on the right the nerve is held down by the next most cranial branchial arch artery, the fourth (there being no fifth) which becomes the subclavian. On the left, the sixth arch artery persists as the pulmonary artery and the ductus arteriosus, and since after birth the ductus becomes the ligamentum, this continues to pin down the left recurrent laryngeal nerve.

The recurrent laryngeal nerves may be involved in lung tumours, resulting in voice changes. Indeed, hoarseness of the voice thus caused may be a presenting sign of a lung tumour. This is more common as a result of a left-sided lesion than a right-sided lesion since there is more scope for lung disease to affect the left recurrent laryngeal nerve, the thoracic course of the nerve being longer on the left than the right.

Having formed the oesophageal plexus, the vagus nerves continue through the oesophageal opening in the diaphragm (vertebral level T10) into the abdomen as the anterior and posterior vagal trunks. The vagus nerve transmits parasympathetic and visceral sensory fibres to and from the heart (cardiac branches), the lungs, the oesophagus and abdominal organs.

Intercostal nerves   (see p. 66; Fig. 10.8)

These lie immediately under the mediastinal pleura between the vertebral column and the point at which they enter the costal groove with the posterior intercostal arteries and veins. The intercostal nerves are connected to the sympathetic chains by means of grey and white rami communicantes.

Intercostal nerves carry:

- motor fibres to intercostal muscles and (in the case of lower intercostal nerves) muscles of the abdominal wall
- sensory fibres from skin, muscle spindles, parietal pleura and (in the case of lower intercostal nerves) parietal peritoneum
- postganglionic sympathetic fibres to blood vessels and sweat glands in the territory of the nerve.

Clinical box

Structures related to the neck of the first rib, Pancoast's tumour

A tumour of the apex of the lung may present with symptoms arising from damage by the tumour to nerves related to the neck of the first rib. These are:

- fibres of T1 nerve which contribute to the brachial plexus to supply the upper limb; involvement of these may mean that the small muscles of the hand are weakened or paralysed, leading to clumsiness and a loss of manual dexterity
- the sympathetic chain; involvement of this may interrupt efferent sympathetic impulses to the head and this would result in Horner's syndrome:
  - pupilloconstriction because of unopposed parasympathetic action
  - facial anhidrosis because of denervation of sweat glands
  - ipsilateral ptosis (drooping of the upper eyelid) because of partial denervation of levator palpebrae superioris muscle.

Such a tumour was described by Professor H K Pancoast and is now commonly known as Pancoast's tumour.

Posterior mediastinum   (Figs 10.30–10.32)

Trachea and oesophagus

The trachea and oesophagus descend in the midline of

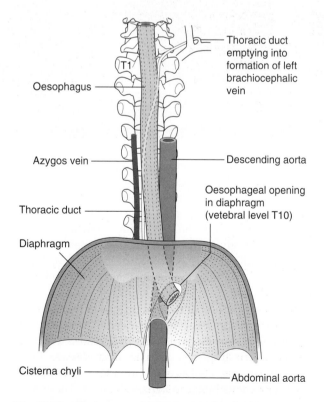

Fig. 10.30   Posterior mediastinum: anterior view.

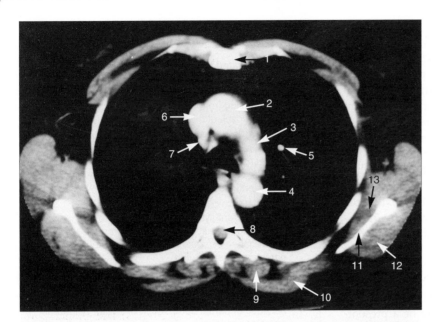

Fig. 10.31 Scan of thorax through the upper part of the manubrium sterni. Note that scans of the trunk are viewed as if from below, with the patient's head in the distance and the feet near the observer (as if the observer is standing at the foot of the bed). The right-hand side of the patient is thus on the left of the image. 1, manubrium sterni; 2, top of ascending aorta; 3, arch of aorta; 4, upper end of descending aorta (so the slice has passed through the aortic arch itself); 5, pulmonary vessel that happens to have been sectioned at right angles to the plane of the scan; 6, superior vena cava; 7, entry of azygos vein to 6; 8, vertebral canal; 9, postvertebral muscles; 10, trapezius; 11, scapula; 12, infraspinatus muscle; 13, subscapularis muscle.

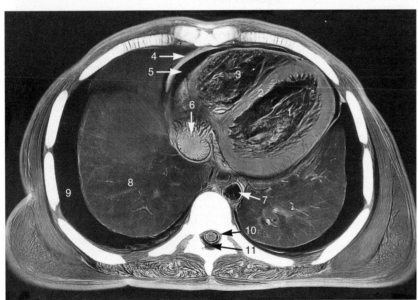

Fig. 10.32 Scan of thorax at the level of the heart. Note that scans of the trunk are viewed as if from below, with the patient's head in the distance and the feet near the observer (as if the observer is standing at the foot of the bed). The right-hand side of the patient is thus on the left of the image. In this case, the 'patient' is an embalmed cadaver, which is why the details are so clearly visible. 1, left ventricle of heart, full of embalmed blood clot; 2, ventricular septum; 3, right ventricle; 4, pericardium (fibrous and parietal layer of serous); 5, pericardial cavity; 6, ascending aorta and blood clot; 7, descending aorta; 8, lung; 9, pleural cavity apparent as a result of lung shrinkage during embalming; 10, vertebral canal – note the detail visible: dura mater, subarachnoid space, grey and white matter of the spinal cord, etc.; 11, extradural (epidural) space.

the superior mediastinum, parting company at the bifurcation of the trachea at about vertebral level T4 (surface marking: sternal angle). At the tracheal bifurcation, the oesophagus is slightly to the left of the trachea and the left main bronchus crosses anterior to it, giving rise to a slight indentation of the anterior wall of the oesophagus. The oesophagus descends to penetrate the diaphragm at vertebral level T10.

The lower portion of the oesophagus in the thorax is the site of anastomosis between systemic venous drainage (to the azygos system) and portal venous drainage (to the liver). It is here that in liver disease these anastomoses may enlarge to provide a roundabout route for venous blood to bypass the liver. These may have important clinical effects (see 11.7, p. 124).

Although the oesophagus meets the diaphragm slightly to the left of the midline, the muscle fibres that surround it arise from the right diaphragmatic crus. These form the gastro-oesophageal sphincter. This may be the site of a hiatus hernia (see Ch. 11, p. 112).

Thoracic duct

This is the main lymphatic channel receiving lymph from the entire body apart from the right arm, right side of the head and neck and right upper thorax. The thoracic duct, or the upper part of the cisterna chyli in the abdomen from which it extends, enters the thorax from below by passing behind the diaphragm with the aorta. It ascends anterior to the azygos system of veins, gradually crosses to the left and at the root of the neck drains into the superior aspect of the junction of the internal jugular and subclavian veins. Abdominal malignancy may give rise to enlarged left supraclavicular lymph nodes (Virchow's node – see Ch. 11, p. 120).

Diaphragmatic orifices

T8   IVC, branches of right phrenic nerve. Note that this orifice is in the central tendon, not a muscular portion, and so the IVC is not compressed with each muscular contraction.

T10   Oesophagus, vagus nerves.

T12   Aorta, tributaries of the azygos venous system, thoracic duct.

The sympathetic chains and splanchnic nerves penetrate the diaphragm independently: you do not need to know the details.

More details of the diaphragm are given with the posterior abdominal wall, from which it arises.

Autonomic nervous system in the thorax

Thoracic sympathetic chain (trunk) and its connections

First, read Chapter 6 again.

The thoracic portion of the sympathetic chain (trunk) on each side runs from the neck of the first rib superiorly to the side of vertebra T12 inferiorly. It continues up into the neck behind the carotid sheath and down into the abdomen. It lies between the intercostal nerves and the parietal pleura. A sympathetic ganglion is present at each segment, grey and white rami communicantes connecting each ganglion to its intercostal nerve. Arising from the ganglia and passing medially and towards the midline are the greater, lesser and least splanchnic nerves. These nerves convey impulses between the sympathetic chains and the abdominal sympathetic plexuses. These will be considered in more detail in Chapter 11 (Autonomic nervous system in the abdomen and pelvis, p. 144).

Sympathetic impulses to heart and lungs

Preganglionic sympathetic impulses to the heart and lungs originate in the lateral grey horns of upper thoracic spinal cord segments. Axons of these neurons pass in the ventral roots of upper thoracic spinal nerves to the spinal nerves themselves and thence through white rami communicantes to the sympathetic chain where some of them ascend to the lowest of the cervical ganglia of the sympathetic chain, the inferior cervical ganglion. From here, and from the upper few thoracic ganglia, they continue into cardiac and pulmonary

branches: in effect the cervical and thoracic splanchnic nerves (although they are not called this). These pass to intercommunicating sympathetic plexuses on and around the great vessels and the bifurcation of the trachea – the cardiac and pulmonary plexuses. The precise location of synapses, whether in the sympathetic chain, in the cardiac plexus, or somewhere between, has not been fully elucidated. Postganglionic fibres pass directly to the heart and lungs.

Parasympathetic impulses to heart

Preganglionic parasympathetic fibres originate from the brain and are conveyed in the vagus (tenth cranial) nerve. They leave the vagus nerve in the neck and travel down as cardiac branches of the vagus to contribute to the cardiac and pulmonary plexuses before reaching the heart. Synapses are generally found in the wall of the destination organ: postganglionic parasympathetic fibres are very short.

Important vertebral levels in the mediastinum

T2   Suprasternal (jugular) notch, formation of brachiocephalic veins, highest point of arch of aorta.

T3   Junction of brachiocephalic veins to form SVC.

T4   Sternal angle (of Louis), bifurcation of trachea, aortic impression on oesophagus.

T5 (about)   Left main bronchus impression on oesophagus.

T8   IVC passes through diaphragm.

T10   Oesophagus passes through diaphragm.

T12   Aorta, thoracic duct and azygos system pass behind diaphragm.

10.5 Breast   (Figs 10.33–10.35)

Overview

The postpubertal female breast is composed of 15–20 independent exocrine secretory units opening around the nipple. It overlies ribs 2–6. It is part of the superficial layer of the chest wall and should not be firmly tethered to underlying muscle. Its arterial supply comes from branches of the subclavian and axillary arteries, and its lymph drains principally to the axilla. Accessory breast tissue may be found in a line from axilla to groin.

Learning Objectives

You should:

- know the surface anatomy of the postpubertal female breast

- know its disposition and relations on the chest wall

- know which arteries supply it

- know its lymph drainage, and the importance of this.

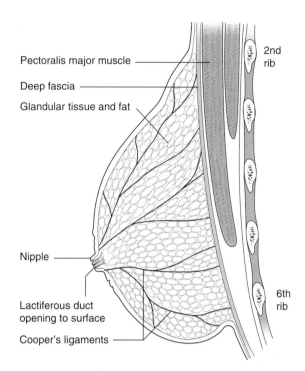

Fig. 10.34 Section through chest wall and breast.

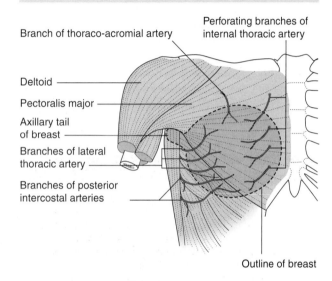

Fig. 10.33 Breast: position and blood supply.

Position and structure

The breast (mammary gland) is a group of 15–20 exocrine glands arranged radially around the nipple.

These individual units are separated by fibrous septa and the duct of each opens independently. The nipple is surrounded by an area of pigmented skin about 3 cm in diameter, the areola. On it are numerous small swellings, Montgomery's tubercles, which become prominent and reddened in pregnancy but are otherwise of no great clinical significance.

The maximum extent of the breast is roughly circular, overlying ribs 2–6 vertically, and sternal edge to midaxillary line horizontally, but an axillary tail (of

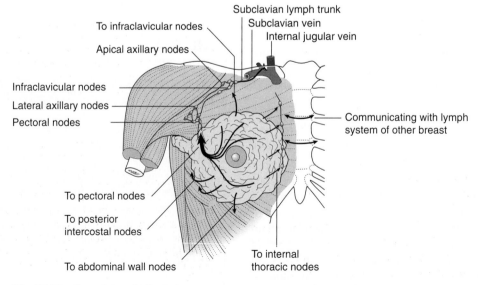

Fig. 10.35 Breast: lymphatic drainage.

Spence) extends upwards and laterally into the axilla. The glandular tissue is confined to the superficial layers of the chest wall, but the axillary tail may penetrate the deep fascia.

The glandular tissue overlies pectoralis major and serratus anterior muscles but, being confined to the superficial fascia, is not attached to these muscles. Any clinical indication of its tethering to these muscles should be treated with the utmost seriousness: it may well be an indication of malignant disease. Asking the patient to raise the arm and observing the way in which the breast moves may reveal tethering. The breast tissue is, however, connected to the overlying skin by fibrous strands, the suspensory ligaments of Cooper. These are more numerous in the upper part of the breast than in the lower. These may become stretched with advancing years and fat deposition.

Arteries and veins (Fig. 10.33)

Arterial blood supply comes mainly from branches of the subclavian artery: the internal thoracic supplies the medial portion, the lateral thoracic the lateral portion. Other arteries that contribute are the thoracoacromial and intercostal arteries 2–5. Venous drainage is by corresponding veins to the subclavian and brachiocephalic veins.

Lymph (Fig. 10.35)

The lymph drainage of the breast is of great importance. It obeys the general rule that lymphatic drainage mirrors arterial supply.

There are two main lymph plexuses in the breast:

- subareolar, immediately under the skin around the nipple
- submammary (or retromammary), between breast and pectoralis major muscle. It is involvement of this that may tether the breast to the muscle.

There are numerous connecting channels running between these two plexuses, each with many tributaries. From these plexuses, lymph drains as follows:

- From the lateral two-thirds: to axillary lymph nodes, thence in lymph vessels alongside the axillary artery to the terminations of the thoracic ducts.
- A small amount of lymph passes to posterior intercostal nodes, and some to nodes of the anterior abdominal wall.
- From the medial portion: to parasternal nodes along the internal thoracic artery, thence up alongside the artery to the terminations of the thoracic ducts. It is possible for lymph from the medial side of one breast to drain to the opposite side, which means

that malignant disease of the medial portion of the breast may spread to the other side.

Blockage of lymph channels in the breast (for example by a tumour) can lead to engorgement of the breast tissue by lymph unable to drain away and a particular appearance of the skin of the breast 'stretched' over the engorged tissue. This is known as *peau d'orange* appearance because of its similarity to orange skin with its multiple pits.

Clinical examination of the breast is not complete without palpation of the axilla and the breast of the other side. Axillary lymph nodes are often removed during surgery and this may result in lymph flow from the upper limb being disrupted.

Nerve supply

The skin over the breast is supplied by intercostal nerves T2–6, which also convey postganglionic sympathetic fibres to the vessels within the breast.

Clinical box

Male breast and age changes in the female breast
The male breast and the prepubertal female breast are much the same: the glands are rudimentary. It is possible for carcinoma of the male breast to arise. It is much less common than carcinoma of the female breast, but its survival rate is poorer, probably because the possibility of this condition is overlooked and so by the time the condition has been diagnosed, it will have spread elsewhere.

At puberty in the female, fat deposition takes place together with some proliferation of the secretory units and at lactation there is substantial proliferation of the secretory components. After the menopause, secretory units atrophy and fat deposition continues. Most breast lumps are innocent tumours of fatty tissue: lipomas.

Cooper's ligaments and disease
Involvement of Cooper's ligaments in malignant disease may lead to their shortening as they become caught up in the tumour. This can cause dimpling of the overlying skin or even, in extreme cases, inversion of the nipple (but note that inversion of the nipple is by no means always a sign of disease).

Accessory nipples
Breast tissue in other mammals is found along a line extending from axilla to groin, the milk or mammary line. In humans breast tissue is limited to one organ on each side. Nevertheless, accessory nipples, and even accessory breast tissue, are found in both sexes anywhere along the mammary lines, most commonly in the thorax and abdomen. Accessory nipples are harmless but may be confused with a mole or suspected as a melanoma; they were once most definitely life-threatening: the unfortunate possessor was regarded as a witch.

Self-assessment: questions

Multiple choice questions

1. Concerning the lungs and pleural cavities:
   a. At the hilum, the bronchi are posterior.
   b. Lung tissue normally occupies the costodiaphragmatic recess.
   c. The right lower lobe has five bronchopulmonary segments.
   d. An inhaled object is more likely to enter the left main bronchus than the right.
   e. The pleural cavities extend above the clavicles.

2. Concerning the heart:
   a. The right ventricle forms most of the inferior border of the heart.
   b. The oblique sinus of the pericardial cavity lies between the left atrium and the oesophagus.
   c. All the heart valves are retrosternal.
   d. The mitral valve is the outflow valve of the right atrium.
   e. The mitral valve is best heard at the left sternal edge.

3. Concerning the coronary vessels and conducting system:
   a. The anterior interventricular artery is a branch of the left coronary artery.
   b. The coronary sinus runs in the posterior interventricular groove.
   c. Blockage of a coronary artery may cause referred pain in the neck.
   d. The atrioventricular node is found near the entry of the superior vena cava to the right atrium.
   e. The moderator band contains the right bundle branch.

4. Concerning the mediastinum:
   a. The vagus nerves pass anterior to the hila of the lungs.
   b. The right main bronchus indents the oesophagus.
   c. Serous pericardium has visceral and parietal layers.
   d. The vagus is the eleventh cranial nerve.
   e. The azygos vein empties into the inferior vena cava.

5. The breast:
   a. Is firmly attached to pectoralis major muscle.
   b. Has lymphatics which drain entirely to the axilla.
   c. Receives blood only from internal thoracic arteries.
   d. Does not extend inferiorly below the fourth rib.
   e. Accessory nipples may be found between axilla and groin.

6. An intercostal nerve:
   a. Is formed by the main trunk of a thoracic segmental nerve.
   b. Is formed by the ventral root of a thoracic segmental nerve.
   c. Is formed by the ventral ramus of a thoracic segmental nerve.
   d. Runs between external and internal intercostal muscles.
   e. Gives a collateral branch which runs on top of the rib below.

7. The anterior interventricular (anterior descending) artery of the heart:
   a. Supplies both right and left atria.
   b. Runs approximately parallel to the internal thoracic artery of the chest wall.
   c. Supplies the ventricular septum.
   d. Is a branch of the left coronary artery.
   e. Is accompanied by the great cardiac vein.

8. The mitral valve:
   a. Is best heard at the left sternal edge.
   b. Is known as the bicuspid valve.
   c. Forms the outflow from the chamber that is closest to the oesophagus.
   d. Is the most superior cardiac valve.
   e. If incompetent, would allow the passage of blood during diastole.

9. The right atrium:
   a. Has the fossa ovalis evident on the septal wall.
   b. Receives blood from the superior vena cava.
   c. Receives pulmonary veins.
   d. Has the sinoatrial node in its wall.
   e. Receives blood from the coronary sinus.

10. The greater splanchnic nerve:
    a. Is in the posterior mediastinum.
    b. Contains preganglionic fibres.
    c. Passes into the abdomen.
    d. Arises from the thoracic sympathetic chain.
    e. Supplies voluntary muscle.

Matching item questions

Questions 1–5

Match the numbered item to the lettered response. Each lettered response may be used once, more than once, or not at all.

    a. on the diaphragmatic surface of the heart
    b. left coronary artery
    c. right coronary artery
    d. superior vena cava
    e. circumflex artery

1. coronary sinus
2. supplying sinoatrial node
3. above anterior cusp of aortic valve
4. above left posterior cusp of aortic valve
5. marginal artery

Questions 6–10

Match the numbered item to the lettered response. Each lettered response may be used once, more than once, or not at all.

    a. left fifth intercostal space, midaxillary line
    b. left fifth intercostal space, midclavicular line
    c. retrosternal about level of fourth costal cartilage
    d. bifurcation of trachea
    e. suprasternal notch

6. position of mitral valve
7. best place to listen to mitral valve
8. normal position of cardiac apex beat
9. vertebral level T4
10. sternal angle of Louis

Questions requiring short answers

1. List the bronchopulmonary segments of the right lung. How do they differ on the left? Which segments are most likely to be affected in a bedridden supine patient who develops pneumonia?

2. Describe or draw:
    a. the surface markings of the right lung, and its fissure(s)
    b. the surface markings of the heart and the heart valves. Indicate where you would place your stethoscope to listen to these valves.

3. Where might you insert a chest drain? Explain your choice. What would the needle penetrate? What would happen if you inserted a needle into a normal pleural cavity?

4. A 65-year-old man develops cancer of the oesophagus at about vertebral level T4 which invades neighbouring structures. What is at risk? Why might such a patient in the advanced stages of the disease cough up fluid that had been drunk?

5. Describe or draw the arterial supply and venous drainage of the heart.

6. List the chambers and valves of the heart in order as a blood cell makes its way from the superior vena cava to the right subclavian artery. Explain the terms incompetence and stenosis as applied to heart valves.

7. Describe the conducting system of the heart. What is the significance of the fibrous skeleton of the heart in this context?

8. You note on a routine chest radiograph that the ribs have much larger than normal costal grooves. How may this be relevant to a narrowing of the aorta, and which other arterial channels may be enlarged? In such a patient, what would you expect to find when you palpated simultaneously the femoral and radial pulses?

9. A 45-year-old woman tells you she has had a lump in the breast which has been present for several months, is hard and is getting larger. Upon examination you note that the skin over the lump is dimpled and that lymph nodes in the axilla are enlarged. Explain the dimpling, explain the enlarged lymph nodes, state which other lymph nodes might be involved and explain why you wish to know if the breast is fixed to pectoralis major muscle. Add any other information you like.

Self-assessment: answers

Multiple choice answers

1. a. **True.**
   b. **False.** They are normally empty, with diaphragmatic pleura and costal pleura separated only by a thin layer of pleural fluid. Lung tissue may enter the recesses in deep inspiration, but even then it does not completely fill the available 'space'.
   c. **True.** They are: apical basal, medial basal, anterior basal, lateral basal, and posterior basal – AMALP.
   d. **False.** It is more likely to enter the right main bronchus: it is wider.
   e. **True.** The apex of the lung is vulnerable in the supraclavicular region.

2. a. **True.**
   b. **True.**
   c. **True.** PAMT 3344 (see text).
   d. **False.** It is the outflow valve of the left atrium.
   e. **False.** It is best heard at the apex.

3. a. **True.**
   b. **False.** It runs in the atrioventricular groove.
   c. **True.** Cardiac pain may also be felt in the chest and left arm.
   d. **False.** This is the SA node.
   e. **True.**

4. a. **False.** The vagus passes posterior to the hilum, the phrenic anterior.
   b. **False.** The left main bronchus indents the oesophagus.
   c. **True.** Serous pericardium is equivalent to pleura and peritoneum.
   d. **False.** The vagus is the tenth cranial nerve.
   e. **False.** It empties into the superior vena cava.

5. a. **False.** It should never be. If it is, it is likely that malignant disease has caused it to be.
   b. **False.** Lymphatics drain most importantly to the axilla, but not entirely. Lymph also drains to the parasternal nodes (with the internal thoracic arteries) and various others.
   c. **False.** The breast also receives blood from lateral thoracic and thoracoacromial arteries. In any case, a question in which the words 'only', 'always', 'never' appear is always (!) false. Nothing is ever so definite.
   d. **False.** It extends usually to the level of the sixth rib.
   e. **True.** They may be found on the milk lines.

6. a. **False.** It is formed by the ventral ramus of the main trunk (this is a 'nit-picking' question, but you will meet plenty of these).
   b. **False.** It is formed by the ventral ramus, not root. This is not so 'nit-picking' because ventral roots carry motor fibres, whereas the nerve itself carries both sensory and motor fibres: clinically, a lesion of the roots causes symptoms distinguishable from those of a lesion of a nerve.
   c. **True!**
   d. **False.** It runs between the internal and innermost intercostal muscles (who cares?).
   e. **True.**

7. a. **False.** It gives no branches to the right atrium.
   b. **True.** The internal thoracic may be anastomosed to a diseased left anterior descending artery.
   c. **True.**
   d. **True.**
   e. **True.**

8. a. **False.** It is best heard at the apex.
   b. **True.**
   c. **True.** This is the outflow valve of the left atrium.
   d. **False.** The pulmonary valve is the most superior.
   e. **False.** It is open during diastole. If it were incompetent, it would allow blood to pass during systole.

9. a. **True.**
   b. **True.**
   c. **False.** Pulmonary veins drain to the left atrium.
   d. **True.**
   e. **True.**

10. a. **True.**
    b. **True.**
    c. **True.**
    d. **True.**
    e. **False.** Autonomic impulses supply involuntary muscle.

Matching item answers

1. a.
2. c (usually).
3. c.
4. b.
5. c.
6. c.
7. b.
8. b.
9. d.
10. d.

Short answers

1. The bronchopulmonary segments of the right lung are: upper lobe – apical, posterior, anterior; middle lobe – lateral, medial; lower lobe – apical basal, medial basal, anterior basal, lateral basal, posterior basal (APALM, AMALP). The medial basal lobe is absent on the left. Lateral and medial segments of the right middle lobe are replaced on the left by the superior and inferior lingular segments, part of the left upper lobe, which thus has five segments. In a bedridden patient lying on his back, fluid is most likely to drain to the most dependent parts: these would be, in this position, the apical basal and posterior basal segments of the lower lobe. This is why regular physiotherapy and bronchial hygiene in seriously ill patients who can not be moved from the supine position is so important.

2. a. The lobes of the right lung are demarcated by two fissures:
   - oblique fissure: a line from the spine of vertebra T2 or T3 round the chest wall to the sixth costal cartilage (there are other ways of describing this)
   - horizontal fissure: a line from about the fourth costal cartilage laterally until it meets that for the oblique fissure.
     What this means is that when you place your stethoscope on the right anterior chest wall, you are listening to the upper and middle lobes, but not the lower lobe. On the left, of course, it is all upper lobe at the front.
   b. Heart surface markings are: (a) second intercostal space at the left sternal edge, to (b) third space at the right sternal edge, to (c) sixth space at the right sternal edge, to (d) left fifth space in the midclavicular line (apex), back to (a). Heart valves are all retrosternal: from top to bottom, pulmonary, aortic, mitral, tricuspid – levels respectively third costal cartilage, third space, fourth cartilage, fourth space (PAMT 3344). They are best heard, though, elsewhere, since sounds are transmitted by blood flow: aortic – second space, right sternal edge; pulmonary – second space, left sternal edge; tricuspid – lower sternal edge, the side depending upon the condition; mitral – apex.

3. A chest drain is usually inserted into the second intercostal space in the midclavicular line, or the fourth or fifth space in the midaxillary line. You must avoid the heart at the front, so you need to remain fairly high. At the side, you need to avoid the axilla and arteries and nerves in that region, so not too high, but on the other hand you need to avoid the risk of damage to abdominal structures, so not too low or too far posterior. If a needle is inserted into a normal pleural cavity, air will enter the cavity, pushing the visceral and parietal layers of pleura leading to a pneumothorax. Chest drains are normally used to drain fluid that has collected in the pleural cavity, or, in a pneumothorax, the drain will be attached to a vacuum so that the air in the cavity will be sucked out.

4. At and around vertebral level T4 the oesophagus is related to the arch of the aorta and the left main bronchus as well as the azygos venous system and the thoracic duct. Erosion of the tumour into the bronchial tree will result in ingested fluids passing into the bronchi, initiating coughing and/or causing pneumonia. Erosion into the arch of the aorta may result in death by massive haemorrhage into the oesophagus.

5. See Figures 10.20 (p. 80) and 10.21 (p. 81).

6. The blood cell travels as follows: SVC – RA – tricuspid valve – RV – pulmonary valve – pulmonary trunk, lungs, pulmonary veins – LA – mitral valve – LV – aortic valve – aorta – brachiocephalic artery – right subclavian artery. In valvular incompetence the valves do not close properly, leading to leakage of blood. In stenosis the valves do not open fully.

7. The pacemaker node is the SA node in the right atrial wall at the top of the crista terminalis, to the left of the SVC orifice. There are no specialised conducting fibres in the atrial walls. The electrical impulse spreads to the AV node in the lower end of the atrial septum beside the coronary sinus opening. From here, Purkinje fibres form the bundle of His, which penetrates the fibrous cardiac skeleton separating atria from ventricles, enters the ventricular septum, and divides about half way down the ventricular septum into right and left bundle branches. The left bundle branch passes to the apex and up the left side of the heart. The right bundle branch crosses to the inferior side of the ventricle in the septomarginal (moderator) band. The fibrous skeleton does not conduct electrical impulse except where pierced by the bundle of His. If the skeleton is damaged (disease), it may allow electrical impulse back into the atria (re-entry phenomena), thus initiating extra beats (extrasystoles).

8. This is notching of the ribs and it is a sign of enlarged intercostal arteries. This may indicate that the intercostal arteries are being used as part of a pathway bypassing a blocked aorta. Blood would pass as follows: ascending aorta – subclavians – scapular anastomosis – intercostals (retrograde flow) – descending aorta. Other bypass channels that may develop include the internal thoracic-superior and inferior epigastric channel (see Fig. 10.25, p. 86). In a normal person the femoral and radial pulses are approximately synchronous, their being similar distances from the heart. But in patients with an aortic coarctation, the femoral pulse is weaker and later than the radial.

9. This sounds like a breast tumour that involves suspensory ligaments (of Cooper) leading to shortening of the ligaments and dimpling of the overlying skin. It also sounds like a malignant tumour, and enlargement of the axillary lymph nodes lends weight to this opinion. Other lymph nodes that might be involved are: parasternal (not normally palpable), nodes of the anterior abdominal wall and possibly even inguinal nodes (if the tumour is low in the breast). A tumour that had involved the pectoralis major muscle would result in fixation of the breast to the muscle – most definitely abnormal and suspicious of malignant disease.

Introduction

The abdominal or peritoneal cavity is separated from the thorax by the diaphragm, and from the perineum below by the pelvic diaphragm or levator ani muscle. It is supported by the vertebral column, rib cage, and the bony pelvis formed by the two hip bones and the sacrum. Upper abdominal organs (e.g. liver, stomach, spleen, kidneys) are to some extent protected by the rib cage, while others low down (e.g. bladder, uterus, prostate) are protected by the bony pelvis. It follows from this that organs most closely related to bone may be damaged by injuries to these bones: for example fractures of the left tenth rib may damage the spleen.

Abdominal walls

The abdominal walls between rib cage and bony pelvis are formed by muscles and fascia. Details of the posterior abdominal wall are of no great clinical importance, and they are considered only briefly in 11.9. The anterior abdominal wall, on the other hand, being so often inspected, palpated and incised, needs a section of its own.

11.1 Anterior abdominal wall

Overview

The anterior abdominal wall is divided into nine regions or four quadrants. The regions are in the midline from top to bottom, epigastrium, umbilical and hypogastrium, and the lateral regions are, from top to bottom, hypochondrial, lumbar and iliac fossa or inguinal. The quadrants are right upper, right lower, left upper and left lower. Muscles of the abdominal wall are external oblique, internal oblique, transversus abdominis and rectus abdominis. The blood supply and innervation of the anterior abdominal wall are relevant to trauma, disease and surgery.

Learning Objectives

You should:

- know the nine regions and four quadrants and the principal organs and structures that lie deep to them and which can be palpated in those regions

- know the muscular components of the anterior abdominal wall

- know the blood supply and innervation of the anterior abdominal wall.

Surface anatomy and regions

The nine descriptive regions of the anterior abdominal wall (Fig. 11.1) are demarcated by two vertical and two

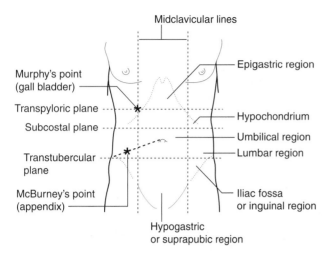

Fig. 11.1 Surface anatomy of the anterior abdominal wall.

horizontal planes. The vertical planes are the right and left midclavicular lines, and the horizontal planes the transpyloric (by most people, although some prefer the subcostal) and transtubercular planes.

- Transpyloric plane: vertebral level L1. This intersects the rib cage at the tip of the ninth costal cartilage. It is about halfway between the suprasternal notch and the pubic symphysis, or about halfway between the xiphoid process and the umbilicus, and it marks the position or level of several internal structures (e.g. pylorus, gall bladder, renal hila, origin of superior mesenteric artery).
- Subcostal plane: vertebral level L2/3. This is the plane marking the lowest point of the rib cage. In an ill, bedridden patient it can be difficult to find, particularly if the patient is obese.
- Transtubercular plane: vertebral level L3. The tubercles of the iliac crests are palpable some distance behind the anterior superior iliac spines (ASIS). In practice, the ASIS is easier to feel than the tubercles and the plane of the ASIS may be substituted for the transtubercular plane. In any case, these lines are only rough guides.

Superficial and deep fascia

Between the skin and the muscles of the abdominal wall is the superficial (Camper's) fascia: thin in a lean person, and thick in a fat person. The deep (Scarpas's) fascia is a tough membrane on the external aspect of the muscles.

Muscles of anterior abdominal wall
(Fig. 11.2)

- Rectus abdominis muscle which lies on either side of the midline.
- The sheet muscles: three anterolateral muscle sheets: external oblique, internal oblique and transversus abdominis muscles.

Rectus abdominis muscle

This runs from rib cage and sternum to the pubic bones. On contraction, it compresses the abdominal contents and is a flexor of the spinal column. Transverse tendinous

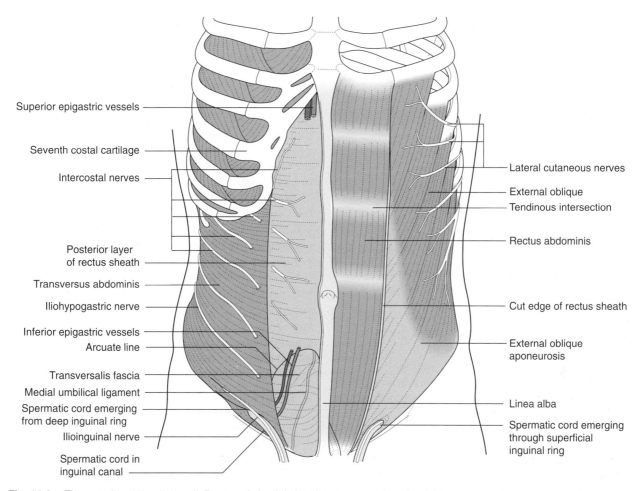

Superior epigastric vessels

Seventh costal cartilage

Intercostal nerves

Posterior layer
of rectus sheath

Transversus abdominis

Iliohypogastric nerve

Inferior epigastric vessels

Arcuate line

Transversalis fascia

Medial umbilical ligament

Spermatic cord emerging
from deep inguinal ring

Ilioinguinal nerve

Spermatic cord in
inguinal canal

Lateral cutaneous nerves

External oblique

Tendinous intersection

Rectus abdominis

Cut edge of rectus sheath

External oblique
aponeurosis

Linea alba

Spermatic cord emerging
through superficial
inguinal ring

Fig. 11.2 The anterior abdominal wall. Rectus abdominis has been removed on the right.

intersections are (in a lean person) visible and palpable above the umbilicus. They are of little significance except that when cut they bleed profusely.

- Linea semilunaris. This is the lateral margin of the rectus abdominis. It meets the rib cage at or near the ninth costal cartilage (vertebral level L1, transpyloric plane). It can be made more obvious (to either hand or eye) by asking the supine patient to raise the head, causing rectus abdominis to contract.
- Linea alba. This is in the midline between the rectus muscles and is usually palpable as a slight depression. Weaknesses in the linea alba may result in midline herniation of abdominal contents, often at the umbilicus.

Sheet muscles: external and internal obliques, transversus abdominis

The sheet muscles are attached to lumbar fascia posteriorly (don't bother with details), to the ribs and costal cartilages superiorly, to the hip bones inferiorly and the inguinal ligament (from ASIS to pubic tubercles) inferiorly. Medially, muscle fibres give way to broad, flat tendons

(aponeuroses) which form the rectus sheath around the rectus abdominis muscle. Fibres of these muscles run in different directions, reinforcing each other, and inferiorly they form the inguinal canal through which the spermatic cord in the male, and the round ligament of the uterus in the female, pass from abdomen to scrotum or labia majora respectively. The inguinal canal is an important area (see 11.2, below).

- External oblique muscle. From the lower eight ribs, fibres pass downwards and medially to the linea alba, pubic region and inguinal ligament, and inferiorly to the anterior superior iliac spine and iliac crest. The aponeurosis of external oblique contributes to the anterior wall of the rectus sheath. Along a line from the anterior superior iliac spine to the pubic tubercle, the aponeurosis is thickened to form the inguinal ligament, where the deep fascia of the thigh is attached to the external oblique aponeurosis.
- Internal oblique muscle. From the lateral part of the inguinal ligament, the iliac crest and the lumbar fascia, these fibres pass upwards and medially to the costal margin and the linea alba. The aponeurosis of

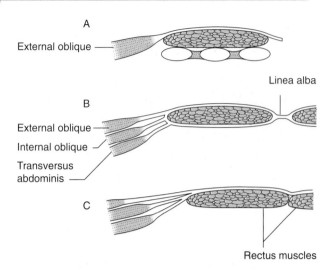

A

External oblique

Linea alba

B

External oblique

Internal oblique

Transversus abdominis

C

Rectus muscles

Fig. 11.3 Rectus sheath: **(A)** above the costal margin; **(B)** between umbilicus (approx.) and costal margin; **(C)** below the arcuate line.

internal oblique splits to contribute to both anterior and posterior walls of the rectus sheath (Fig. 11.3). The lowest fibres, arising from the inguinal ligament, arch down to attach medially with similar fibres of transversus abdominis to the pubic tubercle as the conjoint tendon (see 11.2).

- Transversus abdominis muscle. From the six lowest ribs, lumbar fascia, iliac crest and the lateral part of the inguinal ligament, fibres run across to the linea alba contributing to the rectus sheath (Fig. 11.3). As with internal oblique, the lowest fibres arch down to attach to the pubic tubercle as the conjoint tendon.
- Transversalis fascia. This layer of connective tissue separates the muscles of the anterior abdominal wall from the parietal peritoneum.

Rectus sheath

The usual pattern is shown in Figure 11.3, although there is considerable variation. Inferiorly, since the aponeuroses of all three sheet muscles pass anterior to rectus abdominis, the only tissue separating rectus abdominis from the parietal peritoneum is transversalis fascia. Above this on the posterior aspect of rectus abdominis is the arcuate line – the free lower extremity of that part of the rectus sheath that passes posterior to rectus abdominis.

Action of the muscles as a whole

The sheet muscles and rectus abdominis are active in trunk movements: flexion, lateral flexion and twisting. They compress the abdominal contents during defecation and provide support and stability during lifting. Asymmetrical spasm of these muscles during youth and adolescence has been implicated in cases of scoliosis (twisted spine).

Nerve supply of anterior abdominal wall
(Fig. 11.2)

This is from segmental nerves T7–L1. Intercostal nerves leave the costal grooves where the ribs turn superiorly, and continue into the abdominal wall. T12 segmental nerve is the subcostal nerve. L1 segmental nerve divides into two: the more cranial is the iliohypogastric, which principally supplies the abdominal wall, the more caudal the ilioinguinal, which is diverted to the anterior scrotum or labia majora, and the medial thigh.

Segmental nerves T7–12 travel in the abdominal wall between transversus abdominis and internal oblique, sending branches through these muscles to more superficial structures (e.g. skin) and internally to the peritoneum. The iliohypogastric and ilioinguinal nerves (L1) posteriorly are found between transversus and internal oblique, but in the region of the anterior superior iliac spine they penetrate internal oblique and run between internal and external obliques. This apparently trivial detail is relevant to inguinal anatomy and to incisions near McBurney's point, for example for appendicectomy (see later).

- Sensory fibres in the nerves supply abdominal skin, wall and peritoneum (as well as thoracic skin and pleura). Cell bodies of sensory fibres are in the dorsal root ganglion of the appropriate nerve. See dermatome map (Fig. 6.6, p. 36). Note that the dermatome over the xiphoid process is (usually) T8, over the umbilicus T10, and over the pubic symphysis T12/L1.
- Motor fibres in the nerves supply the sheet muscles and the rectus abdominis. The cell bodies of the motor neurons are in the ventral horn of grey matter of the appropriate segment of the spinal cord.

Blood supply and lymph drainage of anterior abdominal wall

Arteries

- Intercostal arteries, part of the intercostal neurovascular bundles, approach from the lateral aspect.
- Epigastric arteries. Posterior to rectus abdominis muscle are:
  - superior epigastric artery: a continuation of the internal thoracic artery from the subclavian
  - inferior epigastric artery: a branch of the external iliac/femoral.

    These freely anastomose and this may become a bypass channel for an aortic blockage (e.g. coarctation, see Fig. 10.25, p. 86).
- Branches of segmental lumbar arteries supply the posterior abdominal wall.

Veins

Intercostal veins drain to the azygos system. Lumbar (segmental) veins drain to the veins of the posterior abdominal wall and the azygos system (details not necessary), and the superior and inferior epigastric veins drain to subclavian and femoral veins respectively. Anastomoses between these venous channels may provide a bypass for a blockage of the inferior vena cava.

Lymph

The lymph drainage of the anterior abdominal wall is roughly in quadrants: superiorly to right and left axillary nodes, and inferiorly to right and left inguinal nodes.

Clinical box

Abdominal incisions
- Median incisions. The linea alba is a nerveless and comparatively bloodless plane.
- Paramedian incisions. Nerves enter rectus abdominis muscles from the lateral aspect, so in paramedian incisions, the anterior layer of the rectus sheath is incised and the rectus abdominis muscle displaced laterally so as not to tear the nerves. It is better to avoid incisions through the tendinous intersections, if possible: they bleed profusely.
- Incisions through the sheet muscles, e.g. a gridiron incision near McBurney's point for appendicectomy. Muscle fibres need only be separated to give sufficient access, but it is worth noting that the L1 nerves (ilioinguinal and iliohypogastric) are in the vicinity of an incision over McBurney's point, and that damage to the iliohypogastric nerve might weaken the muscles of the anterior abdominal wall in the inguinal region, increasing the possibility of a subsequent inguinal hernia.

11.2 Inguinal canal, scrotum, testis, inguinal hernias   (Figs 11.4, 11.5)

Overview

The inguinal canal is a weak spot in the anterior abdominal wall. In the male it transmits structures to and from the testis; in the female it is much smaller. The internal aspect of the canal is the deep inguinal ring; the external aspect is the superficial ring. In embryonic life the testis migrates from the abdomen to the scrotum. It is covered in the scrotum by three layers of fascia, and most intimately, by the tunica vaginalis, the cavity of which is a part of the peritoneal cavity that becomes detached during development. The abdominal origin of the testis is reflected in its vascular supply, and also its lymph drainage to para-aortic nodes, unlike that of scrotal skin to inguinal nodes.

Learning Objectives

You should:

- know how the inguinal canal is constructed
- understand the anatomy of the testis and its coverings in the scrotum
- understand the descent of the testis to the scrotum
- know the anatomy of inguinal hernias.

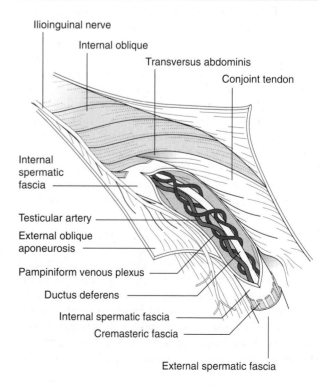

Ilioinguinal nerve
Internal oblique
Transversus abdominis
Conjoint tendon
Internal spermatic fascia
Testicular artery
External oblique aponeurosis
Pampiniform venous plexus
Ductus deferens
Internal spermatic fascia
Cremasteric fascia
External spermatic fascia

Fig. 11.4 Right inguinal canal: external aspect after division of external oblique aponeurosis. The ilioinguinal nerve has been displaced to show the spermatic cord.

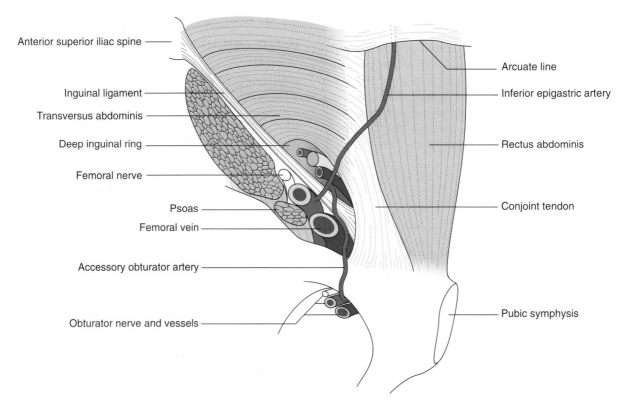

Fig. 11.5 Left inguinal region: internal aspect. This view of the canal is important for the laparoscopic repair of inguinal hernias.

The inguinal canal

The inguinal canal is a passage through the lowest part of the anterior abdominal wall for transmission of the spermatic cord in the male and the round ligament of the uterus in the female. In the male fetus it is the pathway through which the testis descends into what will become the scrotum. The spermatic cord is much larger than the round ligament in the female, and consequently the inguinal canal is more significant in the male than in the female. This matters in that any defect in the musculature of the anterior abdominal wall constitutes a potential weak spot, and since the canal is bigger in the male, the potential weakness is greater in the male. Inguinal hernias result from this weakness. This description will concern inguinal anatomy in the male, with notes on the female as necessary.

Imagine the developing testis inside the abdomen trying to make its way out. It must first penetrate the transversalis fascia: the defect in this layer so caused is the:

Deep (internal) inguinal ring. This is roughly circular and its surface marking is about 2 cm above the femoral pulse at the inguinal ligament, the pulse being roughly halfway between the anterior superior iliac spine and the pubic tubercle. The deep ring is immediately lateral to the inferior epigastric artery passing up on the posterior surface of the rectus abdominis muscle.

Emerging from the deep inguinal ring, the testis makes its way downwards and medially, roughly parallel to and slightly above the inguinal ligament, through (in order) transversus abdominis and internal oblique to arrive at a defect in external oblique, the:

Superficial (external) inguinal ring. This is a triangular defect in external oblique, the base of which is medial to the pubic tubercle, and the apex of which points up and laterally so that most of the superficial ring is more-or-less directly above the pubic tubercle.

Inguinal canal – the pathway between the two rings   (Figs 11.4, 11.5)

- The floor of the canal is formed by the inguinal ligament.
- The anterior wall is formed by external oblique aponeurosis throughout, reinforced laterally (over the deep ring) by internal oblique.
- The posterior wall is formed by transversalis fascia throughout, reinforced medially (deep to the superficial ring) by the conjoint tendon (united internal oblique and transversus abdominis) attached to the pubic tubercle.
- The roof of the canal is made up of the fibres of internal oblique arching over the contents of the inguinal canal to form the conjoint tendon.

In coughing, straining and lifting, the muscles of the anterior abdominal wall contract and the diaphragm is fixed so that abdominal contents (e.g. bowel) might be forced through the potential weak spot of the inguinal region. This is minimised by the way in which the muscles move when contracting which results in the arching fibres of internal oblique being pulled inferiorly to cover the anterior aspect of the deep inguinal ring, thereby reinforcing it and reducing the size of the potential weakness.

Spermatic cord

As the testis 'pushes' its way through the inguinal canal towards the scrotum, it drags with it the ductus deferens, arteries, veins and nerves passing to the testis. These structures constitute the spermatic cord, which acquires coverings that to some extent reflect the layers of the abdominal wall through which they have passed. From inside out these are:

- the internal spermatic fascia
- the cremasteric fascia and cremaster muscle
- the external spermatic fascia.

    The spermatic cord also includes:

- the testicular artery, on each side a direct branch of the aorta
- the pampiniform plexus of veins which form the testicular vein draining on the right to the inferior vena cava and on the left to the renal vein
- testicular lymphatics passing to para-aortic nodes (the lymph drainage of the testis thus reflecting its arterial supply)
- the genital branch of the genitofemoral nerve (L1, 2) which supplies cremaster muscle with involuntary motor fibres – cremaster muscle retracts the testis
- sympathetic nerve fibres
- blood vessels serving the ductus deferens.

Ilioinguinal nerve L1

This supplies anterior scrotal and penile skin. It enters the inguinal canal *not* through the deep inguinal ring, but from the lateral aspect. In the region of the anterior superior iliac spine it lies between internal and external obliques, and so, as it runs down parallel to the inguinal ligament it is joined in the inguinal canal by the structures which have entered through the deep inguinal ring. The ilioinguinal nerve passes through the superficial inguinal ring on the surface of the spermatic cord.

Scrotum (Fig. 11.6)

The scrotum is equivalent to the labia majora in the female. It is a body wall structure, so:

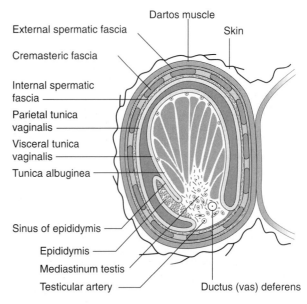

Fig. 11.6 Left scrotum and testes: transverse section.

- its arterial supply is from body wall arteries (pudendal, femoral)
- its venous drainage is to body wall veins (pudendal, great saphenous)
- its lymph drainage is mainly to inguinal lymph nodes (very important)
- its cutaneous sensory nerve supply is from ilioinguinal (L1), genital branch of genitofemoral (L1, 2) and scrotal branches of the pudendal (S2, 3, 4) nerves.

Scrotal skin is thin and contains smooth muscle fibres – dartos, supplied by sympathetic fibres – which contract in the cold to cause wrinkling.

Testis (Fig. 11.6)

In the scrotum, each testis is invaginated into its serous membrane, the tunica vaginalis, much as the lung is invaginated into the pleura. The serous cavity around the testis was in fetal life continuous with the peritoneal cavity through the processus vaginalis (the tunica vaginalis and peritoneum being exactly equivalent), but as the muscles of the anterior abdominal wall are formed and become stronger, the processus becomes separated from the main peritoneal cavity. Attached to the lateral surface of the testis is the epididymis, into which the seminiferous tubules of the testis converge and eventually unite to form at its lower, and narrower end, the ductus (vas) deferens. The recess between the epididymis and the testis is the sinus of the epididymis. The covering of the testis, between it and the visceral layer of tunica vaginalis, is the tunica albuginea.

Unlike the scrotum, the testis is an organ of the posterior abdominal wall, like the kidney, and therefore:

- testicular arteries come directly from the aorta
- testicular veins drain to the IVC on the right and the renal vein on the left
- and, most importantly, lymphatic drainage is to nodes around the abdominal aorta, para-aortic nodes, and *not* to inguinal nodes like scrotal skin.

Clinical box

Testicular descent
The testis develops high on the posterior wall of the embryonic coelom and subsequently descends through the inguinal canal so that at or soon after birth it should be in the scrotum. Its descent may be arrested at any stage. It may take a wrong turn after it has come through the inguinal canal: such ectopic testes are fairly easy to place in the scrotum since the spermatic cord is long enough. More difficult to deal with is the testis which has not travelled far enough to have a sufficiently long spermatic cord for the testis to be placed in the scrotum. Testes which are allowed to remain ectopic are inclined to malignant change.

Retractile testes
The testis may be retracted into the abdomen, out of harm's way (presumably) – this is cremaster in action. The cremaster reflex may be elicited by gentle stimulation of the skin of the scrotum or anterior thigh, and plunging into cold water may cause retraction, although it is not usual for a man to retract his testes at will. It is of clinical significance in the young boy: a testis which has retracted in shock (as it were) because the hand palpating the scrotum is cold may be mistaken for an undescended testis.

Testicular malignancy and lymph drainage
If you suspect a testicular malignancy and find the inguinal nodes are enlarged, it is reasonable to assume that the malignancy has already spread from the testis to invade neighbouring scrotal skin, whence it has spread further to the inguinal nodes. Testicular malignancy is potentially lethal and it is as well for men to examine their testes as women do their breasts.

Testicular torsion
The testis may twist upon the spermatic cord resulting in occlusion of the blood supply. This is painful and is an emergency: the cord needs to be untwisted before the testis dies.

Vasectomy
This is ligation and removal of a short length of the ductus (vas) deferens, usually for the purposes of birth control.

Swellings arising in the testis
- Hydrocele. There may be a build-up of serous straw-coloured fluid between the layers of the tunica vaginalis (compare with pleural effusion). This is usually innocent: it simply needs to be drained by needle aspiration.
- Varicocele. Varicose veins of the pampiniform plexus and testicular veins may arise, more commonly (inexplicably, despite several theories) on the left than the right.
- Spermatocele. This is a fluid-filled cyst of the epididymis containing spermatozoa. It is uncommon.

Inguinal hernias   (Fig. 11.7)

A hernia is a condition in which internal structures are forced out through a weakness in the wall. In the inguinal region, abdominal contents (e.g. intestines, fat) may pass through the inguinal canal – a potential weak spot in the anterior abdominal wall. Since the canal is larger in the male than the female, inguinal hernias are commoner in the male.

Types of inguinal hernia

- Indirect inguinal hernia. Abdominal contents pass through the deep inguinal ring and into the canal. They may be so large that they continue through the superficial ring, above and medial to the pubic tubercle, and present as a scrotal swelling. The neck (internal opening) of the hernia in this case would be through the deep inguinal ring, lateral to the inferior epigastric artery.
- Direct inguinal hernia. Abdominal contents bulge through the anterior abdominal wall between the deep inguinal ring and the midline, usually owing to a weak conjoint tendon. In this case, the neck of the hernia would be medial to the inferior epigastric artery.

  It is not usually possible to distinguish these two hernias on clinical examination alone, except that a large scrotal hernia is more likely to be an indirect hernia.
- Congenital inguinal hernia. The potential space between the two layers of the tunica vaginalis may remain in continuity after birth with the peritoneal cavity. This is a congenital inguinal hernia: coils of intestine may surround the testis in the scrotum.

Clinical box

Is it an inguinal hernia or a scrotal swelling?
It may be difficult to distinguish between a scrotal swelling of testicular origin and a large inguinal hernia extending into the scrotum. If it is possible to 'get above' the swelling, it is not an inguinal hernia but something confined to the scrotum, for example a hydrocele.

Inguinal region in the female

Everything in the inguinal region of the female is much the same as in the male, except that it is all smaller and, as noted, inguinal hernias are less common in the female (but see Ch. 13; Femoral hernia, p. 193). The structure in the female which passes through the inguinal canal is the round ligament of the uterus, an insignificant structure derived from the gubernaculum (see an Embryology text for details). The labia majora of the

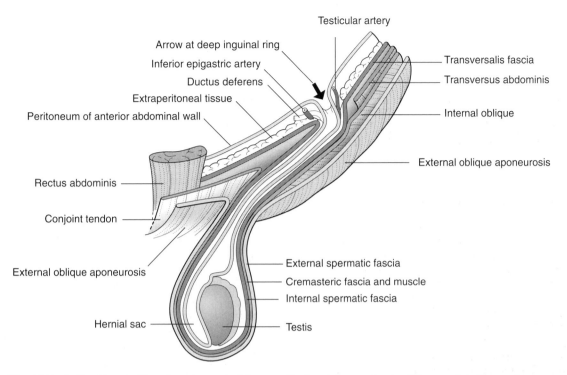

Fig. 11.7 Indirect inguinal hernia: scheme. In this case, the hernial sac extends all the way into the scrotum leaving the way open for peritoneal contents to occupy this entire space. It is virtually a re-establishment of the fetal processus vaginalis.

female share the same blood supply (femoral, pudendal), nerve supply (genitofemoral, pudendal) and lymph drainage (mainly to inguinal nodes) as the scrotum in the male.

11.3 Arrangement of the gut tube in the abdominal cavity

Overview

The intestines and associated organs were originally connected to the posterior abdominal wall by an elongated hilum, the dorsal mesentery. Subsequent changes in the disposition of abdominal viscera result in a complex arrangement of mesenteries and omenta. The transverse colon divides the abdominal cavity into supracolic and infracolic compartments. The areas on either side of the ascending and descending colons are the paracolic gutters. Other important areas of the peritoneal cavity are the lesser sac, the hepatorenal pouch and the subphrenic spaces.

Learning Objectives

You should:

- understand the basic arrangement of the peritoneal cavity

- understand the terms mesentery and omentum

- know the position of: supracolic and infracolic compartments, paracolic gutters, lesser sac, hepatorenal pouch, subphrenic spaces.

Some embryological considerations

Think of the gut tube and associated organs as pushing their way into the peritoneal cavity from behind, much as the lung pushes its way into the pleural cavity. The 'hilum' of the gut tube, where the parietal and visceral peritoneal layers meet, is elongated into a structure which connects the entire length of the gut tube to the dorsal body wall, and through it pass blood vessels, nerves, and lymphatics. This is the dorsal mesentery (Fig. 11.8).

In the embryo, the gut tube enters the abdomen from the thorax passing behind a mass of mesoderm called the septum transversum, which subsequently becomes part of the diaphragm, liver and the connections between them and the ventral body wall. The upper part of the

A

VENTRAL

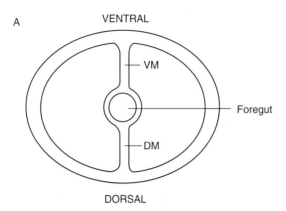

DORSAL

B

VENTRAL

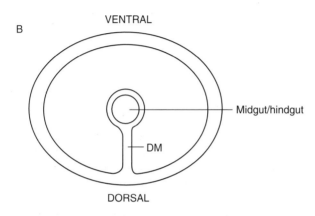

DORSAL

C

VENTRAL

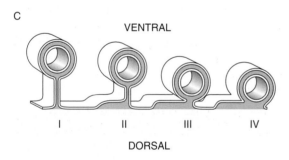

DORSAL

Fig. 11.8 Mesenteries. **(A)** Embryonic foregut attached to both dorsal and ventral body walls by dorsal mesentery (DM) and ventral mesentery (VM). **(B)** Embryonic midgut and hindgut attached to dorsal body wall only by dorsal mesentery (DM). **(C)** How to lose a mesentery. In the progression I to IV, the gut tube falls to the right and the dorsal mesentery which at first is merely lying on the dorsal body wall becomes part of it. In each diagram, dorsal is at the bottom.

abdominal gut tube is attached not only to the dorsal body wall by the dorsal mesentery, but also to the ventral body wall by these derivatives of the septum transversum, which form the ventral mesentery (Fig. 11.8). This part of the gut tube is foregut and it extends distally as far as what will be the mid-portion of the duodenum. The remainder of the gut tube, midgut and hindgut, is connected to the dorsal body wall only by

the dorsal mesentery, known simply as the mesentery: there is no ventral mesentery here.

This simple layout of the gut tube in the peritoneal cavity is subsequently complicated by two factors. First, the tube elongates spectacularly and coils on itself within the abdomen; and secondly some parts of the gut tube then adhere to the dorsal body wall, thus losing their mesentery and becoming apparently retroperitoneal, an adjective meaning that the dorsal mesentery has been lost (Fig. 11.8). Clinically, this means that those parts of the alimentary canal that remain mesenteric are more mobile and may twist or herniate into other areas, while those that are retroperitoneal are more or less fixed. The final layout is shown in Figure 11.9.

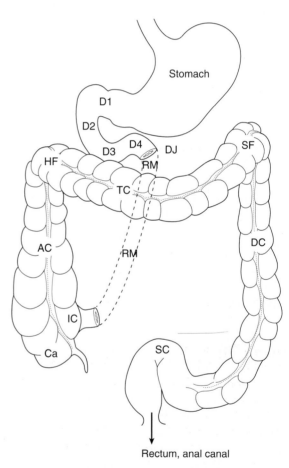

Rectum, anal canal

Fig. 11.9 Layout of gut tube in abdominal cavity: anterior view. D1, first part of duodenum; D2, second part of duodenum; D3, third part of duodenum; D4, fourth part of duodenum; DJ, duodenojejunal junction or flexure; RM, root of the mesentery of the small intestine; IC, ileocolic junction; Ca, caecum; AC, ascending colon; HF, hepatic flexure or right colic flexure; TC, transverse colon; SF, splenic flexure or left colic flexure; DC, descending colon; SC, sigmoid colon. The two circles at either end of RM, marked at DJ and IC, are the respective places where the duodenum becomes mesenteric as the jejunum, and the ileum becomes retroperitoneal again as the caecum and ascending colon. The jejunum and ileum are not shown.

In the peritoneal cavity …

Strictly speaking, nothing is in the peritoneal cavity except a thin layer of peritoneal fluid. Yet, you will hear: 'the stomach is in the peritoneal cavity' as you hear 'the lungs are in the pleural cavities' and 'the heart is in the pericardial cavity'. The function of the peritoneal cavity is, like the pleural and pericardial cavities, to permit movement of the gut tube (postural, peristalsis, etc.) independent of movement of the body wall.

Names – caution!

Abdominal cavity = peritoneal cavity. That part of the peritoneal or abdominal cavity that is within the pelvis is sometimes called the pelvic cavity, although it should more properly be the pelvic part of the peritoneal cavity.

Mesenteric = omental = epiploic = ligamentous (not to be confused with other uses of ligament). Which of these terms is used in any given situation is merely traditional.

Parts of the peritoneal cavity

- Supracolic compartment: superior to the transverse colon. This is usually taken to include the oesophagus, stomach, most of the duodenum, liver and biliary system.
- Infracolic compartment: inferior to the transverse colon. This includes the jejunum, ileum, caecum, ascending, descending and sigmoid colon, and rectum.
- Paracolic gutters: lateral to ascending and descending colons.
- Paravertebral gutters: between ascending and descending colons and the vertebral column.
- Hepatorenal (Morison's) pouch: the superior end of the right paracolic gutter between liver and kidney, also known as the right subhepatic (subdiaphragmatic) space.
- Subphrenic (subdiaphragmatic) and subhepatic spaces (Fig. 11.10). The liver and diaphragm developmentally are different parts of the same thing (septum transversum) and they remain attached to each other at the so-called bare area of the liver. The recesses of the peritoneal cavity partially separate the two structures. Naming of these is not consistent, but the system given here is as good as any:
  - Posterior subphrenic space: posterior to the liver, between it and the posterior diaphragm. It is continuous with Morison's pouch.
  - Anterior subphrenic space: anteriorly between the liver and the diaphragm.

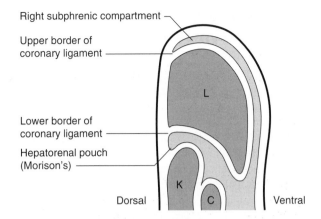

Right subphrenic compartment
Upper border of coronary ligament
Lower border of coronary ligament
Hepatorenal pouch (Morison's)
L
K
C
Dorsal
Ventral

Fig. 11.10 Subphrenic (subdiaphragmatic) spaces: sagittal diagram through the upper abdomen: L, liver; K, kidney; C, transverse colon.

The anatomy of the liver, mainly a right-sided organ, means that these spaces are on the right side of the body.
- Lesser sac. Developmental changes mean that that part of the peritoneal cavity to the right of the (originally midline) stomach becomes at first behind the stomach (as the ventral surface of the stomach is displaced to the right), and then almost completely isolated from the rest of the peritoneal cavity as a result of the duodenum becoming adherent to the dorsal body wall. This is the lesser sac of the peritoneal cavity, behind the stomach, and the small communication between it and the rest of the peritoneal cavity is the epiploic foramen of Winslow (see later). The rest of the peritoneal cavity, with its supracolic and infracolic compartments, is the greater sac.

Clinical box

Pouches and disease
These pouches and sacs may be the sites of collection of inflammatory fluid which, particularly around the diaphragm, may go undiagnosed unless they are deliberately excluded – that is to say unless you think about the possibility of their involvement, you will miss them. This is particularly true of the areas between liver and diaphragm, and Morison's pouch which, in a patient lying supine in bed, is the most dependent part of the peritoneal cavity. Fluid may collect here unless appropriate physiotherapy and regular postural changes are instituted.

11.4 Great vessels of the abdomen, sympathetic chain

Overview

The aorta and inferior vena cava are on the posterior abdominal wall. Aortic branches serve the body wall (lumbar arteries), kidneys (renal arteries), gonads (ovarian and testicular arteries), and the gut tube (coeliac, superior mesenteric, inferior mesenteric arteries). The aorta divides into the common iliac arteries that supply pelvic organs and the lower limbs. The inferior vena cava is formed by the union of the common iliac veins and passes up on the right of the aorta to the liver where it is joined by hepatic veins, before penetrating the diaphragm and opening into the right atrium of the heart.

Learning Objectives

You should:

- know the main branches of the aorta and their territories
- know the disposition of the main veins in the abdomen.

Aorta

The aorta enters the upper abdomen slightly to the left of the midline behind the diaphragm at vertebral level T12. It passes down to about vertebral level L3/4 where it divides (surface marking: just below and to the left of the umbilicus in a recumbent patient) into the common iliac arteries. It is easily palpated in the upper abdomen between the umbilicus and the rib cage.

Branches of the aorta (Fig. 11.11)

- Lumbar segmental arteries. There are paired, body wall branches, equivalent to the intercostals in the thorax. They are of no significance except that they give branches that pass into the vertebral canal to supply the spinal cord. Damage to the larger ones, for example in abdominal aortic surgery, may lead to spinal cord lesions.
- Renals, adrenals, gonadals. These are paired arteries, anomalous arrangements of which are common. The renals arise at about vertebral level L1 and you should study radiographs of them. The origin of the

gonadals is more variable, but is usually about vertebral level L2/3.

- Mesenteric. These single, unpaired branches arise ventrally. There are three:
  - Coeliac. Vertebral level T12. Supplies abdominal foregut (up to duodenal papilla) and structures which develop in foregut mesenteries: stomach, liver, spleen, most of the pancreas, duodenum as far as the papilla, greater omentum, lesser omentum.
  - Superior mesenteric. Vertebral level T12/L1 (that is, immediately below the coeliac). Supplies midgut: distal duodenum, uncinate process of pancreas, jejunum, ileum, caecum, appendix, ascending colon, transverse colon, associated mesenteric structures.
  - Inferior mesenteric. Vertebral level L3 (but more variable). Supplies hindgut: descending colon, sigmoid colon, rectum and upper part of anal canal.
- The common iliac arteries pass down and laterally towards the lower limbs. At the pelvic brim they divide to give external and internal iliac arteries.

Inferior vena cava   (Fig. 11.12)

The inferior vena cava is slightly to the right of the midline. It is formed from the two common iliac veins and passes upwards through the liver and diaphragm (at vertebral level T8) to enter the thorax. Its main tributaries are the renal, gonadal, adrenal and hepatic veins. Venous anatomy is in general much more variable than arterial anatomy, and anomalies are frequently encountered. A study of its complex embryology, though certainly not essential, will help to explain why. Suffice it here to say that the inferior vena cava may begin on the left and cross over the aorta to the right, or there may even be bilateral cavas up as far as the renal veins.

Segmental veins drain eventually to the azygos system and the superior vena cava; they have nothing to do with the inferior vena cava.

Sympathetic chain

- The right sympathetic chain passes down from the thorax and comes to lie posterolateral to the inferior vena cava.
- The left sympathetic chain comes to be posterolateral to the aorta. Below the aortic bifurcation the chains continue over the pelvic brim in front of the sacrum and they unite to form the ganglion impar (unpaired). See 11.13 (p. 144).

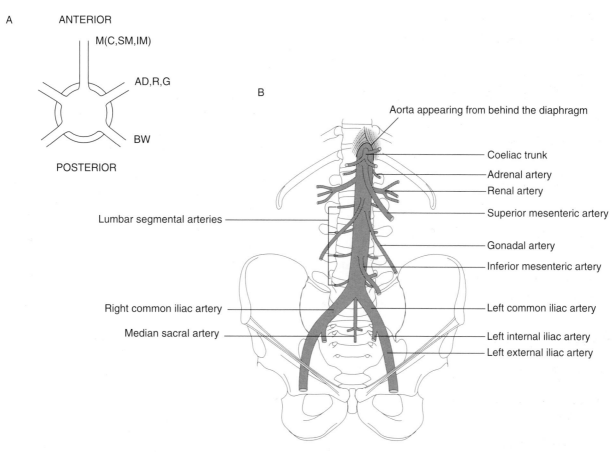

Fig. 11.11   Branches of the aorta: **(A)** diagrammatic layout of branches; **(B)** anterior view. BW, body wall branches; AD, R, G, adrenal, renal, gonadal branches; M, mesenteric branches – C, coeliac, SM, superior mesenteric, IM, inferior mesenteric.

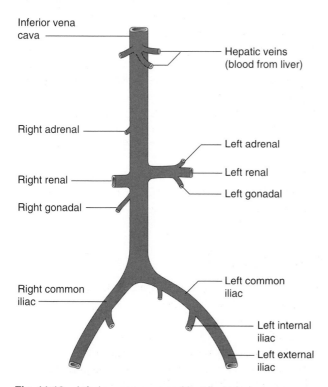

Fig. 11.12   Inferior vena cava and its tributaries.

11.5 Foregut and associated structures: pancreas, spleen, liver, gall bladder

Overview

Abdominal foregut extends from the oesophagus to the second part of the duodenum. The stomach has two curvatures, greater and lesser, to which are attached the greater and lesser omenta. Arterial supply comes from the coeliac artery and venous blood drains to the portal vein. The duodenum is intimately related to the head of the pancreas, which extends to the left where its tail is in contact with the spleen. The liver occupies the right upper abdomen. The biliary system opens into the duodenum at the duodenal papilla with the main pancreatic duct. Blood to the liver comes from the common hepatic artery (freshly oxygenated) or the portal vein (from the intestinal bed). Lymph from foregut structures drains to coeliac nodes. Upper abdominal malignancy is sometimes associated with an enlarged lymph node (Virchow's node) in the left supraclavicular area.

Learning Objectives

You should:

- know the parts, position, vertebral levels and surface markings of the stomach and duodenum

- know the position, vertebral levels and surface markings of the pancreas, spleen, liver and gall bladder

- understand the greater and lesser omenta and the lesser sac

- understand the flow of blood through the liver and the effect of its impairment

- understand the biliary tree and the flow of bile, and the effect of its impairment

- know the lymph drainage of foregut structures.

Oesophagus

The oesophagus enters the abdomen behind the diaphragm at vertebral level T10 slightly to the left of the midline surrounded by fibres from the *right* diaphragmatic crus forming a sphincter mechanism: the cardio-oesophageal sphincter. See 11.9 (p. 126).

Clinical box

Hiatus hernia
This arises when part of the stomach pushes its way up into the thorax through the oesophageal opening in the diaphragm. The two types, rolling and sliding, are dealt with in clinical texts. Hiatus hernias may give rise to epigastric discomfort. This is not the same as a congenital diaphragmatic hernia in which there is a defect in one or both sides of the diaphragm.

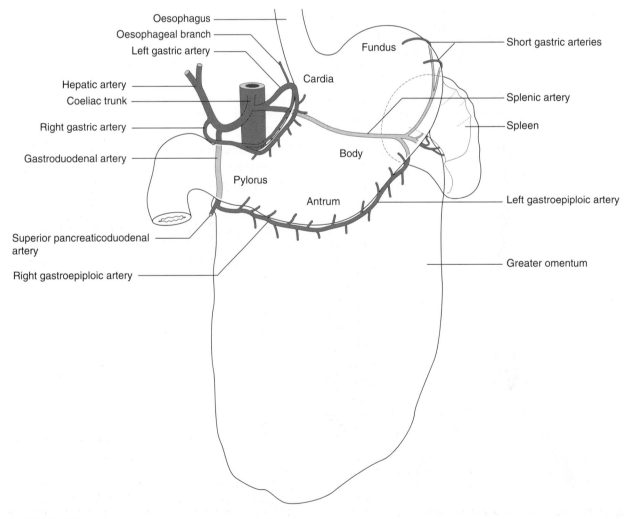

Fig. 11.13 Stomach.

Stomach   (Figs 11.13, 11.14)

The size and position of the stomach vary depending upon body shape, degree of distension, and posture. The five areas of the stomach (do not worry about the precise boundaries) are:

- cardia (around the oesophageal opening)
- fundus (above the level of the oesophageal opening)
- body (central portion)
- antrum (lower part)
- pylorus (the most distal part), the thickened sphincter mechanism controlling passage of stomach contents to the duodenum. The pylorus normally lies at about vertebral level L1, the transpyloric plane.

The left border is the greater curvature and the right the lesser curvature.

Radiology of the stomach   (Fig. 11.14)

The alimentary canal can be demonstrated radio-graphically with the use of radio-opaque barium compounds. A barium swallow demonstrates the mouth, pharynx and oesophagus. In a barium meal the stomach and small intestines are displayed after an appropriate time interval.

Lesser omentum and lesser sac
(Fig. 11.15)

As explained earlier, the original ventral border of the

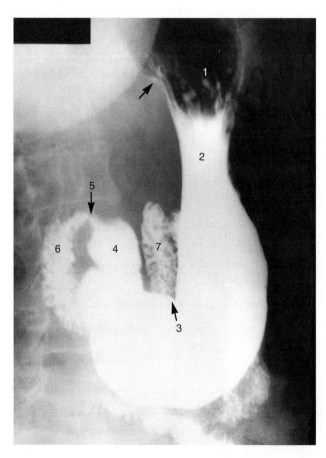

Fig. 11.14   Barium meal showing the stomach: 1, fundus; 2, narrowing of body caused by muscular contraction; 3, incisura angularis: a radiological finding demonstrating the acute angle in the lesser curvature as a result of stomach contraction; 4, antrum; 5, first part of duodenum; 6, second part of duodenum; 7, fourth part of duodenum.

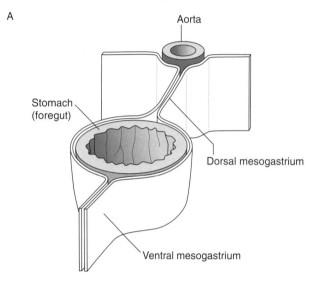

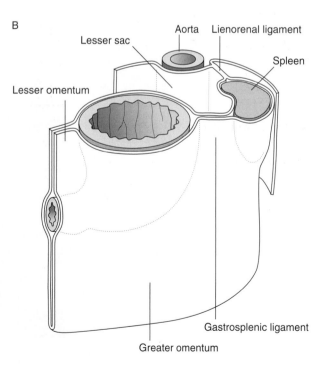

Fig. 11.15   Omenta: **(A)** the primitive embryonic state; **(B)** the later stage as the stomach rotates and part of the original right side of the abdominal cavity becomes trapped as the lesser sac.

stomach is attached to the ventral body wall by the ventral mesogastrium. This border becomes the lesser curvature, and the ventral mesogastrium (mesogastrium = mesentery of the stomach) becomes, from stomach ventrally, lesser omentum, liver and falciform (sickle-shaped) ligament. The lesser omentum moves during development so that by the time of birth it lies in a more-or-less coronal plane, and behind it and the stomach is the lesser sac of the peritoneal cavity, which opens into Morison's pouch of the greater sac through the epiploic foramen of Winslow.

Greater omentum, gastrosplenic ligament and splenorenal (lienorenal) ligament   (Fig. 11.15)

The original dorsal border of the stomach, later the greater curvature, is attached to the dorsal body wall by the dorsal mesogastrium. The spleen develops in this, dividing it into two portions: dorsal body wall to spleen, and spleen to stomach. During development, part of the dorsal mesogastrium adheres to the dorsal body wall so that its dorsal attachment comes to overlie the left kidney, giving rise to that part between dorsal body wall and spleen being named the splenorenal, or lienorenal, ligament (lien = spleen).

Between spleen and stomach the mesentery is known by two names. Above, it is the gastrosplenic ligament. Below, it grows down to form a double layer of omental (mesenteric) tissue partly covering the intestines – the greater omentum. This is, amongst other things, a fat store and may become very large – regrettably so in some middle-aged people (including the author). The greater omentum is, with the stomach and lesser omentum, part of the anterior wall of the lesser sac, and, again in development, it becomes adherent to the mesentery of the transverse colon – the transverse mesocolon – so that the transverse colon is attached to the under surface of the greater omentum.

Duodenum   (Fig. 11.16)

This is like three and a half sides of an approximate rectangle, inside which is the head of the pancreas. There are four parts.

- First part. This passes backwards and horizontally, becoming retroperitoneal (i.e. loses its mesentery). It passes anterior to the common bile duct and the gastroduodenal artery. Posterior duodenal ulcers may erode this, causing haemorrhage.
- Second part. This is retroperitoneal and passes inferiorly, overlying the hilum of the right kidney. It

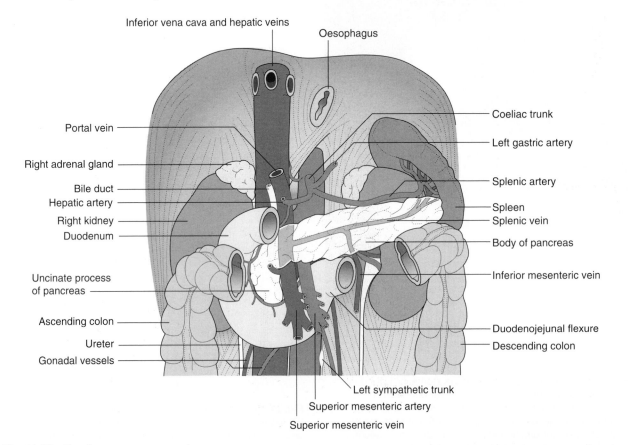

Fig. 11.16   Duodenum, pancreas, spleen.

receives the (common) entry of the biliary and pancreatic ducts about halfway down its left border, the common bile duct having already passed behind the first part of the duodenum in its descent from the liver. The duodenal papilla marks this entry and it indicates the end of the embryonic foregut, the remainder of the duodenum, including the distal region of the second part, being from midgut.

- Third part. This is retroperitoneal and passes horizontally to the left at about vertebral level L2/3, crossing the midline in front of the abdominal aorta below the origin of the superior mesenteric artery. Disease of either duodenum or aorta can result in an aortoduodenal fistula presenting as bleeding into the intestine.
- Fourth part. This, also retroperitoneal, turns upwards on the left side of the midline and at about vertebral level L1 turns to the left and once again becomes mesenteric as the jejunum: this is the duodenojejunal flexure ('d-j flexure') or junction. It is anchored (some say) by a few smooth muscle fibres in the so-called ligament of Treitz which passes down from the diaphragm to the duodenojejunal junction.

Pancreas   (Fig. 11.16)

Parts of the pancreas are, from left to right, tail, body, neck, head and uncinate process, the last two being enclosed by the first three parts of the duodenum. Behind the neck is the formation of the portal vein, and the tail of the pancreas, the only part of the organ that is not retroperitoneal, extends into the splenorenal ligament to reach the hilum of the spleen. The splenic artery runs its tortuous course through, or along the upper border of, the pancreas and gives several branches to supply it. Endocrine secretory units – islets of Langerhans – are scattered throughout the pancreas.

Duct system   (Figs 11.16, 11.17)

The exocrine acini secrete into a duct system that begins in the tail and proceeds to the right. As it enters the head it turns inferiorly to join the common bile duct and enters the duodenum at the papilla. There may be an accessory pancreatic duct opening above the main duct.

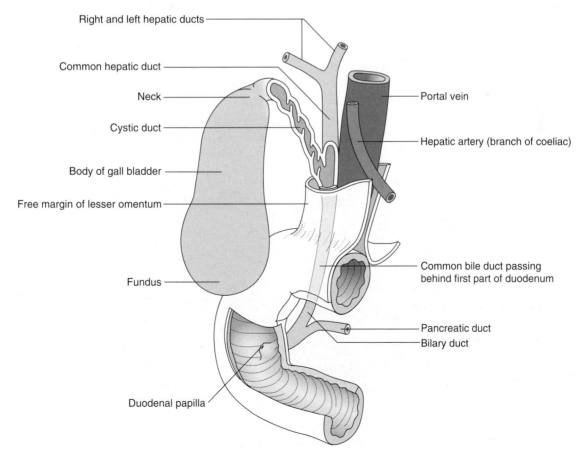

Fig. 11.17   Biliary tree, duodenal papilla.

Blood supply

This is from branches of the coeliac and superior mesenteric arteries (see later).

Clinical box

Pancreatic disease
- Pancreatic pain is often felt in the back as well as generally in the abdomen anteriorly.
- Inflammation of the pancreas (pancreatitis) may result in a collection of inflammatory fluid in the lesser sac – a pancreatic pseudocyst.
- Cancer of the head of the pancreas may result in blockage of the common bile duct as it approaches the duodenal papilla.
- The pancreas develops from two outgrowths of foregut which, after some rotation around the gut tube, fuse. Congenital anomalies include a condition in which pancreatic tissue forms a ring around the duodenum – annular pancreas. This may cause duodenal obstruction.

Spleen   (Fig. 11.16)

This is situated at the back (not the side) on the left, related to ribs 9, 10 and 11. It extends between vertebral levels T12–L2 under the left dome of the diaphragm. It is anterior to the left costodiaphragmatic recess of the pleural cavity. It does not normally extend any further anteriorly than the midaxillary line and is therefore not normally palpable. It is about the size of a clenched fist and, having developed in the dorsal mesogastrium, is attached to the dorsal body wall by the splenorenal ligament and to the stomach by the gastrosplenic ligament. At its hilum (vertebral level L1, transpyloric plane) it is in contact with the tail of the pancreas, which extends into the splenorenal ligament, through which the splenic vessels pass between the posterior abdominal wall and the spleen.

Clinical box

Splenic injury and disease
The spleen is in danger from trauma to the left lower rib cage, particularly ribs 9, 10 and 11. A ruptured spleen may cause fatal haemorrhage since, as part of the haematological policing system of the body, it has a profuse blood supply. It may become enlarged in haematological conditions or liver disease. As it enlarges it becomes palpable at the left subcostal margin, but you should note that by the time it does so it is already about three times larger than normal. It may enlarge further diagonally down towards the right iliac fossa. Such a huge spleen may be found in haematological diseases (e.g. sickle cell anaemia, leukaemia), and, lacking a palpable border in the place where it might be expected because it is so large, it may escape detection.

Liver and biliary system   (Figs 11.18–11.21)

Position and surface anatomy

The liver occupies the right and central upper abdomen, roughly from the fourth intercostal space (nipple in a lean male) to the costal margin. A very

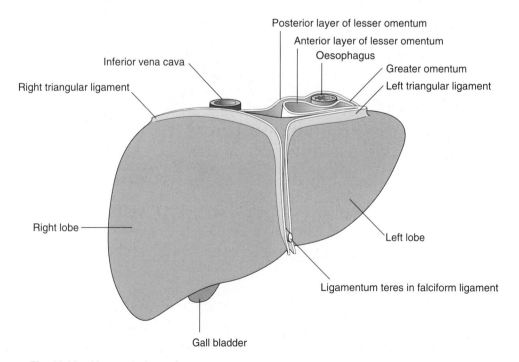

Inferior vena cava

Right triangular ligament

Right lobe

Gall bladder

Posterior layer of lesser omentum

Anterior layer of lesser omentum

Oesophagus

Greater omentum

Left triangular ligament

Left lobe

Ligamentum teres in falciform ligament

Fig. 11.18   Liver: anterior surface.

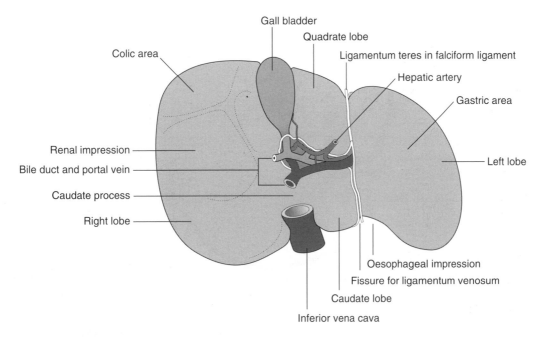

Fig. 11.19   Liver: visceral surface. The anterior border of the liver is at the top, and the posterior at the bottom.

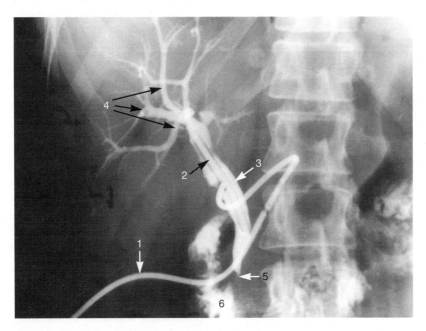

Fig. 11.20   T-tube cholangiogram showing biliary tree: 1, catheter inserted into the common bile duct; 2, one arm of the T-tube in 3, the common bile duct; 4, dilated intrahepatic biliary tree; 5, position of blockage in the common bile duct, as it passes through the pancreas; 6, contrast medium in the duodenum. The fact that contrast medium has passed into the duodenum may indicate that the obstruction at 5 is periodic rather than complete (e.g. a mobile gallstone rather than cancer of the head of the pancreas).

rough approximation is to draw a triangle whose angles are the two nipples and the tenth costochondral junction. Posteriorly, it is somewhat smaller: to map its surface projection, join the two inferior angles of the scapulas to the midpoint of the right eleventh rib.

Diaphragmatic and peritoneal attachments of the liver, bare area

The liver and most of the diaphragm develop from the septum transversum, and part of the liver remains in

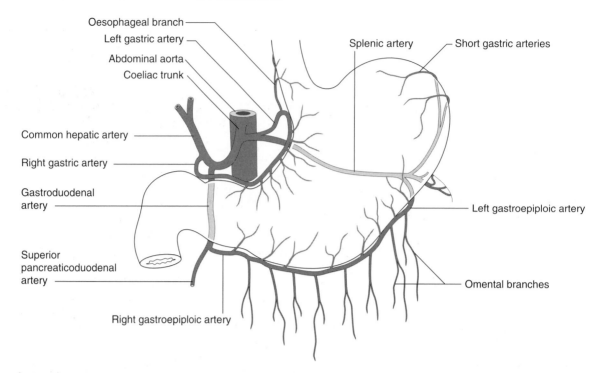

Oesophageal branch
Left gastric artery
Abdominal aorta
Coeliac trunk

Splenic artery   Short gastric arteries

Common hepatic artery

Right gastric artery

Gastroduodenal
artery

Left gastroepiploic artery

Superior
pancreaticoduodenal
artery

Omental branches

Right gastroepiploic artery

Fig. 11.21   Foregut blood supply.

direct contact with the diaphragm with no intervening peritoneum: this is the bare area. The margins of the bare area, where the hepatic visceral peritoneum is reflected on to the under surface of the diaphragm, are known as the coronary ligament, and the right and left extremities of this are the right and left triangular ligaments.

Posteriorly, the liver is supported mainly by the inferior vena cava and the hepatic veins. Anteriorly (Fig. 11.18) it is connected to the anterior abdominal wall by the falciform ligament which has a free lower border extending from the internal aspect of the umbilicus to the inferior surface of the liver. This border contains the ligamentum teres – the obliterated umbilical vein that in fetal life conveyed oxygenated blood from the placenta to the fetus.

Parts of the liver

There are four anatomical lobes: right, left, quadrate and caudate. Their boundaries are not demarcated on the anterosuperior surface of the liver, but are clearer on the inferior, or visceral, surface (Fig. 11.19). This surface displays an H-shaped group of fissures. The crossbar of the H is the porta hepatis, the area anterior to it the quadrate lobe and posterior to it the caudate lobe.

- The left sided limb of the H is a deep fissure receiving:
  - the falciform ligament (with the ligamentum teres in its free edge), and

  - part of the lesser omentum from the stomach, attached deep in this fissure to the obliterated ligamentum venosum (a continuation in the fetus of the umbilical vein).
- The right limb of the H is made up of two fossas, anteriorly for the gall bladder and posteriorly for the inferior vena cava.
- The caudate lobe forms part of the anterior wall of the lesser sac and the superior margin of the epiploic foramen (of Winslow), the only communication between the greater and lesser sacs.
- The quadrate lobe lies between the falciform ligament and the fossa for the gall bladder.

Physiologically and functionally, these anatomical lobes are of no significance. Functionally, the liver is divided into lobes and segments similar to the broncho-pulmonary segments of the lung, each with its own branches of the hepatic artery and portal vein, and each with its own tributaries of the hepatic vein and the biliary tree. Knowledge of these is useful for surgeons but is not required for undergraduates.

Inferior vena cava and the liver

The inferior vena cava passes through the bare area of the liver and the diaphragm (vertebral level T8) to enter the thorax and the right atrium of the heart. In this region the right adrenal gland is posterior to the IVC and intimately related to the bare area of the liver.

Biliary tree and gall bladder (Fig. 11.17)

The biliary tree conveys the exocrine products of the liver (bile) to the duodenum. The gall bladder is a blind diverticulum of the biliary tree for the purposes of bile storage. The right and left hepatic ducts unite to form the common hepatic duct. The cystic duct from the gall bladder joins this to form the common bile duct. There is some variation in the layout of this duct system: the important thing is that the common bile duct passes down in the free edge of the lesser omentum, then posterior to the duodenum and into the substance of the head of the pancreas. It turns to the right and unites with the pancreatic duct. There is then a small widening, the ampulla of Vater, before the sphincter mechanism (sphincter of Oddi) which protrudes slightly into the left side of the second part of the duodenum as the duodenal papilla.

Clinical box

Biliary obstruction, obstructive jaundice (Fig. 11.20)
This arises when the normal passage of bile into the duodenum is blocked, either partially or wholly. It may arise within the liver (intrahepatic) or outside it (extrahepatic). Extrahepatic causes include gallstones which find their way into the common bile duct and then block it, or cancer of the head of the pancreas, compressing the common bile duct from the outside as it passes through the head of the pancreas. In these cases with severe or complete blockage of the biliary tree, bile pigments will not reach the duodenum so the faeces will be lighter coloured than normal; biliary enzymes will not reach the intestines so that fat will be poorly digested and the faeces will be fatty (steatorrhoea) and float in the toilet bowl; bile pigments, instead of being in the intestines, will be absorbed into the bloodstream, so the patient appears yellow, and bile pigments are excreted in the urine, so the urine is dark. The combination of pale stools and dark urine means obstructive jaundice. Associated with episodes of excruciating pain, it probably means gallstones in the duct; associated with lassitude and weight loss it probably means cancer of the head of the pancreas.

Blood supply of foregut derivatives: oesophagus, stomach, proximal duodenum, liver, gall bladder, pancreas, spleen – coeliac artery (Fig. 11.21)

The coeliac artery arises from the aorta at vertebral level T12, and supplies all the abdominal foregut and derivatives. There are three branches: splenic, hepatic, left gastric.

- Splenic: passes in the posterior wall of the lesser sac through or along the top of the pancreas (giving branches to it) and through the lienorenal ligament to the spleen. Near the spleen it gives short gastric arteries that pass in the gastrosplenic ligament to the fundus of the stomach, and the left gastroepiploic, which supplies the greater omentum and the greater curvature of the stomach.
- Common hepatic (usually simply hepatic): passes to the liver in the free edge of the lesser omentum. It gives:
  - right gastric: lesser curvature
  - gastroduodenal: passes inferiorly, behind the first part of the duodenum, and divides into the right gastroepiploic (for the greater curvature) and the superior pancreaticoduodenal which runs between the head of the pancreas and the duodenum, supplying them both
  - cystic: to the gall bladder
  - right and left hepatic arteries (terminal branches).
- Left gastric: lesser curvature and terminal oesophagus.

Variations in this arrangement are found, and rarely the hepatic artery may be a branch of the superior mesenteric rather than the coeliac artery.

Note that the duodenum distal to the duodenal papilla is a midgut derivative. It is therefore supplied by branches of the superior mesenteric artery, in particular the inferior pancreaticoduodenal, which runs in the groove between pancreas and duodenum, anastomosing with the superior pancreaticoduodenal.

Boundaries of the epiploic foramen (of Winslow)

- Anterior – structures in the free edge of the lesser omentum: portal vein (behind), common hepatic artery (front left), common bile duct (front right).
- Superior – caudate lobe of liver.
- Posterior – inferior vena cava.
- Inferior – duodenum (first part).

Clinical box

Bleeding from the liver, Pringle's manoeuvre
All blood passing to the liver enters through either the hepatic artery (freshly oxygenated, from the aorta) or the portal vein (from the intestinal bed). Both these vessels pass in the free edge of the lesser omentum. Bleeding from the liver, therefore, can be stemmed by compressing the free edge of the lesser omentum (Pringle's manoeuvre). Should bleeding continue, it is likely that the inferior vena cava has been damaged.

Lymph drainage of foregut: stomach, liver, spleen, pancreas, duodenum, Virchow's node

Lymph from foregut structures drains to coeliac nodes, although in reaching them other structures may be involved. The lymph drainage of the stomach is particularly important because of stomach cancer and, as elsewhere, it mirrors the arterial supply:

- lymph from the greater omentum passes to splenic and pancreatic nodes before reaching coeliac nodes
- as well as draining to the coeliac nodes, lymph from the lesser curvature may pass retrogradely to the liver, leading to hepatic involvement – this is not uncommon.

From the coeliac nodes, lymph passes to the cisterna chyli, the thoracic duct and its termination in the formation of the left brachiocephalic vein. In some cases of upper abdominal malignant disease, particularly stomach cancer, involvement of left supraclavicular nodes may occur, presumably because of their proximity to the termination of the main thoracic duct. This, when present, is known as Virchow's node.

11.6 Midgut and hindgut

Overview

Midgut and hindgut extend from the second part of the duodenum to the anal canal. They receive blood from the superior and inferior mesenteric arteries, and venous blood drains to the portal system. Lymph drains to mesenteric nodes, thence to preaortic nodes and the cisterna chyli.

Learning Objectives

You should:

- know the disposition of the jejunum and ileum
- know the disposition and surface anatomy of the caecum, ascending colon, transverse colon, descending colon and sigmoid colon
- understand the blood supply of midgut and hindgut and the importance of the marginal artery.

Midgut

The midgut extends from the duodenal papilla to (roughly) the distal end of the transverse colon (splenic flexure), and hindgut extends from there to the pectinate (dentate) line of the anal canal. For the third and fourth parts of the duodenum, see above.

Small bowel: jejunum and ileum

At the duodenojejunal flexure, the gut tube once again becomes mesenteric and the first (about) two-fifths of the mesenteric small bowel is the jejunum, the remainder the ileum. Anatomically they may be differentiated by the pattern of arteries in the mesentery, and the jejunal walls are somewhat thicker, but neither of these matters to anyone except surgeons. The mesentery of the jejunum and ileum is known simply as 'the mesentery'. Originally in the midline, it has shifted during development so that it runs from above left to bottom right. Branches of the superior mesenteric vessels pass in it.

Inside the jejunum, the mucosa forms prominent folds: the plicae circulares.

Clinical box

Meckel's diverticulum
Within about 1 metre or so of the distal end of the ileum is the site of the embryonic vitellointestinal duct attachment, and a remnant of this duct may persist: Meckel's diverticulum. It is clinically important in that it may contain ectopic gastric mucosa, which secretes acid and causes bleeding from the intestinal mucosa. It should be included in the differential diagnosis of anyone with otherwise unexplained blood loss, especially children.

Peyer's patches
These are aggregations of lymphoid tissue in the wall of the small intestine. In certain conditions (e.g. lymphomas) these may enlarge and cause intestinal obstruction.

Carcinoid tumour
Tumours of the small intestine are rare, but occasionally the neuroendocrine cells scattered throughout the epithelium undergo neoplastic change resulting in overproduction of pressor (causing blood pressure to increase) amines. This may present as episodes of increased bowel movements, diarrhoea and hypertension and other cardiovascular effects.

Large bowel

Caecum and appendix

The ileocaecal junction is marked by a valve. The surface marking of the caecum and base of the appendix is McBurney's point. The appendix is of variable length and position: it usually lies retrocaecally but may extend down into the pelvis and give rise, when inflamed, to pelvic pain. See 'Appendicitis and pain' (11.8, p. 125).

Palpating the caecum

A hard mass in the right iliac fossa is strongly suggestive of caecal disease (e.g. cancer).

Colon

There are four parts:

- ascending
- transverse
- descending
- sigmoid.

The colon is distinguished by the concentration of longitudinal muscle in its wall into three broad bands, the taenia coli. They converge at the appendix. They are responsible for powerful peristaltic movements that convey the increasingly solid faeces towards the anus. They are responsible for another characteristic feature of the colon – it is as if they are shorter than the colon itself, so the colon is 'gathered' to form sacculations or haustrations.

The ascending, transverse and descending colons form three sides of a rectangle, the two angles being the hepatic and splenic flexures. The ascending and transverse (or most of it) are midgut derivatives, so are supplied by the superior mesenteric artery. The descending colon is a hindgut derivative and is supplied by the inferior mesenteric artery. Ascending and descending colons are retroperitoneal and so are not usually mobile, but the transverse colon has a mesentery – the transverse mesocolon – that may be sufficiently extensive for the transverse colon to loop down for some distance. The descending colon is often palpable on the left side of the abdomen, particularly if it contains faecal matter.

The sigmoid colon has a mesentery (the sigmoid mesocolon) and meets the rectum in front of the body of S3, as the gut tube loses its mesentery and once again becomes retroperitoneal. This junction is known as the rectosigmoid junction, recto- coming first because clinically it is usually considered from the bottom up, as when viewed through a sigmoidoscope or at a barium enema radiographic examination.

Rectum

The rectum and anal canal are considered with other pelvic and perineal structures (see 11.12).

Clinical box

Diverticular disease
Repeated straining at stool, such as may result from a diet lacking fibre, may cause small out-pouchings of the colonic lumen through weak spots in the muscular coat of the colon. These diverticula may be apparent on barium examination of the colon (diverticulosis) and may become inflamed (diverticulitis) with episodes of abdominal pain.

Radiology of the large bowel   (Fig. 11.22)

The colon and rectum may be demonstrated radiologically by a barium enema: barium is injected through the anal canal and pumped up to, usually, the caecum.

Blood supply of midgut and hindgut
(Fig. 11.23)

The midgut artery is the superior mesenteric (origin: vertebral level T12/L1). The hindgut artery is the inferior mesenteric (origin: about vertebral level L3).

Superior mesenteric artery: main branches

- Inferior pancreaticoduodenal: as name suggests.
- Right colic: ascending colon.
- Jejunal and ileal: as names suggest. Since coils of ileum hang down into the pelvic cavity, on an

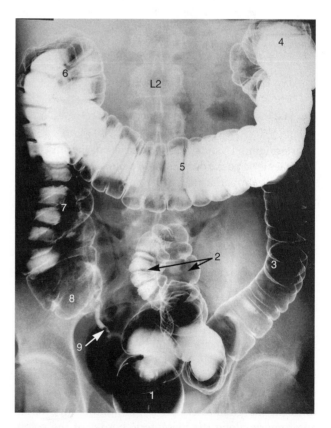

Fig. 11.22   Radiograph of barium enema and colon. Barium sulphate preparation (radio-opaque) was introduced through the anal canal and forced backwards along the alimentary canal. Subsequently, air was introduced to dilate the intestines. 1, rectal ampulla; 2, sigmoid colon; 3, descending colon; 4, splenic (left) flexure of colon; 5, transverse colon ('suspended' on transverse mesocolon); 6, hepatic (right) flexure of colon; 7, ascending colon; 8, caecum; 9, appendix. Note the haustrations (sacculations) of the colon.

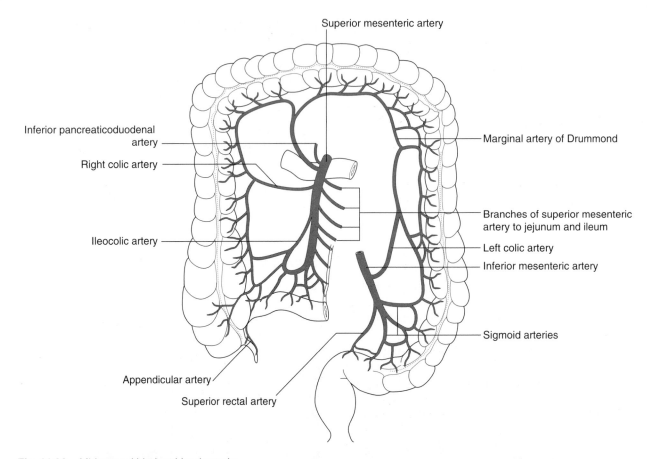

Fig. 11.23 Midgut and hindgut blood supply.

arteriogram it appears as if branches of the superior mesenteric pass down into the pelvis.

- Ileocolic, appendicular: as names suggest.
- Middle colic: transverse colon.

Inferior mesenteric artery: main branches

- Left colic: descending colon.
- Sigmoid colic: sigmoid colon.
- Superior rectal or superior haemorrhoidal: rectum and upper part of anal canal.

Marginal artery

Branches to the colon from both mesenteric arteries form the marginal artery (of Drummond) – an arterial anastomosis along the mesenteric border of the colon that allows the descending colon and sigmoid colon to receive sufficient arterial blood from the superior mesenteric artery even if the inferior mesenteric artery is ligated. The converse does not hold: the inferior mesenteric artery does not supply enough blood to the marginal artery to allow the ligation of the superior mesenteric artery.

Lymph drainage of midgut and hindgut

Midgut: duodenum, small intestine, ascending and transverse colons

This is to nodes in the mesentery, and preaortic nodes around the origin of the superior mesenteric artery from the aorta. It then passes to the cisterna chyli and thoracic duct.

Hindgut: descending and sigmoid colons, rectum, upper part of anal canal

This is to nodes in the posterior abdominal wall and the sigmoid mesentery, and preaortic nodes around the origin of the inferior mesenteric artery from the aorta. It then passes to the cisterna chyli and thoracic duct.

11.7 Portal venous system: venous drainage of the gut tube and associated organs (Fig. 11.24)

Overview

All venous blood from the intestinal bed drains to the liver through the portal vein. Liver disease that impairs this may induce anastomoses between the portal and systemic venous systems.

Learning Objectives

You should:

- know the basic arrangement of the portal venous system

- know the anatomy of the portal vein in the free edge of the lesser omentum

- understand how portosystemic anastomoses arise, and where they are most often found.

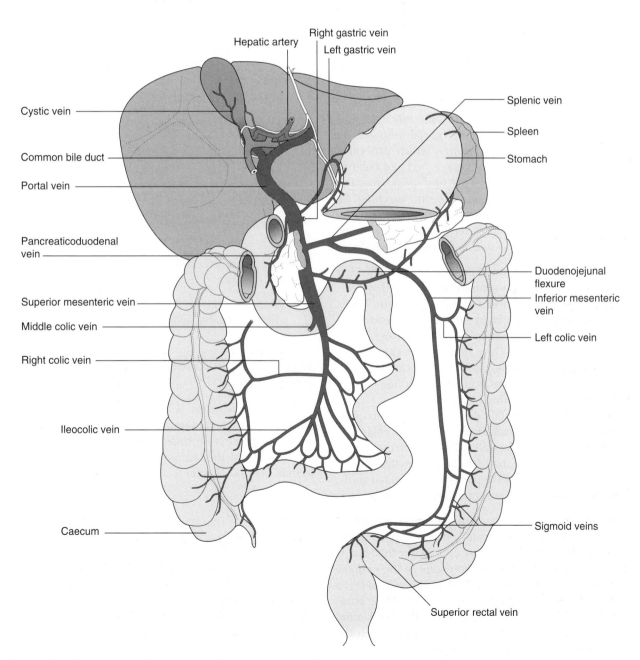

Fig. 11.24 Portal vein and its tributaries. The liver has been lifted so that the visceral surface is shown.

Portal system, portal hypertension, portosystemic anastomoses

Venous blood from the abdominal gut tube, spleen and pancreas passes in the inferior and superior mesenteric veins and the splenic vein, which unite to form the hepatic portal vein (usually known simply as the portal vein) behind the neck of the pancreas. The portal vein then passes in the free edge of the lesser omentum to the liver, dividing into right and left branches before branching to reach all parts of the liver. By this means, all nutrients absorbed through the intestinal mucosa pass first to the liver.

Blood which enters the liver, whether by portal vein or hepatic artery, passes through the hepatic sinusoids to the central veins. These unite to form (usually) three hepatic veins opening directly into the inferior vena cava as it passes through the liver on its way to the right atrium of the heart. In liver disease in which blood flow through the sinusoids is either impaired or blocked (e.g. certain forms of cirrhosis) this leads to a build-up of back pressure in the portal vein and its tributaries – portal hypertension – which can cause engorgement of the intestinal venous bed and enlargement of the liver and/or spleen (hepato/spleno/megaly). In extreme cases this may lead to blood 'searching' for alternative channels to pass from portal vein to inferior vena cava. These anastomoses between portal veins and systemic veins (portosystemic anastomoses) include:

- Vessels at the lower end of the oesophagus when left gastric veins normally draining to the portal system connect with tributaries of the azygos system. These anastomoses are important since they can lead to enlarged veins in the oesophageal submucosa: oesophageal varices. These may rupture causing haematemesis (vomiting blood) which can be fatal.
- Connections between veins in and around the falciform ligament, including a recanalised ligamentum teres (umbilical vein), and the veins of the anterior abdominal wall. These can result in enlarged veins of the abdominal wall radiating from the umbilicus: caput Medusae (read Greek mythology).
- Other anastomoses of the posterior abdominal wall and bare area of the liver: clinically insignificant.

Occasionally, surgeons may manufacture an artificial portosystemic anastomosis to relieve severe portal hypertension. There are several options for this: one is to make a communication in the region of the epiploic foramen (of Winslow) between the portal vein and the inferior vena cava: this is a portocaval shunt or anastomosis. Of course, this means that all the material absorbed from the intestines fails to pass through the liver and much of it is toxic. It is a palliative procedure, not a curative one.

11.8 Nerve supply of the gut tube, gut pain

Overview

The intestines are innervated by the autonomic nervous system, which modulates the intrinsic neural activity of myenteric plexuses. Pain from the gut tube passes centrally in autonomic neurons and enters the spinal cord in dorsal roots of thoracic spinal nerves, so pain is referred to anterior abdominal wall skin: from foregut structures to the epigastrium, from midgut structures to the umbilical region, and from hindgut structures to the hypogastrium. In addition, upper abdominal disease can irritate the diaphragm giving rise to referred pain in the shoulder as a result of the cervical origin of the phrenic nerve.

Learning Objectives

You should:

- know the basic arrangement of gut tube innervation
- know the sites of referred pain from stomach, ileum, caecum and colon
- understand why gall bladder disease can cause shoulder pain
- understand why the pain of appendicitis often shifts from central umbilical to right iliac fossa.

Myenteric plexuses, autonomic influences

A plexus of neurons is situated in and around the smooth muscle layers of the gut wall. These myenteric plexuses possess intrinsic neural activity which is modulated by the action of the autonomic nervous system. Revise Chapter 6.

Sympathetic

Lateral horn cells (preganglionic) of the thoracolumbar spinal cord give rise to axons which pass through the ventral root of thoracolumbar spinal nerves, to white rami communicantes, the sympathetic chain (no synapse) and the splanchnic nerves to arrive at the pre-aortic group of plexuses: coeliac, superior mesenteric, etc. Here they synapse and postganglionic fibres pass with the arteries to their destination. For nerves to hindgut, see later.

Parasympathetic

Foregut and midgut: the vagus nerves in the abdomen. The vagus nerves enter the abdomen with the oesophagus. They form anterior and posterior trunks which pass close to the lesser curvature in the lesser omentum. Vagal branches pass to the liver and to the pyloric sphincter. Section of these (vagotomy) may be performed to reduce the secretion of gastric acid, but this operation interferes with the sphincter mechanism and disrupts gastric emptying, so a gastrojejunostomy (making a communication between stomach and jejunum) may be required. Pyloric and antral branches of the vagus are known as nerves of Latarjet, the French physician who described them. It is questionable how much vagal activity passes beyond the pyloric sphincter, and it is now accepted that the myenteric plexuses in the gut tube walls form a kind of gut brain; this has its own intrinsic activity which is capable of being modified by sympathetic and (perhaps) parasympathetic activity from elsewhere.

Hindgut: pelvic splanchnic nerves. Cell bodies (preganglionic) in grey matter of S2, 3, 4 segments give rise to axons which pass through the ventral roots of S2, 3, 4 and form the pelvic splanchnic nerves. These pass to the hypogastric plexus where they (probably) synapse, postganglionic fibres passing with branches of the inferior mesenteric artery to their destinations.

Clinical box

Hirschsprung's disease
This is a rare inherited condition in which neurons of the hindgut (descending and sigmoid colon) myenteric plexuses, normally formed by neural crest cells, are absent. There is thus no intrinsic muscular activity present here and the colon remains narrow and incapable of peristalsis. It presents as intestinal blockage fairly soon after birth and the affected part of the colon must be removed.

Gut pain
- Foregut. Pain from foregut structures is referred to the epigastrium. However, when the disease or inflammation also spreads to involve body wall structures (e.g. parietal peritoneum), pain may also be perceived over the region concerned. Furthermore, gall bladder pain may also be referred to the right shoulder, presumably because of local irritation of the diaphragm as it attaches to the rib cage anteriorly, and since the sensory innervation of the diaphragm is from the phrenic nerve, C3, 4, 5 pain is referred to those dermatomes.
- Midgut and hindgut. Pain from midgut structures is referred to the umbilical region, and from hindgut structures is referred to the hypogastric (suprapubic) region. Again, when the disease or inflammation also spreads to involve body wall structures (e.g. parietal

---

Clinical box (*cont'd*)

peritoneum), pain may also be perceived over the region concerned.

Appendicitis and pain
The classic picture is one of central abdominal (periumbilical) pain that after some time appears to shift to the right iliac fossa. The explanation usually given is that initially the inflammation involves only the appendix, which becomes distended, and the resulting midgut visceral sensation is referred to the umbilical region. As the disease progresses, the inflamed appendix enlarges and inflammation spreads to the parietal peritoneum of the anterior abdominal wall. This is then perceived as body wall (somatic) pain – well localised and sharp. Why does the appendix become inflamed? Is appendicitis always appendicitis? Ask a pathologist how often a removed appendix is, in fact, normal.

11.9 Posterior abdominal wall, diaphragm and associated structures

Overview

The erector spinae muscle group behind the rib cage helps to maintain our upright posture. Muscular components of the posterior abdominal wall inside the abdomen are psoas major muscle (hip flexor) and the attachments of the diaphragm. Related to these are the aorta, inferior vena cava, and the lumbar plexus and the nerves arising from it.

Learning Objectives

You should:

- know the sites and vertebral levels of penetration of the diaphragm by the inferior vena cava, oesophagus and aorta
- know the innervation of the diaphragm
- understand how the lumbar plexus is formed
- know the root values of the branches of the lumbar plexus, particularly the femoral and obturator nerves.

Lumbar vertebrae

Revise Chapter 5. Lumbar vertebrae:

- are bigger than thoracic vertebrae, increasing in size from L1 to L5

- lack facets for rib articulations
- possess several other processes for the attachment of muscles particularly associated with the maintenance of the upright posture (the details of these need not concern you).

Posterior abdominal wall

The posterior abdominal wall is formed by muscles and fascia on either side of the vertebral column. The lumbar fascia surrounds these muscles and extends laterally, providing attachment for the sheet muscles of the anterior abdominal wall.

- Postvertebral muscles: erector spinae (more properly sacrospinalis) muscle: the muscle mass behind the rib cage, responsible for our upright posture. You do not need to know details of their construction. They are supplied by dorsal rami of regional nerves and are covered posteriorly by latissimus dorsi muscle attaching the upper limb to the trunk (see Ch. 12).
- Psoas (major and minor). This is attached to the lumbar vertebrae and intervertebral discs and passes down and laterally, deep to the inguinal ligament, to attach to the lesser trochanter of the femur. It is the main hip flexor and is supplied by direct twigs from ventral rami of lumbar nerves 2, 3 and 4. Running on its anterior surface is the genitofemoral nerve (L1, 2). For meat eaters, psoas is better known as a fillet steak.
- Quadratus lumborum muscle: twelfth rib to posterior part of ilium (quadratus lumborum is a lateral flexor of the spinal column).

Diaphragm

The diaphragm is attached posteriorly to both sides of vertebrae T12, L1 and to the right side of L2. In the midline, fibres from both sides arch (median arcuate ligament) over the aorta as it passes down from the thorax. Passing laterally, fibres arch over psoas (medial arcuate ligament) to the transverse process of vertebra L1, and from there they arch over quadratus lumborum (lateral arcuate ligament) to the tip of the twelfth rib. Laterally and anteriorly, diaphragmatic muscle fibres are attached to the internal aspects of ribs, costal cartilages and the sternum.

The peripheral portions are muscular, and the central portion is tendinous.

Orifices

- Vertebral level T8: the inferior vena cava passes through the central tendon. This means that the IVC remains open when the diaphragm contracts and intra-abdominal pressure rises.
- Vertebral level T10: the oesophagus and vagus nerves pass through the muscular portion, and this means that when the diaphragm contracts and intra-abdominal pressure rises, the cardio-oesophageal sphincter closes.
- Vertebral level T12: aorta, cisterna chyli and tributaries of the azygos vein pass behind the diaphragm.

Nerve supply

- Motor: phrenic nerve C3, 4, 5.
- Sensory: phrenic nerve centrally and branches of local intercostal nerves peripherally.

The diaphragm may be irritated by disease of abdominal organs, leading to referred pain in the shoulder tip (because of C3, 4, 5 innervation). Typically, gall bladder disease may give referred pain in the right shoulder region.

Clinical box

Abdominal CT and MRI scans (Fig. 11.25)
A scan is a widely used way of 'looking into' the abdomen to assess the anatomy and seek any abnormality. Figure 11.25 shows an example of a scan, in effect a horizontal section at vertebral level L1 (although of course scans can be taken at any level and in any plane). Now that you have covered a good deal of abdominal anatomy you will be able to understand what you see in this scan.

Nerves of the posterior abdominal wall: lumbar plexus (Fig. 11.26)

These arise form the ventral rami of T12–L5, which form the lumbar plexus.

The nerves are, in order of importance:

- Femoral (L2, 3, 4): knee extension, hip and knee joints, anterior thigh sensation.
- Obturator (L2, 3, 4): hip adduction, hip and knee joints, medial thigh sensation.
- Lateral cutaneous nerve of the thigh (L2, 3). Sensory, lateral thigh. This passes close to the anterior superior iliac spine where it may be damaged by trauma or belts that are too tight.
- Ilioinguinal and iliohypogastric (L1): lower anterior abdominal wall.
- Genitofemoral (L1, 2): anterior scrotum, labia, cremaster.

Relationship of these nerves to the psoas muscle

- Lateral to psoas, from below upwards:
  - femoral nerve, which is formed within psoas muscle

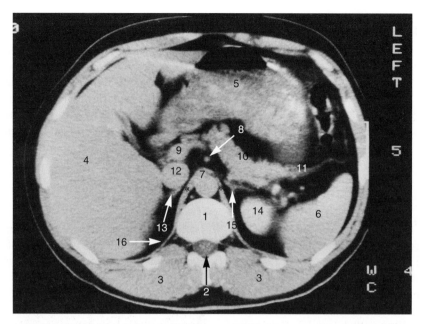

Fig. 11.25 Scan through abdomen at vertebral level L1. Note that scans of the trunk are viewed as if from below, with the patient's head in the distance and the feet near the observer (as if the observer is standing at the foot of the bed). The right-hand side of the patient is thus on the left of the image. 1, vertebral body; 2, vertebral canal; 3, postvertebral muscles; 4, liver; 5, stomach, full; 6, spleen; 7, aorta with crura of the diaphragm (marked *) on either side; 8, branch of superior mesenteric artery descending and sectioned at right angles to the plane of the scan; 9, head of pancreas; 10, body of pancreas; 11, tail of pancreas; 12, inferior vena cava; 13, right adrenal gland; 14, left kidney, upper pole; 15, left adrenal gland; 16, diaphragm.

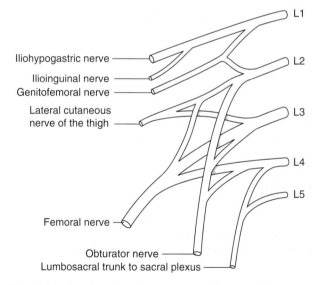

Iliohypogastric nerve
Ilioinguinal nerve
Genitofemoral nerve
Lateral cutaneous nerve of the thigh
Femoral nerve
Obturator nerve
Lumbosacral trunk to sacral plexus

L1 L2 L3 L4 L5

Fig. 11.26 Lumbar plexus.

- lateral cutaneous nerve of the thigh: this aims for the anterior superior iliac spine
- ilioinguinal, iliohypogastric, subcostal: often with connections between them.
- Anterior to psoas: genitofemoral nerve.

- Medial to psoas, between psoas and the lumbosacral junction:
  - obturator
  - lumbosacral trunk, which passes into the pelvis to contribute to the sacral plexus.

11.10 Kidneys, ureters, adrenals

Overview

The kidneys are retroperitoneal organs posterior to, on the right, the colon and duodenum, and on the left, the colon, spleen and stomach. Behind them are the costodiaphragmatic recesses of the pleural cavities and the lowest one or two ribs. Anomalies of the renal vessels are common. The ureters descend from the renal pelvis to the bladder, passing over the pelvic brim at the sacroiliac joint. There are three sites of ureteric narrowing at which renal stones may stick: the pelviureteric junction, crossing the pelvic brim, and traversing the bladder wall. The adrenal glands are related to the superior poles of the kidneys.

Learning Objectives

You should:

- know the position and relations of the kidneys
- know what types of injury may damage the kidneys
- know the course of the ureter and the sites of its narrowing.

Kidneys (Fig. 11.27)

Position and relations

The kidneys are retroperitoneal. They are higher than you think. Although the right kidney (under the liver) is slightly lower than the left, the hilum of each is at about vertebral level L1 (transpyloric plane). The upper pole is approximately level with T12 vertebra and the lower pole approximately with L2 or L3. Remember, though, that the kidneys move up and down with breathing, and at body temperature the perinephric fat which surrounds them is more liquid than solid so these levels are only guides. Each kidney is surrounded by a tough capsule, which is firmly attached to the fascia over the renal vessels, best seen in a butcher's shop. Adult human kidneys are not usually lobulated, unlike those of other species (also readily seen at the butcher's) and also unlike fetal human kidneys, although fetal lobulation persists into childhood and, occasionally, adulthood.

- The important posterior relations of the kidney are the diaphragm and the costodiaphragmatic recess of the pleural cavity. An inexpertly performed renal biopsy, or injection into the kidney, may first enter the pleural cavity and cause a pneumothorax.
- Important anterior relations of the kidney are different on the two sides: they include ascending colon, splenic flexure and duodenum on the right, and spleen, stomach, splenic flexure and descending colon on the left.

Vessels and anomalies

Both renal arteries arise from the aorta at vertebral level L1. The left renal artery is short but that on the right is longer, passing posterior to the inferior vena cava.

The right renal vein is very short but the left receives both adrenal and gonadal veins before crossing anterior to the aorta immediately below the origin of the superior mesenteric artery.

The kidneys develop low down and ascend during fetal life. This may be arrested and thus a kidney may be lower than its normal position. As the kidneys ascend they acquire new blood vessels and accessory renal vessels are common, especially at the lower poles of the kidneys.

Renal arteries are end-arteries: that is to say their territories do not communicate significantly, so accessory renal arteries should not be tied. Accessory renal veins, however, may be tied since there are significant connections between the territories of individual veins.

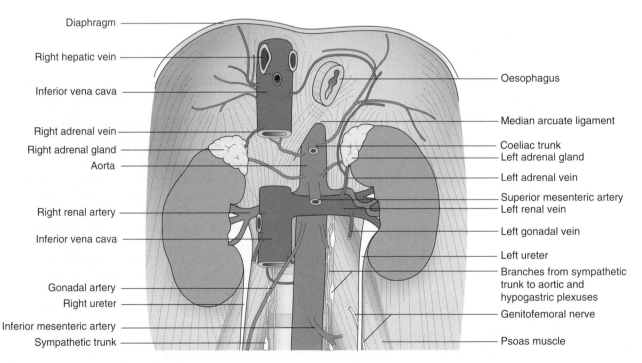

Fig. 11.27 Kidneys and associated organs.

Renal pelvis, ureter   (Fig. 11.28)

The collecting ducts of the renal tubular system open into:

- minor calyces, which then form
- major calyces, which open into
- the renal pelvis, not to be confused with bony pelvis or pelvic part of the abdominal cavity. This is the most posterior of the structures at the renal hilum: it rapidly narrows to become
- the ureter: this descends approximately in line with the tips of the transverse processes of lumbar vertebrae (an important landmark radiologically), crossing the pelvic brim anterior to the sacroiliac joint and the bifurcation of the common iliac arteries. It then turns forwards and medially to enter the bladder at the level of the ischial spine – also important radiologically.

Clinical box

Renal injuries
The kidneys are at risk from penetrating injuries to the lower rib cage and from trauma (e.g. sports injuries, kicks, etc.) in the renal angle – the inferior angle between the twelfth rib and the vertebral column.

Ureteric constrictions, stones
There are three sites of narrowing where kidney stones are particularly likely to be stuck. They are:

- pelviureteric junction
- as the ureter crosses the pelvic brim
- as the ureter passes through the bladder wall.

Adrenal glands

These retroperitoneal structures are related to the upper poles of both kidneys. The asymmetry of the great vessels in the upper abdomen means that it is relatively easy to gain access to the left adrenal, but the right adrenal is partly posterior to both the inferior vena cava and the bare area of the liver, making access very difficult. The gland produces steroids from the cortex and catecholamines from the medulla, the two parts having distinct embryological origins: cortex from (steroid-producing) intermediate mesoderm and the medulla from (amine-producing) neural crest. The medulla may be involved in multiple endocrine neoplasia with medullary tumours (phaeochromocytomas) leading to abnormalities in the production of pressor amines. Because of the fact that veins of the adrenal gland communicate with lumbar veins leading to the azygos system, high levels of pressor amines in these conditions may be found in the superior as well as the inferior vena cava.

Lymph from the kidneys and adrenals

This drains to para-aortic nodes. It is not particularly clinically important.

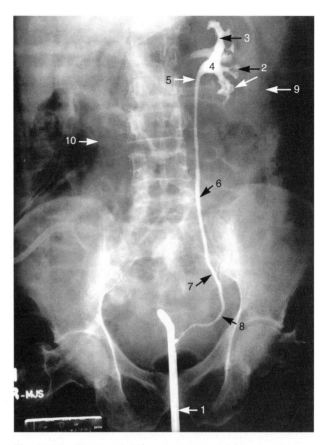

Fig. 11.28   Retrograde left ureterogram: 1, instrument in urethra and bladder, through which radio-opaque die is injected up the left ureter; 2, minor calyces; 3, major calyx; 4, renal pelvis; 5, pelviureteric junction; 6, ureter related to tips of transverse processes of lumbar vertebrae; 7, ureter related to sacroiliac joint; 8, ureter related to ischial spine; 9, border of left kidney; 10, lateral margin of psoas major muscle.

11.11 Pelvis

Overview

The pelvic girdle is made up of the hip bone, the sacrum and various ligaments. Immediately inside the pelvic walls are the nerves of the sacral plexus contributing to the innervation of the lower limb. Pelvic organs include the sigmoid colon, rectum, internal genital organs, bladder and prostate. The pelvis is bounded inferiorly by the pelvic diaphragm (levator ani muscle), which separates the pelvis above from the perineum below. Pelvic structures are supplied by the internal iliac artery and its branches, and innervated by branches of lumbar nerves and by pelvic extensions of the abdominal sympathetic plexuses. The pelvic diaphragm is important in the maintenance of faecal continence, and is also responsible for helping to maintain the integrity of the pelvic floor, particularly supporting the uterus.

Learning Objectives

You should:

- know the bones of the pelvic walls and the anatomy of the pelvic diaphragm

- understand the arrangement of the sacral plexus and its main nerves: sciatic and pudendal

- know the anatomy of the rectum

- know the disposition of the female internal genitalia and the factors responsible for their support

- understand the relationship between the vagina and the rectouterine pouch of Douglas

- know the disposition of the ureters, bladder, prostate and male genital ducts in the pelvis.

- know how pelvic disease may involve the vertebral column and spinal nerves.

General disposition

The pelvis and perineum contain organs of the reproductive system, and the caudal terminations of the alimentary and urinary systems. There are, nevertheless, separate anatomical components, as below:

- the caudal or pelvic part of the peritoneal cavity
- a muscular diaphragm (pelvic diaphragm or levator ani muscle) which:
  - limits the abdominopelvic cavity inferiorly
  - provides support for internal organs (e.g. uterus, bladder, rectal ampulla)

  - is penetrated by the distal portions of the alimentary, urinary and reproductive systems; and
  - contributes to the sphincter mechanisms for gut tube and urinary system
- the perineum: the area caudal or inferior to the pelvic diaphragm.

The perineum is concerned largely with the external genitalia, and the effluent and sphincters of the gut tube and urinary system. Perineal structures are cloacal derivatives (Latin: *cloaca* = sewer), and are supplied by the (internal) pudendal artery and the pudendal nerve (S2, 3, 4).

Beware!

The term pelvis can mean:

- the bony pelvis or pelvic girdle: the two hip bones, with or without the sacrum
- the pelvic part of the abdominal or peritoneal cavity
- the renal pelvis.

Bony pelvis, pelvic girdle   (Fig. 11.29)

This is made up of the hip bones, sacrum, and ligaments and muscles associated with them.

- Hip (innominate) bone. Made up of three bones, ilium, ischium and pubis, which fuse together during adolescence.
- Sacrum. Five fused vertebrae, coccyx attached caudally.

The articulated pelvic girdle looks like a narrow bowl with, on top, two large flattened 'handles' or wings.

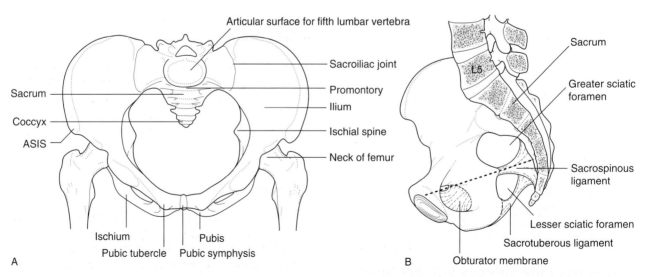

Fig. 11.29   Bony pelvis: **(A)** from above; **(B)** right hemipelvis from the left. The broken line indicates the position of the outer margin of the pelvic diaphragm.

The area above the wings is the greater or false pelvis (terms of little use) and the bowl is the true pelvis. The ridge forming the border between the two is the pelvic brim and marks the pelvic inlet. The inferior extent of the true pelvis is marked by the pelvic outlet, made up of the two inferior pubic rami, the ischial tuberosities, the sacrotuberous ligaments and the sacrum and coccyx. Between the inlet and outlet is the birth canal, so-called for obvious reasons.

Sexing the pelvis

Compared with the female, the male pelvis has:

- a more acute subpubic angle (in the female it is similar to that between thumb and index finger in a hand in neutral position; in the male it is similar to the angle between index and middle fingers)
- more inturned ischial spines
- a sacrum that projects more anteriorly.

It can be difficult to pronounce on the sex of an isolated pelvis, and it is a skill that is unnecessary unless you are concerned with archaeology or forensic science. You may be asked to give an opinion based on a radiograph; my tip is to look for the soft tissue shadow of the penis since this is usually a fairly reliable guide to the sex of the individual.

Pelvic diameters

These terms used in obstetrics are shown in Figure 11.30.

Surface anatomy

- The iliac crests are palpable throughout their length. You should be able without hesitation to put your

fingers on the anterior superior iliac spine and identify it on radiographs and the skeleton. The posterior superior iliac spine marks the posterior end of the crest: it is always marked by a skin dimple, no matter how fat the person.
- The pubic symphysis is palpable in the midline, and the pubic tubercle is about 1.5 cm lateral to it. The pubic symphysis and the pubic tubercles are used in the examination of the inguinal region.

Posteriorly, the ischial tuberosity is palpable (this is what you sit on) and the ischial spines are palpable on rectal or vaginal examination.

Vertebral levels

- Anterior superior iliac spines: about vertebral level L5.
- A line joining the highest points of the two iliac crests will intersect the vertebral column between vertebrae L3 and 4. This is a useful guide for the performance of lumbar puncture.

Ligaments and membrane

- Inguinal ligament: anterior superior iliac spine to pubic tubercle.
- Sacrotuberous ligament: sacrum to ischial tuberosity.
- Sacrospinous ligament: sacrum to ischial spine.

The last two ligaments convert two notches on the hip bones, the greater and lesser sciatic notches, into the greater and lesser sciatic foramina (Fig. 11.30).

The obturator foramen, facing anteroinferiorly, separates the superior pubic ramus above from the inferior pubic ramus and ischial ramus below. It is closed by the obturator membrane.

Walls of the pelvis

Pelvic walls consist of the bones and ligaments as above, the obturator internus muscle on the internal aspect of the obturator membrane, and piriformis muscle arising from the anterior aspect of the sacrum and passing to the gluteal region through the greater sciatic foramen.

Sacral plexus (Fig. 11.31)

The nerves forming the sacral plexus are immediately adjacent to (internally) the pelvic walls.

All roots (L4–S3) unite to form the sciatic nerve which is in fact two nerves, the tibial and the common peroneal (note: a word referring to the fibula in the leg – not perineal) or common fibular nerve.

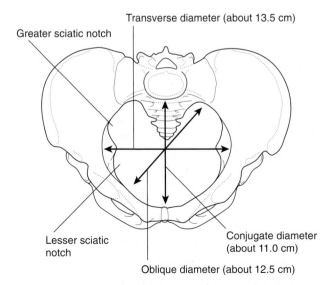

Transverse diameter (about 13.5 cm)

Greater sciatic notch

Lesser sciatic notch

Conjugate diameter (about 11.0 cm)

Oblique diameter (about 12.5 cm)

Fig. 11.30 Pelvic diameters.

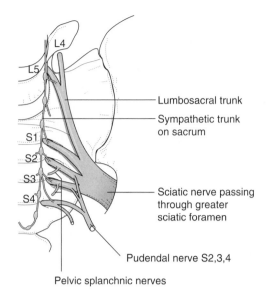

Fig. 11.31 Sacral plexus.

Other branches of the sacral plexus are:

- superior gluteal L4, 5, S1: hip abduction, weightbearing
- inferior gluteal L5, S1, 2: powerful extension
- pudendal S2, 3, 4: the perineum.

Contents of the pelvis

The pelvis contains the sigmoid colon and rectum, the termination of the ureters and the bladder and prostate, the ovaries, Fallopian tubes, uterus and upper part of the vagina, and the main nerves and arteries supplying these organs and the lower limb.

Pelvic diaphragm, perineal body

(Fig. 11.32)

This is a sheet of voluntary muscle, also called levator

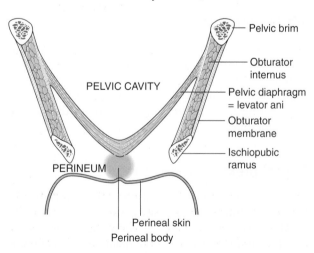

Fig. 11.32 Scheme of pelvis and perineum: coronal section of true pelvis.

ani or the pelvic floor, separating the pelvic part of the peritoneal cavity above from the perineum below. It is a funnel pointing inferiorly, the outer edges of which rest against the pelvic walls in a circle extending from behind the pubic symphysis, over the obturator membrane, ischial spine, sacrospinous ligament and the anterior aspect of the sacrum at about S4 (Figs 11.29B, 11.34). It has several constituent parts, the names of which you do not need to know except for puborectalis which is described with the anal sphincters (p. 144). It is supplied by small branches from sacral nerves.

Besides its function as part of the urinary and anal sphincters, it is important in providing support for pelvic organs, particularly the uterus and bladder.

The apex of the funnel (the most inferior point) is a fibromuscular node known as the perineal body. It is just deep to the skin between the anus and the vaginal opening (female), posterior scrotal skin (male), If this is damaged, the efficiency of the pelvic diaphragm is in doubt and there may be problems with incontinence and prolapse of pelvic organs (uterus, rectum, bladder). Such damage could be caused by falling astride a sharp object, cycling injuries, repeated trauma (e.g. childbirth), inexpertly performed episiotomy (see p. 142).

Blood vessels of the pelvis

Pelvic blood vessels lie inside the plane of the nerves.

Common iliac artery

From the bifurcation of the aorta, the common iliac arteries pass down and laterally. As they cross the pelvic rim, near the sacroiliac joint, they divide into:

- external iliac: this heads for the midpoint of the inguinal ligament and the lower limb
- internal iliac: this supplies all the contents of the pelvis and perineum and sends small branches to the lower limb.

Internal iliac artery and its main branches (Fig. 11.33)

- Branches which supply the body wall (not important): iliolumbar and lateral sacral.
- Visceral branches. It is not necessary to memorise these, simply know that they exist. Think of a pelvic organ and name an artery after it: uterine, superior and inferior vesical, etc. The only pelvic organ not supplied by the internal iliac artery is the gonad (artery from the aorta directly).
- Branches which leave the pelvis:
  – obturator: to medial thigh
  – superior and inferior gluteal: to gluteal region
  – pudendal: to the perineum.

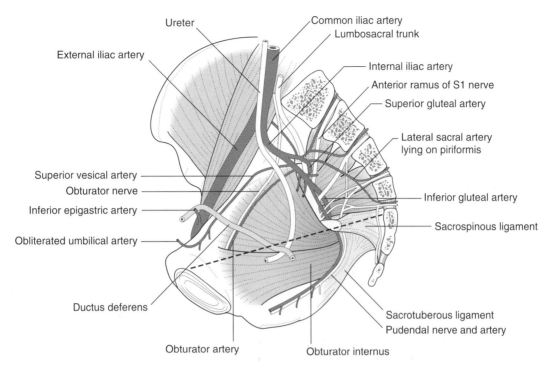

Fig. 11.33 Right male hemipelvis: median sagittal section. The broken line indicates the position of the outer margin of the pelvic diaphragm.

Labels (clockwise from top): Ureter · Common iliac artery · Lumbosacral trunk · Internal iliac artery · Anterior ramus of S1 nerve · Superior gluteal artery · Lateral sacral artery lying on piriformis · Inferior gluteal artery · Sacrospinous ligament · Sacrotuberous ligament · Pudendal nerve and artery · Obturator internus · Obturator artery · Ductus deferens · Obliterated umbilical artery · Inferior epigastric artery · Obturator nerve · Superior vesical artery · External iliac artery

Course of the pudendal neurovascular bundle (Fig. 11.33)

All perineal structures receive arterial blood via the pudendal artery, and are innervated by the pudendal nerve (S2, 3, 4). The pudendal neurovascular bundle leaves the pelvis through the greater sciatic foramen, passes over the external aspect of the ischial spine, and turns medially again through the lesser sciatic foramen. Remember that the outer margin of the funnel-shaped pelvic diaphragm is attached to the internal aspect of the ischial spine and so the pudendal neurovascular bundle has, by this manoeuvre, passed from above the diaphragm to below it without having to penetrate it.

Veins

These mirror the arteries. Tributaries conveying blood from the pelvis and perineum eventually unite to form the internal iliac vein. This unites with the external iliac vein (blood from the lower limb) to form the common iliac vein, and the two common iliac veins unite to form the inferior vena cava. The gonadal veins drain directly to the inferior vena cava on the right, and to the left renal vein on the left.

> **Clinical box**
>
> **Venous connections, spread of malignancy**
> In addition to the named veins, there are numerous connections (Batson's veins) between pelvic veins and the internal vertebral venous plexus. They allow disease to spread readily from pelvic organs to the vertebral column and may result in, for example, cancer of the prostate causing backache and symptoms of lumbar nerve root entrapment.

Pelvic cavity in the female and male
(Fig. 11.34)

In the male the pelvic part of the peritoneal cavity is limited by the side walls of the pelvis, the rectum behind and the bladder and anterior abdominal wall below and in front. It contains coils of ileum.

In the female, the pelvic cavity is partially divided into a smaller anterior portion and a larger posterior portion by a side-to-side fold of tissue projecting up from the pelvic floor. This is the broad ligament, or broad ligament of the uterus. It is formed embryologically by two ingrowths from the sides, which unite in the midline. It contains in the midline the uterus and in its superior margins the uterine or Fallopian tubes extending laterally. Underneath the Fallopian tubes, lateral to the uterus, the broad ligament contains nothing in particular except some embryological remnants of the male

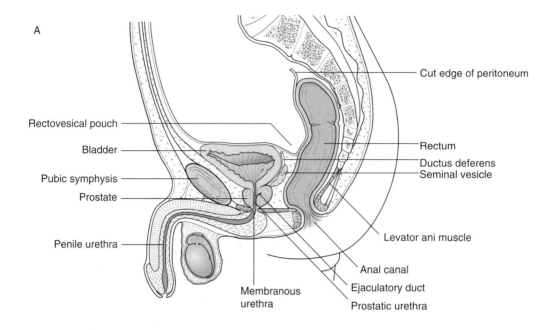

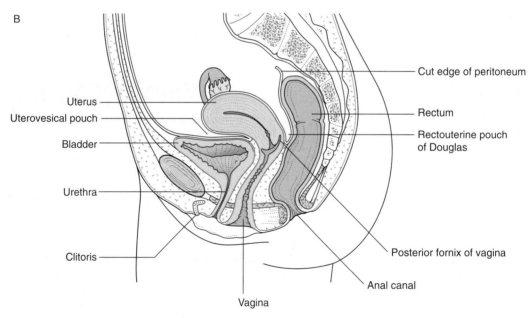

Fig. 11.34   Male and female pelvic organs: median sagittal section through **(A)** male pelvis; **(B)** female pelvis.

genital system that may occasionally become involved in disease (epoöphoron, paroöphoron). Passing from back to front in the base of the broad ligament are the ureters.

Rectouterine pouch of Douglas, uterovesical pouch

The broad ligament is angled forwards so that the

posterior surface is more superior, and the anterior surface more inferior. That part of the cavity behind and above the ligament is the rectouterine pouch of Douglas which contains coils of ileum.

In front of (inferior to) the broad ligament is the uterovesical pouch. It is normally empty, that is to say its peritoneal surfaces are in contact with each other, and insignificant.

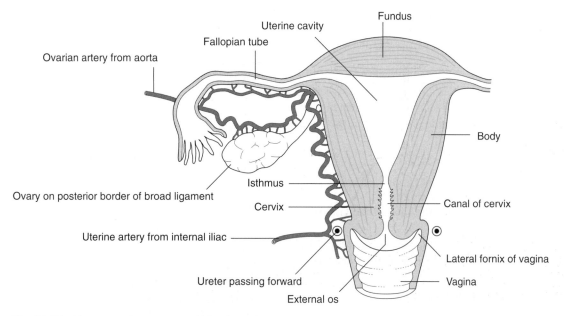

Fig. 11.35 Uterus, vagina, ovary and blood supply.

Uterus and vagina (Fig. 11.35)

These are midline structures. The uterus has three parts:

- cervix, which projects into the vagina
- body, the main bulk
- fundus, that part between and above the entry of the two Fallopian tubes.

The vagina is angled upwards and backwards. The cervix of the uterus projects into its upper anterior wall, the recesses around the projecting cervix being the fornices: one anterior, one posterior (superior), and two lateral. An important relation of the lateral fornix is the ureter which is between the lateral fornix and the uterine artery.

The rectouterine pouch of Douglas directly overlies the superior (posterior) vaginal fornix, and abscesses in the pelvic cavity may be drained through the vagina in the female.

External os and cervical smears

This is the opening between the vagina and the cavity of the cervix. Just inside it is the site of the squamo-columnar junction. The spatula used to take a cervical smear is shaped with a long arm to be inserted in the cervical opening for columnar cells, and a short arm which remains outside it for squamous cells. One hopes not to see squamous cells near the tip of the long arm.

The external os in a woman who has not borne children is more or less circular. After the birth of the first child it becomes, and remains, slit-like.

Internal os

This is the opening between the cervical canal and the main part of the uterine cavity.

Mechanical support

The two main factors in the support of the uterus are:

- Pelvic diaphragm which acts as a sling supporting these organs. It clasps the cervix and vagina.
- Ligaments on the upper surface of the pelvic diaphragm:
  – cardinal, or lateral cervical, or Mackenrodt's
  – pubocervical
  – sacrocervical.

Damage to, or stretching of, these structures or of the perineal body (trauma, repeated childbirth) may result in uterine and/or vaginal prolapse which may be so severe that the uterus is palpable or even visible at the vaginal opening.

Anteversion, anteflexion

Another factor in maintaining the position of the uterus is the fact that it is normally bent forwards on the backward-sloping vagina: this is anteversion. Furthermore, the body of the uterus is angled further forwards on the cervix: this is anteflexion. If there is any degree of retroversion or retroflexion, prolapse of the uterus is more likely.

Blood supply

- Fundus of uterus and Fallopian tubes: branches of the ovarian artery (from the aorta).

- Body and cervix of uterus, and vagina: uterine and vaginal arteries (from internal iliac artery).

Nerve supply

Sensory fibres from the uterus pass back to the central nervous system in autonomic nerves. The pathways are not clearly understood. Uterine pain is felt in the lower back and perineum.

Lymph drainage

- From lower vagina: inguinal nodes.
- From upper vagina, cervix and lower body: internal iliac nodes.
- From upper body and fundus: para-aortic nodes (by lymph channels running with the ovarian arteries).

Fallopian or uterine tubes

The Fallopian tubes are extensions of the upper lateral corners of the uterine cavity along the upper margin of the broad ligament. However, before they reach the side walls of the pelvis, they open into the peritoneal cavity on the posterior (superior) surface of the broad ligament. In the female, therefore, there is a potential route for foreign organisms to enter the peritoneal cavity from the external environment. This is not so in the male, where the peritoneal cavity is entirely sealed.

The Fallopian tube has four parts, from medial to lateral:

- interstitial or intramural: in the thickness of the uterine wall
- body: lateral to that
- ampulla: slightly wider, fertilisation normally takes place here
- fimbriated end: the opening into the peritoneal cavity. This is mobile.

Ovaries

The ovaries are attached to the posterosuperior surface of the broad ligament by the mesovarium through which branches of the ovarian vessels pass to and from the ovary. Although on the back of the broad ligament, the ovaries are sufficiently close to the side walls of the pelvis for an inflamed ovary to irritate the tissue supplied by the obturator nerve on its way to the obturator foramen. Pain from ovarian disease, or even a heavy menstrual period, may be referred to the territory of the obturator nerve: hip and medial thigh.

Ovarian vessels

The ovary develops high up in the primitive coelomic cavity. During development it is pulled down by the gubernaculum until it is arrested by coming into contact with the broad ligament. The ovary retains its blood supply from the aorta, the ovarian arteries arising just below the renals at about vertebral level L2.

Ovarian veins show a similar pattern, the right passing directly to the inferior vena cava, and the left to the left renal vein (as with the testis).

Lymphatics. Ovarian lymphatics, together with those from the fundus of the uterus and the Fallopian tubes, pass directly to para-aortic nodes.

Round ligaments: gubernaculum in the female

- The round ligament of the ovary is a cord-like thickening on the posterior (superior) aspect of the broad ligament between the ovary and the junction of the Fallopian tube and the uterus.
- The round ligament of the uterus is a similar thickening on the anterior (inferior) aspect of the broad ligament from the same part of the uterus to the deep inguinal ring; it passes through the inguinal canal to the subcutaneous tissue of the labia majora outside the superficial inguinal ring.
- They are two different parts of the same thing, the embryological gubernaculum, and are otherwise entirely insignificant.

Ureters, bladder (Fig. 11.36)

The urinary bladder lies between the peritoneum of the anteroinferior pelvic cavity and the pelvic diaphragm, upon which it rests.

The ureters enter the posterior surface of the bladder near the midline. The area of bladder wall bounded by the two ureteric orifices and the single midline urethral orifice is the trigone. It is the part of the bladder that expands least as the bladder fills.

The bladder neck is the term given to the bladder as it narrows down to open into the urethra. In the male, this is surrounded by the prostate gland.

The muscle of the bladder wall is the detrusor muscle. It is involuntary (smooth) muscle.

Nerve supply

Motor supply of the bladder muscle is from the pelvic splanchnic nerves, S2, 3, 4. Sensory fibres pass in the same nerves to enter the same segments of the spinal cord, with their cell bodies in the dorsal root ganglia of S2, 3, 4. The function of sympathetic fibres to the bladder has not been fully elucidated.

Bladder pain is referred to the lower abdomen, perineum and back.

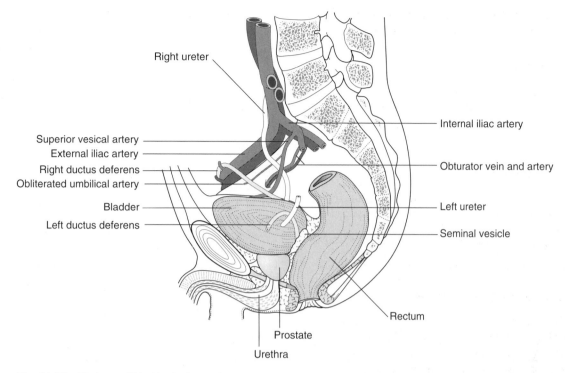

Fig. 11.36 Ureter and bladder in the male.

Blood vessels, medial umbilical ligaments

Superior and inferior vesical arteries (from internal iliac). The superior vesical arteries in fetal life were the umbilical arteries and continued forwards and upwards onto the posterior aspect of the anterior abdominal wall to the umbilicus. These conveyed deoxygenated blood from fetus to placenta. After birth, the portion between the bladder and the umbilicus degenerates to become the medial umbilical liga-ments (the obliterated umbilical arteries). Note: lateral umbilical ligament is the name some people give to the elevation on the back of the anterior abdominal wall raised by the inferior epigastric artery. This does not, of course, pass to the umbilicus, and so the name is inappropriate.

Venous blood and lymph vessels

These drain to the internal iliac veins and nodes.

Median umbilical ligament, patent urachus

Extending in the midline from the bladder to the umbilicus is the obliterated remnant of the urachus, itself the successor of the allantois. Should this fail to close before birth, a patent urachus will result in urine leaking from the umbilicus of the newborn.

Prostate gland, seminal vesicle, ductus deferens   (Fig. 11.36)

These are reproductive organs, secreting fluid into the urethra to provide sustenance for the great journey that the spermatozoa must undertake.

In the male, the prostate gland surrounds the neck of the bladder and rests upon the pelvic diaphragm. The seminal vesicle is a tightly coiled gland above and behind the prostate on the posterior wall of the bladder. As the urethra passes through the prostate, it receives the ejaculatory ducts on each side, each ejaculatory duct formed by the union of the ductus (vas) deferens and the seminal vesicle.

Lobes of the prostate

These are not anatomically or functionally separate lobes, merely different areas.

- Anterior lobe: anterior to the urethra.
- Lateral lobes: lateral to the urethra. Posteriorly, there is a slight midline sulcus that separates the two lateral lobes.
- Posterior lobe: the posterior parts of both lateral lobes.
- Median lobe: the area of the gland in the midline posterior to the urethra, bounded by it and the two ejaculatory ducts.

Prostatic enlargement, palpation of the prostate, rectal examination

Enlargement of the prostate gland may be benign or due to cancer and is common in old men. It may compress the urethra, leading to difficulty in passing urine (urinary retention). This is particularly so if the median lobe is involved.

Insertion of the examiner's finger, suitably protected, into the rectum is a routine part of a full clinical examination. Apart from any anal or rectal disease, it is usually possible to feel the prostate gland, its midline posterior sulcus, and possibly even the seminal vesicle. In a patient with urinary retention, a palpably enlarged prostate is indicative of the root of the problem: if the posterior part of the gland is enlarged, the chances are that the whole gland is also enlarged. Unfortunately, the converse does not hold: the fact that the posterior lobe is not palpably enlarged does not mean that the gland is not the cause, since the median lobe, the most likely culprit, is not palpable.

Prostatic malignancy and the vertebral column

Because of the connections between the pelvic veins and the vertebral venous plexuses, prostatic malignancy may spread to the vertebral column. It may present as a collapsed vertebra as a result of erosion of the vertebral body by secondary deposits, or by shooting pains down the legs, as a result of nerve entrapment resulting from vertebral collapse.

Blood supply and lymph drainage

Prostatic arteries arise from the internal iliac. Veins drain to the internal iliac veins and connect with the vertebral venous plexuses. Lymph vessels drain to internal iliac nodes.

The nerve supply of the prostate is not important.

Ductus (vas) deferens (Fig. 11.36)

From the testis the ductus passes through the inguinal canal. After traversing the deep inguinal ring it passes lateral to the inferior epigastric artery and turns medially and down, crossing the ureter and passing between the bladder and the medial aspect of the iliac vessels and their branches. It approaches the prostate gland from behind, above the seminal vesicle, the duct of which it joins to form the ejaculatory duct entering the postero-lateral aspect of the prostate gland and the urethra.

Rectum (Fig. 11.37)

The rectum begins in front of vertebra S3 where the sigmoid colon loses its mesentery. Like the sacrum, it is concave anteriorly and continues downwards and for-wards on the superior aspect of the pelvic diaphragm. Behind the prostate in the male, or vagina in the female, is the rectal ampulla, a dilatation in which faeces collect

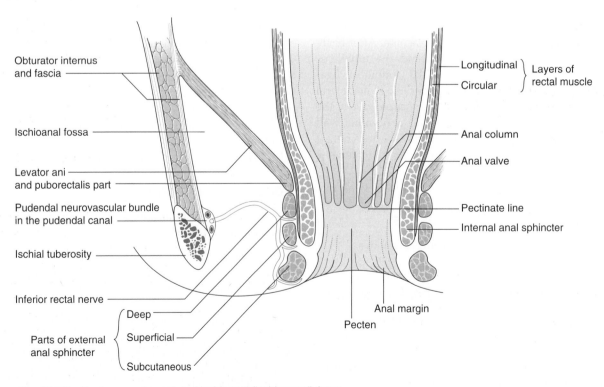

Fig. 11.37 Rectum, anal canal, and ischioanal (ischiorectal) fossa.

before being expelled at defecation. They are kept here by the puborectalis part of levator ani muscle which 'pulls' the rectum forwards so that just beneath the ampulla the rectum turns sharply backwards (approximately 90°) and down through the pelvic diaphragm. This angle and the role of puborectalis are important in the maintenance of faecal continence and damage to the pelvic diaphragm or the perineal body may result in incontinence.

Already you can see that the human rectum is not well named: it is not straight. There are, furthermore, three lateral curvatures with corresponding mucosal folds, sometimes called the valves of Houston. These folds project into the lumen, from above down (or below up), from the left, from the right, and from the left. They are easily torn and so you should be careful when inserting instruments into the rectum.

Blood supply. Being a derivative of hindgut, the rectal blood supply comes from branches of the inferior mesenteric artery. Venous blood drains to the inferior mesenteric vein and the portal vein.

Nerve supply. See later.

Lymph drainage. This is to mesenteric nodes and internal iliac nodes.

Rectoanal junction

Opinions differ about where the rectum becomes the anal canal: my view is that the pelvic diaphragm is the demarcation. The anal canal is considered in 11.12 (p. 143).

11.12 Perineum

Overview

The perineum is the area inferior to the pelvic diaphragm (levator ani muscle). All perineal structures are supplied by the pudendal artery and the pudendal nerve (S2, 3, 4). It contains the anal canal, the ischioanal (ischiorectal) fossa on either side of the anal canal, and the external genitalia. It is partly divided by the urogenital diaphragm between the ischiopubic rami, which contains muscles of the external (voluntary) urinary sphincter (sphincter urethrae). The perineal body, anterior to the anal canal, is a fibromuscular node and focal point for the activity of both pelvic and urogenital diaphragms: damage to it may result in sphincter incontinence and prolapse of pelvic organs.

Learning Objectives

You should:

- know the anatomy of the anal canal in relation to the pelvic diaphragm, and the watersheds of the anal canal
- understand the mechanism of faecal continence
- understand the general arrangement of the perineum
- know the anatomy of the urethra in the male and female, and the anatomy of urinary continence
- know the anatomy of the external genitalia, and how to catheterise the urethra in male and female.

Spatial considerations in the perineum: the ischioanal (ischiorectal) fossa
(Fig. 11.37)

Think of the perineum below the pelvic diaphragm as a space with a sloping ceiling such that it is highest at the sides and lowest in the centre (the perineal body). It is penetrated by the anal canal posteriorly and the space on either side of this is the ischioanal fossa, normally full of fat (this fossa used to be called the ischiorectal fossa – a name still much used, but inaccurate). Anteriorly the ischioanal fossa is divided into an upper storey and a lower storey by a balcony slung between the two inferior pubic rami, the urogenital diaphragm, which meets the perineal body in the middle but otherwise has a free posterior border. The area above this balcony, between it and the pelvic diaphragm, is on each side the anterior recess of the ischioanal fossa. Thus, the fossa is of two storeys in front, and one storey behind, much as a theatre with one balcony of seats.

Pudendal vessels and nerve: course and branches

See Figure 11.33 to remind yourself how clever the vessels are to pass from above the pelvic diaphragm to below it without having to penetrate it. Once in the perineum, the pudendal neurovascular bundle makes its way downwards and forwards on the lateral wall of the ischioanal fossa, which is formed by obturator internus muscle. It is enclosed by a fascial sheath called Alcock's canal (pudendal canal). The nerve and artery give branches to the anal canal and eventually reach the back of the urogenital diaphragm, which they supply (perineal branches). Other branches continue to the external genitalia (dorsal nerve/artery of the penis/clitoris).

Urogenital diaphragm   (Figs 11.38–11.40)

This incomplete shelf of muscle runs between the inferior pubic rami and merges with the perineal body in the midline posteriorly. It is penetrated by the urethra (in both sexes) and, in the female, by the vagina. It consists of, from above down:

- a thin fascial layer with no particular name
- a sheet of voluntary muscle, the perineal muscles, which form the external urinary sphincter and are supplied by the pudendal nerve – this muscle sheet is somewhat rearranged in the female where the vagina passes through it, but you need not worry about this
- a thick fascial layer called the perineal membrane.

Female urethra

From the bladder neck the urethra passes inferiorly through the urogenital diaphragm. Since the inferior layer of the urogenital diaphragm is the perineal membrane, this is sometimes called the membranous portion of the urethra. From here the urethra continues down directly to open at the vestibule.

Male urethra   (Fig. 11.38, 11.39)

- Prostatic urethra. From the bladder neck the urethra enters the prostate gland. It is here quite wide and U-shaped. Below the prostate gland, it passes through the urogenital diaphragm as the:
- Membranous urethra. Immediately below the perineal membrane there is a slight dilatation, the urethral bulb, and it turns forwards to run immediately inferior to the perineal membrane as the:
- Spongy urethra. Here the urethra is surrounded by caverns of venous blood, the corpus spongiosum, or spongy erectile tissue, and smooth muscle fibres, the bulbospongiosus muscle. This forms one of the three tubes of erectile tissue that make up the penis, and it is enlarged at its tip to form the glans penis. The spongy urethra continues forwards in the penis as the:
- Penile urethra. Slightly before its termination there is another slight dilatation, the navicular fossa, in the region of which a mucosal fold projects into the urethra from what would be the superior aspect of the urethra with the penis pointing forwards.

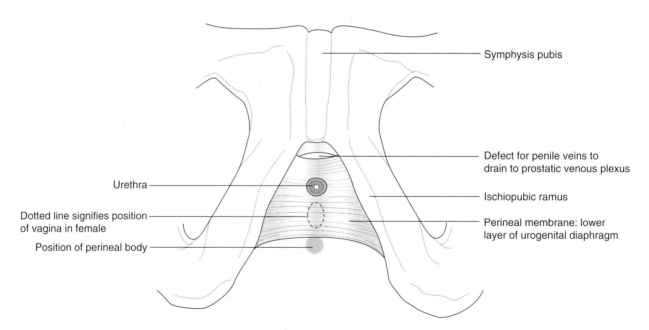

Urethra

Dotted line signifies position of vagina in female

Position of perineal body

Symphysis pubis

Defect for penile veins to drain to prostatic venous plexus

Ischiopubic ramus

Perineal membrane: lower layer of urogenital diaphragm

Fig. 11.38   Urogenital diaphragm in male: from below.

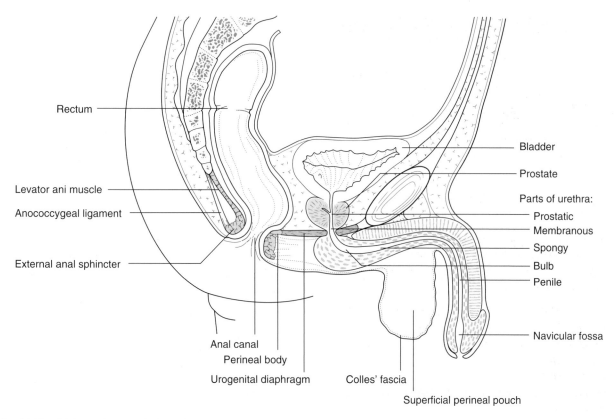

Rectum

Levator ani muscle

Anococcygeal ligament

External anal sphincter

Bladder

Prostate

Parts of urethra:

Prostatic

Membranous

Spongy

Bulb

Penile

Navicular fossa

Anal canal

Perineal body

Urogenital diaphragm

Colles' fascia

Superficial perineal pouch

Fig. 11.39 Male urethra: sagittal section.

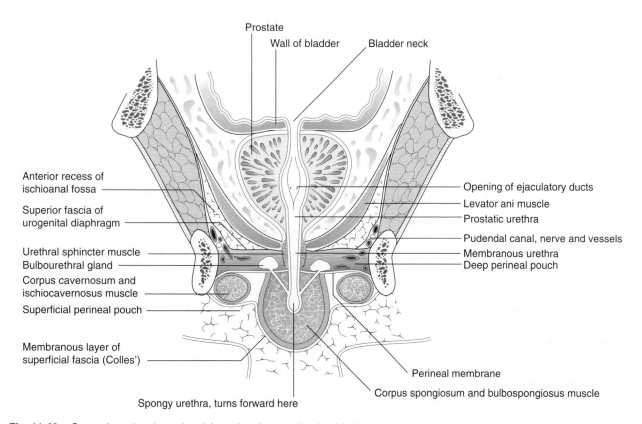

Prostate

Wall of bladder

Bladder neck

Anterior recess of ischioanal fossa

Superior fascia of urogenital diaphragm

Urethral sphincter muscle

Bulbourethral gland

Corpus cavernosum and ischiocavernosus muscle

Superficial perineal pouch

Membranous layer of superficial fascia (Colles')

Opening of ejaculatory ducts

Levator ani muscle

Prostatic urethra

Pudendal canal, nerve and vessels

Membranous urethra

Deep perineal pouch

Perineal membrane

Corpus spongiosum and bulbospongiosus muscle

Spongy urethra, turns forward here

Fig. 11.40 Coronal section through pelvis and perineum showing bladder, prostate, urogenital diaphragm and root of penis

Catheterisation of the male urethra
- First, avoid the mucosal fold near the navicular fossa by aiming the catheter down, assuming the penis is pointing forwards, held in your hand.
- Next, push the catheter gently back until you meet increased resistance. The catheter tip is now at the bulb with the right-angled bend.
- Now turn the penis inferiorly and gently ease the catheter round the corner. If you are rough you may rupture the urethra.
- The next difficult region is the membranous urethra as it penetrates the urogenital diaphragm. Remember that in an old gentleman you are likely to be inserting the catheter because of urinary retention, and so the bladder will be very full and the poor old man will be contracting his urinary sphincter very tightly indeed. This makes it even harder to advance the catheter. After you have managed this, the rest is easy: the prostatic urethra is wide and easily distensible and the catheter will go straight into the bladder. The old gentleman is now very relieved and may well be grateful to you for ever.

Superficial and deep perineal pouches, Colles' fascia

- Deep perineal pouch. This is the area of the urogenital diaphragm between the upper and lower fascial components. It is a silly term, since it is full of perineal muscles.
- Superficial perineal pouch. This is the area inferior to the perineal membrane, bounded posteriorly by the perineal body. Urine may leak into this area if the urethra is ruptured. Such a urinary leak is limited by Colles' fascia – the superficial fascia of the perineum (Figs 11.39, 11.40), and urine may spread up the superficial tissues of the anterior abdominal wall.

Surface anatomy of the perineum

The surface anatomy is usually described as if the patient were in 'lithotomy position': lying on the back, with the lower limbs elevated and the feet in stirrups. A line joining the two ischial tuberosities divides the perineum into two approximate triangles:

- the urogenital triangle anteriorly, roughly coexistent with the urogenital diaphragm internally
- the anal triangle posteriorly.

Female external genitalia: the vulva (Fig. 11.41)

The vulva is the name given to the female external

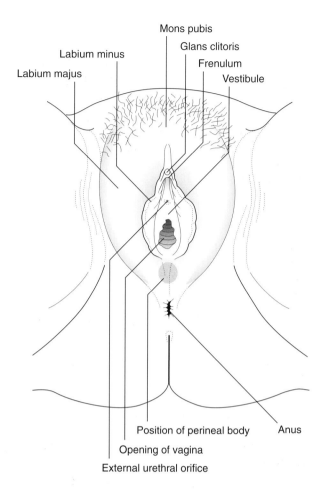

Fig. 11.41 Female external genitalia.

genitalia. The vestibule signifies that area between the two labia majora. Internally, the bulbospongiosus and ischiocavernosus muscles are much as in the male, except smaller. The clitoris has erectile tissue as does the penis. Lymph drains to inguinal nodes.

Episiotomy, perineal tear
Look at Figure 11.41. In order to enlarge the mother's vaginal orifice for the baby's head, an incision is sometimes made posteriorly from the vagina into the soft tissues of the perineum and perineal skin. This is an episiotomy. If it is performed in the midline posteriorly from the vagina, there is a risk of damaging the perineal body, immediately deep to this region. For this reason the procedure is normally performed obliquely. A perineal tear which damages the perineal body may result from direct trauma, or uncontrolled expulsion of the fetal head during birth. It would result in functional loss of both muscular diaphragms associated with the perineal body: urinary incontinence, faecal incontinence and pelvic organ prolapse.

Male external genitalia

- Regard the penis as an enlarged clitoris and labia minora into which the urethra has been diverted.
- Regard the scrotum as the two labia majora that have been stitched together.

This is not simply bizarre fantasy, it is embryological fact. Hypospadias, the commonest penile congenital anomaly, is simply some degree of reversion to the female, or basic, form.

Penis   (Fig. 11.42)

The terms ventral and dorsal are applied to the penis in the erect position, so when the penis is dependent, the dorsal surface is in front. Three tubes of erectile tissue form the penis.

- In the ventral midline is the corpus spongiosum that contains the urethra. This is attached to the under surface of the urogenital diaphragm by the bulbospongiosus muscle and is enlarged at its tip to form the glans. Bulbospongiosus is split into two in the female to form the sphincter vaginae.
- On each side, slightly dorsally, is the corpus cavernosum. Each is attached to the inferior ramus of the pubis by the ischiocavernosus muscle, and terminates just proximal to the glans.

These three chambers of venous caverns communicate with each other: this is evident clinically by the treatment of priapism, a painful condition of perpetual erection caused by venous engorgement, in which incision into one of the chambers usually solves the problem. (Priapus was a Greek fertility imp with an enormous penis. Statues of him abound).

An interesting linguistic snippet
The Latin word *penis* means tail: perhaps its use for the male organ developed as a euphemism so as not to offend the delicate ears of the ladies of Rome. The proper English word is cock, defined in the Compact Oxford English Dictionary (second edition, 1991) as 'a spout or short pipe serving as a channel for passing liquids through'.

Blood supply of external genitalia

Arteries from the pudendal; veins to the prostatic venous plexus and thence to the internal iliacs.

Lymph drainage of external genitalia

- Clitoris, glans penis, penile urethra: inguinal nodes.
- Urethra inferior to the urogenital diaphragm and bulb: external iliac nodes.
- Membranous urethra and above: internal iliac nodes.
- Labia majora and scrotum: inguinal nodes.
- Ovary and testis: para-aortic nodes.

Nerve supply of external genitalia and perineal skin.

- From pudendal nerve and branches:
  - S4 around the anus, vulva, posterior scrotum (the anterior scrotum is part of the anterior abdominal wall and is supplied by lumbar nerves)
  - S3 more laterally between the legs
  - dorsal nerve of the penis or clitoris (mainly S4).
- Twigs from S5 supply a small area at the tip of the coccyx (not important).

Anal canal   (Fig. 11.37)

Opinions differ about anal anatomy, so be prepared for this.

From the puborectalis sling of levator ani (see p. 132), the anal canal passes down and backwards to the anal orifice.

Mucosa of the anal canal, columns, valves, pectinate (dentate) line

- Upper part. The mucosa of the upper part of the anal canal is thrown into between 5 and 10

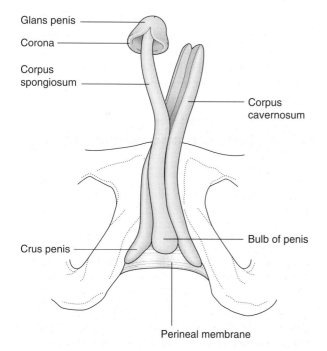

Glans penis
Corona
Corpus spongiosum
Corpus cavernosum
Crus penis
Bulb of penis
Perineal membrane

Fig. 11.42   Components of penis: dissected, viewed from below.

Table 11.1 The 'watersheds' in the anal canal

	Above pectinate (dentate) line	Below pectinate (dentate) line
Epithelium	Columnar (mucosa)	Stratified squamous (skin)
Arteries	Branches of inferior mesenteric, e.g. superior rectal	Branches of internal iliac, e.g. inferior rectal
Veins	To the portal system (inferior mesenteric)	To the systemic system (internal iliac veins)
Lymph drainage	To mesenteric nodes	To internal iliac and inguinal nodes
Nerve supply	Visceral (autonomic): pelvic splanchnic nerves (S2, 3, 4 and sympathetic). Pain is thus dull and poorly defined	Somatic: inferior rectal from pudendal (S2, 3, 4). Pain is thus sharp and well defined

longitudinal mucosal folds, the anal columns. At their lower end, about halfway along the canal, these folds are joined together by mucosal ridges, called valves (not to be confused with valves of the rectum) with a small recess behind, something like a pocket. Mucous glands open into these pockets. The apparent line formed by the valves is the pectinate (dentate) line and it marks the approximate position of several boundaries or watersheds (Table 11.1).

- Middle part. This is lined by skin and is smooth. It is sometimes known as the pecten.
- Lower part (anus). This is lined by hairy skin and is puckered by the sphincters.

Veins

You might suppose that, since the anal canal is a site of anastomoses between the portal and systemic venous systems, it would be involved in the manifestation of liver disease in a way similar to oesophageal varices. You would be wrong: it is not, and nobody knows quite why.

Clinical box

'Piles' – haemorrhoids
These are varicose veins of anal columns. As long as they are confined to the area above the pectinate line, they are relatively painless, although they may be uncomfortable, and they may rupture causing bleeding. As soon as they stray into the territory of the somatic nerve innervation below the line, they become ... ouch!

Anal sphincters (Fig. 11.37)

- Internal sphincter: smooth muscle, autonomic innervation. This is simply the somewhat expanded inferior termination of the circular smooth muscle component of the wall of the gut tube.
- External sphincter: skeletal muscle, voluntary (somatic) innervation (S2, 3, 4). There are three parts. From outside (anus) in, these are:
  - subcutaneous: this is the part that puckers the anal skin
  - superficial: this is level with the inferior edge of the internal sphincter
  - deep: this is level with the anal columns. The posterior part of the deep part is functionally related and merges with the puborectalis sling of levator ani muscles (pelvic diaphragm). This is why damage to the pelvic diaphragm, or to the perineal body, which is a part of the same mechanism, may lead to loss of sphincter control.

Sacral spinal cord and the perineum: sphincters and sex

You have read that the perineum is innervated by sacral segments 2, 3 and 4. Although the sacral nerves emerge through the sacrum, you should remember that the sacral part of the spinal cord itself from which they arise is actually level with vertebrae T11, T12 and L1. A catastrophic injury to the vertebral column in the low thoracic or upper lumbar region may therefore cause loss of S2, 3, 4 function. In two 's' words, these are sphincters and sex, functional implications being incontinence and, in the male, impotence. The sacral nerve roots, like all constituents of the cauda equina, are also liable to injury anywhere between their origin and their foramina of exit from the vertebral canal.

11.13 Autonomic nervous system in the abdomen and pelvis: a review

Revise Chapter 6.

Sympathetic

Preganglionic cell bodies are in the lateral column of grey matter of the thoracolumbar spinal cord. Impulses pass through ventral roots of spinal nerves and white rami communicantes to the sympathetic chain, thence without synapsing to the splanchnic nerves. They arrive at the preaortic group of plexuses, coeliac, superior mesenteric, etc., where they may synapse, postganglionic fibres being delivered to their destinations in the walls of the arteries which supply them. Preganglionic sympathetic impulses to hindgut derivatives pass down the preaortic group of plexuses in front of the aorta and, below the aortic bifurcation, continue into the pelvis as the hypogastric or pelvic plexus, also known as the presacral nerves, synapsing somewhere along the way. In this way sympathetic impulses reach the pelvic organs, postganglionic fibres passing directly to the organs concerned (e.g. bladder, internal genitalia).

The sympathetic chains continue down into the pelvis, uniting as the ganglion impar in front of the sacrum. Between T1 and about L1 or L2 the chain is connected at each segment to spinal nerves by white and grey rami communicantes. Below (and above) this thoracolumbar region, there are only grey rami. Destruction of the sympathetic chains at the lower ends of the aorta and inferior vena cava will interrupt sympathetic outflow to lower lumbar and sacral spinal nerves (for the lower limbs), but will not affect sympathetic outflow to the gut tube or pelvic viscera which parted company with the sympathetic chains higher up through the thoracic (greater, lesser, least) and lumbar splanchnic nerves to gain the preaortic and pelvic plexuses. This procedure is lumbar sympathectomy and is performed to interrupt vasoconstrictor fibres to the lower limbs in the case of peripheral vascular disease.

Parasympathetic

The parasympathetic system in the abdomen supplies only gut tube derivatives: foregut and midgut structures through the vagus, and hindgut (cloacal) structures through fibres originating from segments S2, 3 and 4. These pass into the sacral nerve roots and then, as soon as they have emerged from the sacral foramina, part company with the somatic nerves to form the pelvic splanchnic nerves. Since these are responsible for penile erection, they are also known as the nervi erigentes. You do not need to know the details.

Visceral sensation

These fibres have not been well defined for most abdominal structures, and certainly not for pelvic and perineal structures. They pass back to the spinal cord in nerves which are conveying sympathetic fibres in the opposite direction, or in nerves that convey parasympathetic fibres in the opposite direction, or possibly both. Cell bodies are in the dorsal root ganglion of whichever segment transmits the sensory fibre into the spinal cord and thus pain may be referred to the skin, or other somatic structure, supplied by that segment.

11.14 Summary of surface markings and vertebral levels

(Table 11.2)

Table 11.2 Surface markings and vertebral levels

Surface marking		Vertebral level
Nipple, fourth intercostal space	Liver, upper limit	T7
Xiphoid process		T9 or 10
	Origin of coeliac artery	T12
Ribs 9–11 posteriorly	Spleen	
	Origin of superior mesenteric artery	T12/L1
Tip of ninth costal cartilage, transpyloric plane	Gall bladder, pylorus, duodenojejunal flexure, hilum of kidneys, head of pancreas	L1
Subcostal plane	Origin of gonadal, inferior mesenteric artery (approximate)	L2/3
Umbilicus, just below and to the left	Bifurcation of aorta	L3/4
Highest point of iliac crest (posteriorly)	L3/4 intervertebral disc (for lumbar puncture)	L3/4
McBurney's point, right iliac fossa	Base of appendix, caecum	L4
Midinguinal point, and 2 cm above	Femoral pulse, and deep inguinal ring	Not applicable
Pubic tubercle	Superficial inguinal ring	Not applicable

Self-assessment: questions

Multiple choice questions

1. In the inguinal region and scrotum:
   a. The deep inguinal ring is directly over the femoral artery as it passes posterior to the inguinal ligament.
   b. The conjoint tendon is posterior to the spermatic cord at the superficial inguinal ring.
   c. The lymph drainage of scrotal skin is to para-aortic nodes.
   d. A hydrocele is a collection of fluid in the tunica vaginalis.
   e. The ilioinguinal nerve passes through both superficial and deep rings.

2. The spleen:
   a. May be damaged by fractured left ribs 10 and 11.
   b. Is supplied by the superior mesenteric artery.
   c. May be enlarged as a result of portal hypertension.
   d. Enlarges towards the left iliac fossa.
   e. Is anterior to the left costodiaphragmatic recess.

3. The lesser omentum:
   a. Runs between stomach and liver.
   b. Forms the anterior wall of the lesser sac.
   c. Is attached to the lesser curvature of the stomach.
   d. Is derived from the dorsal mesogastrium.
   e. Has a free edge containing the portal vein and common bile duct.

4. Regarding the pancreas:
   a. It is supplied by both foregut and midgut arteries.
   b. The uncinate process is in contact with the spleen.
   c. Pancreatic pain may be referred to the back.
   d. It is in the posterior wall of the lesser sac.
   e. Cancer of the head of the pancreas may block the common bile duct.

5. The diaphragm:
   a. Receives motor fibres from the thoracic spinal cord.
   b. Sensory impulses enter the thoracic spinal cord.
   c. Is penetrated by the inferior vena cava at vertebral level T10.
   d. Separates the costodiaphragmatic recesses from the upper poles of the kidneys.
   e. Is firmly attached to the liver at the bare area.

6. Vague periumbilical pain is likely to result from disease of the:
   a. Stomach.
   b. Ileum.
   c. Appendix.
   d. Descending colon.
   e. Bladder.

7. The nerve in contact with the ischial spine:
   a. Arises from the sacral segments of the spinal cord.
   b. Runs on the lateral wall of the ischioanal fossa.
   c. Supplies the upper part of the anal canal.
   d. Supplies the labia majora and clitoris.
   e. Supplies the voluntary urethral sphincter.

8. Regarding the prostate:
   a. It surrounds the urethra.
   b. It is above levator ani muscle.
   c. It is supplied by branches of the pudendal artery.
   d. The median lobe may be palpated at rectal examination.
   e. Prostatic veins connect with the internal vertebral venous plexus.

9. The internal iliac artery supplies:
   a. Kidney.
   b. Bladder
   c. Ovary.
   d. Uterus.
   e. Rectum.

10. Trauma at the following sites may have the stated results:
    a. Left eighth rib → ruptured spleen.
    b. Anterior superior iliac spine → sensory loss in the thigh.
    c. Nerve near McBurney's point → direct inguinal hernia.
    d. Perineal body → faecal and urinary incontinence.
    e. Spinal cord section at level of vertebrae T12, L1, L2 in the male → impotence.

11. Structures at about the level of the transpyloric plane include:
    a. Hilum of the kidneys.
    b. Origin of superior mesenteric artery.
    c. Duodenojejunal junction.
    d. Cardio-oesophageal junction.
    e. Ninth costal cartilage.

12. Meckel's diverticulum:
    a. Is a remnant of the vitellointestinal duct.
    b. Is attached to the ileum.
    c. May contain ectopic gastric mucosa.
    d. May cause bleeding.
    e. Is supplied by a branch of the superior mesenteric artery.

13. The radiological landmarks of the ureter include:
    a. Tip of ninth rib.
    b. Tips of transverse processes of lumbar vertebrae.
    c. L4–L5 joint.
    d. Ischial spine.
    e. Sacroiliac joint.

14. Structures posterior to the right kidney include:
    a. Duodenum.
    b. Pancreas.
    c. Adrenal gland.
    d. Costodiaphragmatic recess of pleural cavity.
    e. Subcostal nerve.

15. The left renal vein receives the:
    a. Left adrenal vein.
    b. Inferior mesenteric vein.
    c. Left gonadal vein.
    d. Left colic veins.
    e. Splenic vein.

Matching item questions

Questions 1–5

Match the numbered item to the lettered response. Each lettered response may be used once, more than once, or not at all.
  a. left iliac fossa
  b. epigastrium
  c. umbilical pain
  d. McBurney's point
  e. tip of right ninth costal cartilage

1. base of appendix
2. sigmoid colon
3. stomach cancer
4. fundus of gall bladder
5. transpyloric plane

Questions 6–10

Match the numbered item to the lettered response. Each lettered response may be used once, more than once, or not at all.
  a. T10
  b. T12
  c. L1
  d. L3–4
  e. L5

6. dermatome of umbilical skin
7. dermatome over pubic tubercle
8. vertebral level of oesophageal orifice in diaphragm
9. vertebral level of bifurcation of the aorta
10. vertebral level of highest point of iliac crest

Questions 11–20

Match the numbered item to the lettered response. Each lettered response may be used once, more than once, or not at all.
  a. internal iliac nodes
  b. inguinal nodes
  c. external iliac nodes
  d. para-aortic nodes
  e. coeliac nodes

11. scrotal skin
12. ovary
13. rectum
14. uterine cervix
15. anal canal inferior to pectinate line
16. glans penis
17. lesser curvature of stomach
18. first part of duodenum
19. prostate
20. bladder

Questions requiring short answers

1. In the inguinal canal, what forms (a) the anterior wall; (b) the posterior wall; (c) the roof; and (d) the floor?

2. Describe the testis in the scrotum. Which layer is equivalent to peritoneum? What is the cremasteric reflex? What is a hydrocele?

3. What is the significance of portosystemic anastomoses? What is a caput Medusae? Suggest surgical procedures that might achieve the same purpose. What would be the drawbacks of this?

4. What are the subphrenic spaces? How do they relate to the liver? What is the hepatorenal recess (Morison's pouch)? What other spaces does this communicate with? Why does all this matter?

5. Describe the vagus nerves in the abdomen. What is vagotomy?

6. How is the uterus maintained in position? What is a uterine prolapse and how may it be caused?

7. What is the pouch of Douglas? How would you drain an abscess in it in (a) a female; (b) a male?

Why is this relevant to inexpertly performed abortions?

8. A rugby player is kicked in the back between the left rib cage and the vertebral column. Lower ribs are fractured. There is severe internal bleeding, blood in the urine and the patient is short of breath. Explain.

9. What is the functional significance of the part of levator ani called puborectalis?

10. A 75-year-old man presents with urinary retention, back pain and shooting pains down the legs. Explain.

Self-assessment: answers

Multiple choice answers

1. a. **False.** It is 2 cm above the femoral pulse.
   b. **True.**
   c. **False.** Lymph drainage of scrotal skin is to inguinal nodes; it is drainage of testis that is to para-aortic nodes. This is important.
   d. **True.**
   e. **False.** It passes through the superficial ring, but not the deep.

2. a. **True.**
   b. **False.** The splenic artery is a branch of the coeliac.
   c. **True.**
   d. **False.** It enlarges towards the right iliac fossa.
   e. **True.**

3. a. **True.**
   b. **True.**
   c. **True.**
   d. **False.** It is derived from the ventral mesogastrium. (This is difficult and unimportant.)
   e. **True.** It also contains the hepatic artery.

4. a. **True.**
   b. **False.** The tail is in contact with the spleen; the uncinate process is within the loop of duodenum.
   c. **True.**
   d. **True.**
   e. **True.**

5. a. **False.** It receives motor fibres from C3, 4 and 5.
   b. **True.** Intercostal nerves supply the periphery.
   c. **False.** The IVC penetrates the diaphragm at T8, the oesophagus at T12.
   d. **True.**
   e. **True.**

6. a. **False.** Foregut derivatives would cause epigastric pain.
   b. **True.** Midgut visceral sensation is referred to the umbilical region.
   c. **True.** Midgut visceral sensation is referred to the umbilical region.
   d. **False.** Hindgut/cloacal derivatives would cause suprapubic pain.
   e. **False.** Hindgut/cloacal derivatives would cause suprapubic pain.

7. a. **True.** It is the pudendal nerve, S2, 3, 4.
   b. **True.** It runs in Alcock's (pudendal) canal.
   c. **False.** It supplies the lower part of the anal canal.
   d. **True.**
   e. **True.**

8. a. **True.**
   b. **True.**
   c. **False.** The pudendal artery supplies below levator ani.
   d. **False.**
   e. **True.** This is why cancer can spread to the spine.

9. a. **False.** The renal artery supplies the kidney.
   b. **True.**
   c. **False.** The ovarian artery is a branch of the aorta.
   d. **True.**
   e. **False.** The inferior mesenteric artery supplies the rectum.

10. a. **False.** The spleen is related to ribs 9, 10 and 11, but not 8.
    b. **True.** The lateral cutaneous nerve of the thigh L2, 3 may be damaged.
    c. **True.** Damage to the iliohypogastric nerve increases the possibility of inguinal hernia.
    d. **True.** The perineal body is an integral part of the pelvic diaphragm and associated voluntary anal and urethral sphincters.
    e. **True.** The sacral spinal cord is at the level of these vertebrae. S2, 3, 4 segments give rise to nerve impulses for, amongst other things, penile erection.

11. a. **True.**
    b. **True.**
    c. **True.**
    d. **False.** This is much higher. The oesophageal hiatus in the diaphragm is at vertebral level T10, so the cardio-oesophageal junction would be about T10/T11.
    e. **True.**

12. a. **True.**
    b. **True.**
    c. **True.**
    d. **True.**
    e. **True.**

13. a. **False.** It is irrelevant.
    b. **True.**
    c. **False.**
    d. **True.** It appears to be related to the ischial spines on a PA radiograph.
    e. **True.**

14. a. **False.** This is anterior.
    b. **False.** This is anterior.
    c. **False.** This is superomedial.
    d. **True.** This is important in renal biopsy procedures.
    e. **True.**

15. a. **True.**
    b. **False.** This joins the splenic and superior mesenteric veins to form the portal vein.
    c. **True.**
    d. **False.** These would drain into the inferior mesenteric vein.
    e. **False.** See 15b above.

Matching item answers

1. d.
2. a.
3. b.
4. e.
5. e.
6. a.
7. c.
8. a.
9. d.
10. d. The level of the iliac crests is useful as a landmark in lumbar puncture.
11. b.
12. d.
13. a.
14. a.
15. b.
16. b.
17. e.
18. e.
19. a.
20. a.

Short answers

1. See 11.2 (p. 103) and Figures 11.4 and 11.5.

2. See 11.2 (p. 105). In the scrotum the testis is covered by tunica albuginea and the two layers, visceral and parietal, of the tunica vaginalis (equivalent to peritoneum). Vessels and nerves pass between testis and scrotum through the spermatic cord,

which also includes the cremaster muscle. Contraction of this muscle, such as in the cremasteric reflex elicited, for example, by cold hands, causes testicular retraction. A hydrocele is a collection of serous fluid between the visceral and parietal layers of the tunica vaginalis. A word on the embryology would be appropriate, but not necessary.

3. If blood can not flow through liver sinusoids (e.g. in disease) it will find bypass channels, or portosystemic anastomoses. Veins at the lower end of the oesophagus are important, as also are those resulting from reopening of channels in the falciform ligament (ligamentum teres, umbilical vein) taking blood to the anterior abdominal wall. Veins of the anterior abdominal wall radiate from the umbilicus giving the appearance of Medusa's head. Other connections of clinical significance are in the posterior abdominal wall. Artificial bypass could be provided by connecting the portal vein to the inferior vena cava, but this would mean substances absorbed from the gut tube did not pass through the liver and were not detoxified.

4. Although the liver and diaphragm are attached to each other at the bare area, recesses of the peritoneal cavity extend between them for some distance – the anterior and posterior subphrenic spaces. The right posterior space communicates with the greater sac at the hepatorenal (Morison's) pouch, between liver and kidney on the right, which also communicates with the lesser sac through the foramen of Winslow, and the right paracolic gutter. This matters because fluid can collect in these spaces and be the cause of disease that is difficult to diagnose.

5. The vagus nerve enters the abdomen with the oesophagus through the diaphragm at vertebral level T10. It travels down the lesser curvature in the lesser omentum. Branches pass to the stomach, antrum (nerves of Latarjet) and liver. Vagotomy means that the pyloric sphincter does not function properly and a connection may have to be made between the stomach and jejunum (gastrojejunostomy). Vagotomy is now infrequently performed since the advent of suitable drugs for ulcer treatment.

6. The uterus is supported by levator ani (pelvic diaphragm) and ligaments on its superior surface (pubocervical, sacrocervical, cardinal). These suspend the uterus in a sling and help maintain anteversion (uterus bent forwards on vagina),

along with the broad ligament. Since levator ani is anchored centrally at the perineal body, damage to this will weaken the uterine supports. This may be caused by direct trauma, or wear and tear (e.g. repeated childbirth).

7. The rectouterine pouch = pouch of Douglas. It is full of coils of small intestine and is intimately related to the posterior vaginal fornix, through which an abscess may be drained in the female. In the male, one would have to go through the anterior rectal wall. Back-street abortionists pushed implements straight up the vagina, not knowing about the angle of anteversion, with dire consequences.

8. Rugby is a very dangerous game. The player has been kicked in the renal angle, with resultant kidney damage. Internal bleeding into the pelvis and ureter explains blood in the urine. Fractured ribs cause right pneumothorax with breathing difficulties, and have ruptured the spleen to give massive internal bleeding. All this could be fatal.

9. Puborectalis maintains the angle between the rectal ampulla and anal canal. It is intimately connected with the deep part of the external (voluntary) anal sphincter and so together they are vital in the maintenance of faecal continence.

10. Prostate cancer (like any pelvic cancer) can spread by valveless veins of Batson to the internal vertebral venous plexus and lead to secondary deposits in vertebral bodies. This may cause back pain and lead to collapse of vertebrae, trapping lumbar nerve roots and giving shooting pains, and/or numbness, in the lower limb(s).

12 Upper limb

12.1 The big picture

Beware!

'Arm' means upper limb from shoulder to elbow, not the entire upper limb. 'Forearm' means upper limb from elbow to wrist.

Radial, ulnar, lateral, medial

Particularly in the forearm and hand, the terms radial and ulnar are used in preference to lateral and medial (respectively). This avoids confusion which may arise depending upon the position of the hand. The thumb is always on the radial side, and the little finger always on the ulnar side.

Arteries (Fig. 7.1, p. 44; Fig. 12.1)

Arterial blood to the upper limb comes from the subclavian and axillary arteries.

- Subclavian: extends from its origin to the lateral border of the first rib.
- Axillary: extends from the lateral border of the first rib to the lateral border of teres major muscle.
- Brachial: extends from the lateral border of teres major to the cubital fossa, where it bifurcates to give:

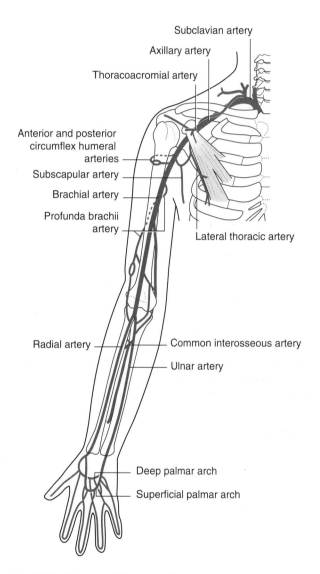

Fig. 12.1   Arteries of the upper limb.

- Radial (lateral) and ulnar (medial) arteries. These pass down the respective sides of the forearm to the hand where they form two anastomoses in the palm:
- Superficial and deep palmar arterial arches.

Veins (Fig. 7.2, p. 45)

Venous blood drains to the subclavian veins, thence to the brachiocephalic veins and the superior vena cava.

- Superficial veins are immediately subcutaneous, superficial to the deep fascia which surrounds the muscles, bones and other deeper structures like a sleeve. These veins are visible or palpable (unless the patient is very fat) and are easily accessible for venepuncture. The pattern of superficial veins is very variable: you need only bother with:
  - the dorsal venous arch on the back of the hand, very variable pattern, from which arise:
    a. the cephalic vein: lateral side of the upper limb to the deltopectoral groove between the deltoid and pectoralis major muscles
    b. the basilic vein: medial side of the upper limb, piercing the deep fascia as it approaches the axilla and contributing to the formation of the axillary vein
  - veins in front of the elbow (often injection sites): these are very variable, but there is usually a median cubital vein (Fig. 12.20, and look at your own).
- Deep veins, within the fascial sleeve, accompany the arteries and are thus named venae comitantes (Latin: accompanying veins). They receive connections from the superficial veins and in the axillary region unite to form the axillary vein, which then becomes the subclavian.

The subclavian vein crosses the superior surface of the first rib, anterior to the attachment of scalenus anterior (the artery is posterior to it). This joins the internal jugular vein behind the sternoclavicular joint) to form the brachiocephalic vein.

Lymph

All lymph drains to axillary nodes.

- From the radial side of the upper limb, lymph drains alongside the cephalic vein to the deltopectoral (infraclavicular) nodes, outposts of the axillary nodes to which they drain. The deltopectoral nodes are the only lymph nodes on this pathway and are the first nodes to be involved in, for example, an infection of the thumb.
- From the ulnar side of the upper limb, lymph drains alongside the basilic vein to the epitrochlear nodes, just above the elbow, thence to the axillary nodes.

Nerves

All nerves come from the ventral rami of C5, 6, 7, 8 and T1, which form the brachial plexus.

Dermatomes and myotomes. In the body wall, the muscles and skin supplied by one segmental nerve are roughly coexistent. This is not so in the limbs. The dermatomes (sensory) are shown in Figure 6.6 (p. 36),

but the muscles supplied by the same spinal segments are often far distant. For example, T1 dermatome is in the axilla, but muscles supplied by T1 are in the hand. An embryology book will explain why.

12.2 Upper thorax, brachial plexus, pectoral girdle, scapula

Overview

The subclavian, axillary and branchial arteries, together with their branches, supply the upper limb. Easily palpable pulses are the brachial, radial and ulnar. Upper limb nerves come from the brachial plexus formed by ventral rami of spinal nerves C5, 6, 7, 8 and T1. Extensor muscles and skin over the posterior aspect of the upper limb are supplied by the radial and axillary nerves and their branches. The principal nerves supplying flexor muscles and anterior skin are the median, ulnar and musculocutaneous. The clavicle and scapula articulate with the thorax at the sternoclavicular joint, and with each other at the acromioclavicular joint, diseases of both joints hindering upper limb movements.

Learning Objectives

You should:

- know the main arterial tree of the upper limb, and the position of the brachial, radial and ulnar pulses
- understand the principles of venous and lymph drainage of the upper limb
- know the formation, position and main branches of the brachial plexus
- know the principal features of the clavicle and scapula, and understand the manner in which they move on the thorax.

Vessels (Fig. 12.1)

Subclavian artery

This is divided into three parts by scalenus anterior muscle.

- Branches of first part (medial to scalenus anterior):
  - internal thoracic: to supply breast, anterior chest wall, anterior abdominal wall, pericardium, diaphragm

- vertebral: to spinal cord, brain stem, brain
- thyrocervical trunk, which gives inferior thyroid, suprascapular (unimportant), transverse cervical (unimportant): to supply thyroid gland, upper scapular region and anterior neck.
- Branches of second part (behind scalenus anterior) and third part (between scalenus anterior and lateral border of first rib):
  - branches are variable and unimportant, but include the costocervical trunk and dorsal scapular artery, the last named contributing to the scapular anastomosis (see later).

Subclavian pulse. The subclavian pulse is palpable above and behind the middle of the clavicle. The artery is deep to the vein here.

Axillary artery

This is divided into three parts by pectoralis minor muscle.

- Branches of first part (medial to pectoralis minor):
  - supreme or highest thoracic (unimportant).
- Branches of second part (behind pectoralis minor):
  - thoracoacromial: to upper chest and acromial region, breast
  - lateral thoracic: to breast and chest.
- Branches of third part (between pectoralis minor and lateral border of teres major):
  - subscapular: to scapular muscles, scapular anastomosis
  - anterior circumflex humeral
  - posterior circumflex humeral.

These last two may arise by a common trunk. They form an arterial circle round the surgical neck of the humerus (Fig. 12.9) and supply the neighbouring bone, muscles and shoulder joint.

Scapular anastomosis

The arterial anastomosis around the shoulder joint receives blood from branches of the subclavian and axillary arteries, and has connections with the intercostals. It may be involved in bypassing a blocked distal subclavian or proximal axillary artery, blood flowing retrogradely up the subscapular to reach the distal axillary; and in bypassing an aortic coarctation (see Fig. 10.25, p. 86).

Veins

All veins from the upper limb, pectoral and scapular regions, together with the external jugular veins from the neck, drain into the subclavian vein. The only details worth committing to memory are:

- The cephalic vein penetrates the clavipectoral fascia (a fascial sheet between the clavicle and pectoralis minor muscle, occupying the deltopectoral triangle) to become deep before it joins the axillary vein. This is one place where central lines (catheters inserted into the heart) may be inserted.
- The subclavian vein is accessible for catheters etc. just behind the middle of the clavicle. Aim the catheter downwards and medially: the vein is superficial here.
- The subclavian vein joins the internal jugular to form the brachiocephalic behind the sternoclavicular joint.

Brachial plexus and main branches
(Fig. 12.2)

Roots and trunks

Roots of the plexus: ventral rami of C5–T1.

- The ventral rami of C5 and 6 join to form the upper trunk.
- The ventral ramus of C7 is the middle trunk.
- The ventral ramus of C8 and T1 join to form the lower trunk.

Branches of roots and trunks, in order of importance

- Long thoracic (supplies serratus anterior), from C5, 6, 7 roots.
- Suprascapular (supplies infra- and supraspinatus), upper trunk C5, 6.

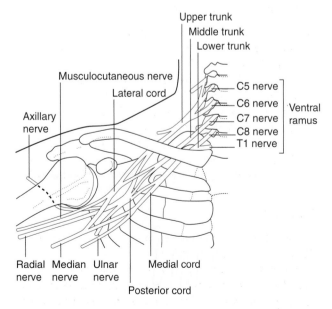

Fig. 12.2 The brachial plexus.

- Dorsal scapular (supplies rhomboids), C5 root; nerve to subclavius, C5, 6 roots (don't bother with either the nerve or the muscle).

Divisions, cords

Each trunk divides into an anterior and a posterior division, the divisions uniting to form cords as described. The cords are named by the position in respect to the axillary artery: posterior, lateral, medial.

Posterior cord and branches   (Fig. 12.3)

Posterior divisions all unite to form the posterior cord, branches of which supply the posterior skin of the upper limb and all the extensor muscles. Its branches are:

- axillary, C5, 6: to deltoid muscle (shoulder abduction), skin over deltoid muscle
- radial, C5–T1: to all extensor muscles, posterior skin of entire upper limb

- other branches: subscapular nerves, thoracodorsal nerves: to posterior scapular muscles and latissimus dorsi.

Lateral cord and branches   (Fig. 12.4)

The anterior divisions of the upper and middle trunks unite to form the lateral cord. Its branches are:

- musculocutaneous nerve, C5, 6, 7: to elbow flexors and lateral skin of the forearm
- contribution to the median nerve (see below)
- lateral pectoral: to pectoral muscles (not important).

Medial cord and branches   (Fig. 12.4)

The anterior division of the lower trunk forms the medial cord. Its branches are:

- ulnar nerve, C7, 8, T1: to a few forearm flexors, most hand muscles, and skin on the ulnar side of the hand

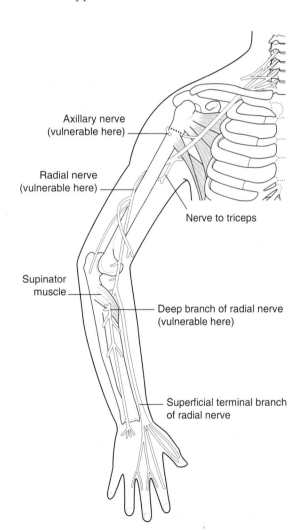

Axillary nerve
(vulnerable here)

Radial nerve
(vulnerable here)

Nerve to triceps

Supinator
muscle

Deep branch of radial nerve
(vulnerable here)

Superficial terminal branch
of radial nerve

Fig. 12.3   Radial and axillary nerves.

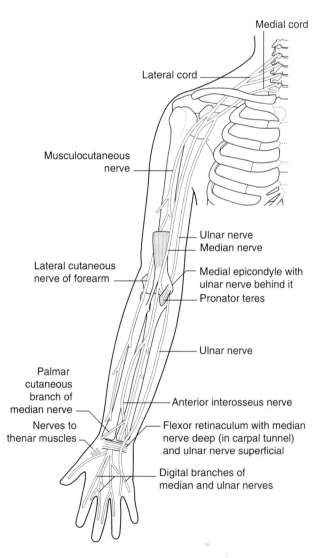

Medial cord

Lateral cord

Musculocutaneous
nerve

Ulnar nerve
Median nerve

Lateral cutaneous
nerve of forearm

Medial epicondyle with
ulnar nerve behind it
Pronator teres

Ulnar nerve

Palmar
cutaneous
branch of
median nerve

Anterior interosseus nerve

Nerves to
thenar muscles

Flexor retinaculum with median
nerve deep (in carpal tunnel)
and ulnar nerve superficial

Digital branches of
median and ulnar nerves

Fig. 12.4   Median, ulnar and musculocutaneous nerves.

- contribution to the median nerve (see below)
- medial pectoral: to pectoral muscles (not important)
- medial cutaneous nerves of the forearm and arm (C8, T1): functions are as their names imply (not particularly important).

Median nerve, plexus position and variations

- The median nerve is formed from all roots, C5–T1. The contributions from the lateral and medial cords may unite within a short distance, or they may remain separate until well down the arm. It supplies most forearm flexors, the thenar muscles of the hand, and skin of the radial side of the palm of the hand.
- The brachial plexus is found at the top of the rib cage. It is behind and beneath the clavicle and first rib, and trauma or disease in the posterior triangle of the neck may damage the upper trunk.
- The plexus may arise from C4–C8 (prefixed), or C5–T2 (postfixed).

Bones of the pectoral girdle

(Fig. 4.1, p. 20; Figs 12.5, 12.6)

Clavicle

The only feature of note is the tuberosity near the lateral end, for the attachment of the coracoclavicular ligaments. The clavicle tends to fracture immediately medial to this ligamentous attachment (see later).

Scapula

- The anterior or costal surface is plain and is the subscapular fossa (sub- because it is 'underneath' in the quadruped).

- The posterior or dorsal surface is divided by the spine into the supraspinous and infraspinous fossas.
- The spine is prolonged laterally to form the acromion, which articulates with the clavicle.
- Projecting from the upper margin is the coracoid process, palpable deep in the deltopectoral groove. It 'articulates' with the acromion by the coracoacromial ligament, and with the clavicle by the coracoclavicular ligaments.
- The glenoid fossa is the articular surface for the head of the humerus.

Movements and muscles of the pectoral girdle

Every time you move your upper limb, you move the

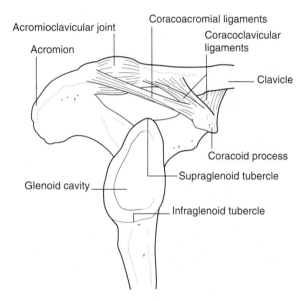

Fig. 12.6 Ligaments and bones of the pectoral girdle: lateral aspect, head of humerus removed.

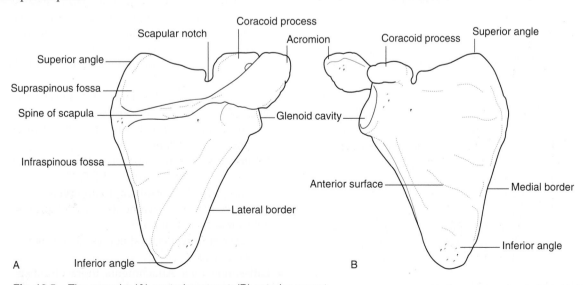

Fig. 12.5 The scapula: (**A**) posterior aspect; (**B**) anterior aspect.

clavicle and scapula. The joints that link them to the trunk are therefore important and disease of them will limit upper limb movement.

Joints and ligaments (Fig. 12.6)

Sternum – clavicle – scapula

- Sternoclavicular joint: synovial. Important relation: immediately posterior is the formation of the brachiocephalic vein from the subclavian and internal jugular veins. This joint sometimes disarticulates, the medial end of the clavicle appearing as a lump. It may or may not be painful, and often happens for no very obvious reason.
- Acromioclavicular joint: synovial.
- Coracoacromial 'articulation'. A strong ligament.
- Coracoclavicular 'articulation'. Strong ligaments, conoid and trapezoid, form an axis around which some rotation of the scapula on the clavicle (or vice versa) takes place, and the union is sufficiently strong for force transmitted up the arm from, say, a fall on the outstretched hand to fracture the clavicle medial to the attachment of the coracoclavicular ligament. The lateral portion of the fractured clavicle is displaced downwards by the weight of the upper limb.

Muscles (Figs 12.7, 12.8)

- Trapezius. Attachments: external occipital protuberance, spines of cervical (through ligamentum nuchae) and thoracic vertebrae – clavicle, acromion and lateral part of spine of

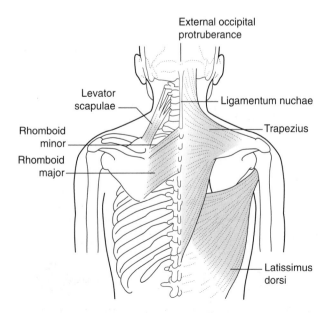

Fig. 12.7 Posterior scapular muscles.

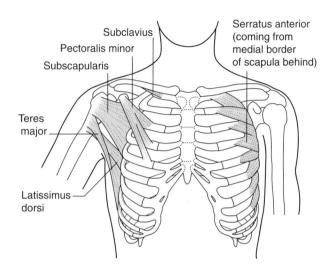

Fig. 12.8 Anterior scapular muscles.

scapula. Upper fibres pass to the clavicle, acromion and lateral end of the spine; lower fibres pass to the medial end of the spine.
  - Nerve supply: accessory (eleventh cranial) nerve. See Neck, page 239.
- Serratus anterior. Attachments: medial border of scapula – upper eight ribs. This runs laterally and anteriorly from the medial border of the scapula, between the scapula and the rib cage. It is important in a quadruped since it is one of the muscles that suspends the trunk from the limbs. Because of the separate digitations to the eight ribs, the anterior border appears serrated, hence the name serratus. (Serratus posterior muscle: don't even think about it.)
  - Nerve supply: long thoracic nerve (of Bell). This nerve runs on the medial wall of the axilla, or, if you prefer, on the lateral surface of the rib cage, and may be damaged in axillary surgery, or by trauma to the chest wall. Paralysis or weakness would result in winging of the scapula in which the medial border of the scapula was no longer closely apposed to the back of the rib cage. Shoulder protraction and abduction would be impaired.
- Levator scapulae. Attachments: C1–4 vertebrae – upper medial border of scapula.
  - Nerve supply: branches from C3, 4, 5 ventral rami. Unimportant.
- Rhomboids. Attachments: medial border of scapula – spines of thoracic vertebrae T2–5.
  - Nerve supply: dorsal scapular nerve.
- Pectoralis minor. Attachments: coracoid process – anterior aspect of ribs 3–5.
  - Nerve supply: pectoral nerves (details not necessary).
- Latissimus dorsi. Attachments: thoracolumbar vertebrae and lumbar fascia – humerus. It is

considered later, but a small portion of it attaches to the inferior angle of the scapula, and so it may be involved in scapular rotation.

– Nerve supply: thoracodorsal nerve from posterior cord.

Movements of the scapula

The scapula moves over the chest wall, but there are no distinct anatomical joints. Instead, muscles pull the scapula forward and backwards (protraction and retraction), and they rotate it so that the inferior angle moves laterally and up, and the superomedial angle medially and down.

- Protraction: serratus anterior, pectoralis minor.
- Retraction: trapezius (lower fibres), rhomboids (latissimus dorsi possibly).
- Rotation: trapezius (upper fibres), serratus anterior. Upper fibres of trapezius pull the acromioclavicular region superomedially, and the lower fibres of serratus anterior pull the inferior angle laterally and forwards. This means that the glenoid cavity faces upwards, and this movement is a necessary accompaniment of shoulder abduction (see later).

12.3 Shoulder region

Overview

The glenohumeral joint, an articulation between scapula and humerus, sacrifices stability for mobility. Movements in all planes are possible, ligaments and the rotator cuff muscles providing stability lacking in the bony conformation. These may be damaged giving rise to limitation of movement. Dislocations of the humeral head, or fractures of the surgical neck of the humerus, may damage the axillary nerve which supplies the principal shoulder abductor, deltoid.

Learning Objectives

You should:

- know the surface anatomy of the shoulder region
- know the principal features of the upper humerus and scapula
- know the main muscle groups producing shoulder movements, and their innervation
- understand how stability is provided at the joint, and the medical conditions that can arise.

Bones and ligaments

Scapula

- Glenoid fossa. This relatively shallow articular surface is made deeper by a circumferential lip of cartilage, the glenoid labrum. Above and below the fossa are two areas, the supra- and infraglenoid tubercles, to which the long heads of, respectively, biceps and triceps are attached.

Upper humerus   (Figs 12.9, 12.10)

- Head. This articulates with the glenoid fossa of the scapula.
- Anatomical neck. This is immediately distal to the head. Unimportant.
- Greater (lateral) and lesser (anteromedial) tuberosities provide attachments for muscles and are separated by the intertubercular sulcus or groove which, because it transmits the tendon of the long head of biceps is also known as the bicipital groove (the name used in this text).
- Surgical neck. This is important since it is a site of fracture and is related to the axillary nerve that passes from medial to lateral behind the surgical

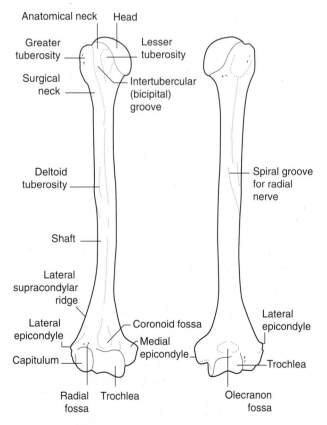

Fig. 12.9   Humerus: (**A**) anterior aspect; (**B**) posterior aspect.

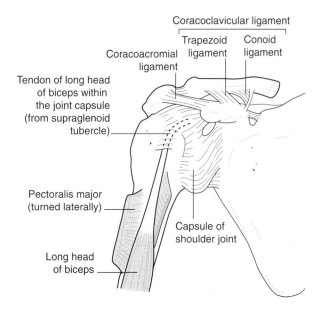

Fig. 12.10 Anterior view of shoulder joint.

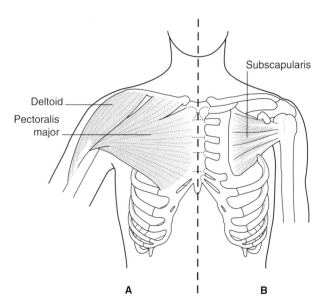

Fig. 12.11 Shoulder muscles attached to the humerus, anterior view: (**A**) muscles attached to the front of the rib cage and sternum; (**B**) muscles attached to the anterior aspect of the scapula, behind the rib cage.

neck. It may be damaged in surgical neck fractures or by shoulder dislocations. The circumflex humeral arteries are also related to it.

- Deltoid tuberosity. This is a roughness just above midway down the lateral aspect of the humerus. Deltoid muscle is attached here.
- Spiral groove. You will see a 'spiral' impression running from the upper medial aspect of the bone, behind the shaft and appearing on the lower lateral aspect. This is formed by the attachments of triceps muscle, but its importance lies in the fact that the radial nerve is close to the bone throughout the length of the groove. Mid-shaft fractures of the humerus may damage the radial nerve leading to paralysis or weakness of all extensor muscles distal to the injury. See later: wrist drop (12.8, p. 158).

Muscles of the shoulder region

- Pectoralis major (Fig. 12.11). Attachments: medial half of clavicle (the clavicular head) and sternum, ribs and external oblique aponeurosis (the sternocostal head) –
lateral lip of the bicipital groove of the humerus. The two heads can work separately. To demonstrate this, put your hand in front of your chest underneath a desk surface and pull up, feeling the muscle. Now put your hand on top of the desk and push down. Despite its size, we could live well enough without it. It flexes the shoulder (bringing the humerus in front of the chest) and adducts it (although gravity more often than not does this). It is large in creatures that swing from tree to tree and some athletes.
  - Nerve supply: medial and lateral pectoral nerves.

- Latissimus dorsi and teres major (Fig. 12.12). Latissimus dorsi attachments: lumbosacral fascia, spines of vertebrae L5 up to T7 – floor of the bicipital groove of the humerus. It has an extensive trunk attachment but a small humeral attachment. It is the posterior counterpart of pectoralis major, and extends and adducts the shoulder. As it sweeps past the inferior angle of the scapula it is joined by some fibres attached to that bone. It is very closely associated with teres major muscle.

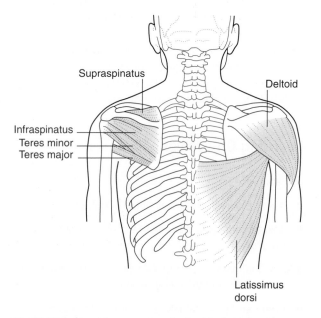

Fig. 12.12 Shoulder muscles attached to the humerus: posterior view.

Teres major attachments: lower lateral part of the scapula – medial edge of the bicipital groove of the humerus.

- Nerve supply of both muscles: branches of the posterior cord of the brachial plexus (as befits extensors), the nerve to latissimus dorsi being the thoracodorsal nerve.

● Deltoid (Figs 12.11, 12.12). Attachments: lateral end of spine of the scapula, acromion, acromioclavicular joint, lateral clavicle – deltoid tuberosity of the humerus.

- Nerve supply; axillary nerve C5, 6. This muscle is often the site of intramuscular injections. If you insert the needle within 4 cm of the acromion you are unlikely to damage the axillary nerve as it enters the muscle from behind the surgical neck of the humerus. If you go lower than this, you deserve to be prosecuted for incompetence.

● Rotator cuff muscles (Figs 12.12, 12.13). The four muscles of the rotator cuff form a protective sheath for the shoulder joint behind, on top and in front. They are, from back to front:

- Teres minor: lateral aspect of scapula (above teres major) – posterior surface of greater tuberosity of humerus. It is really a slightly detached part of the infraspinatus. Nerve supply: axillary nerve (C5, 6).

- Infraspinatus: infraspinous fossa of the scapula – greater tuberosity of humerus. Nerve supply: suprascapular nerve (C5, 6).

- Supraspinatus: supraspinous fossa of the scapula – upper part of greater tuberosity of humerus. Nerve supply: suprascapular nerve (C5, 6).

- Subscapularis: anterior (costal) surface of scapula (subscapular fossa) – lesser tuberosity of

humerus. Nerve supply: subscapular nerves from posterior cord of brachial plexus.

● Biceps and coracobrachialis (Fig. 12.14). Biceps has two heads: the long head is attached to the supraglenoid tubercle of the scapula; the short head is attached to the coracoid process. The tendon of the long head originates within the shoulder joint capsule and passes between the capsule and the synovium to emerge at the bicipital groove of the humerus through which it runs. The two bellies of biceps unite inferiorly to attach to the radius and to the fascia over forearm flexor muscles. Biceps crosses two joints, shoulder and elbow, flexing them both. It is also considered in relation to the elbow joint (see 12.5, p. 167).

Coracobrachialis (unimportant): coracoid process of the scapula – upper humerus.

Both muscles contribute to shoulder flexion.

- Nerve supply: musculocutaneous nerve (C5, 6) which, having supplied these muscles, continues distally with a new name: the lateral cutaneous nerve of the forearm (Fig. 12.4).

● Triceps (Fig. 12.15). Attachments: scapula and humerus – ulna. Triceps has three heads:

- long, from the infraglenoid tubercle of the scapula

- lateral, from the back of the humerus, above and lateral to the radial groove (more superficial than lateral)

- medial, from the back of the humerus, below and medial to the radial groove (more deep than medial).

The radial nerve runs through the muscle in the spiral groove of the humerus between the lateral and medial heads.

- Nerve supply: radial nerve (C7, 8).

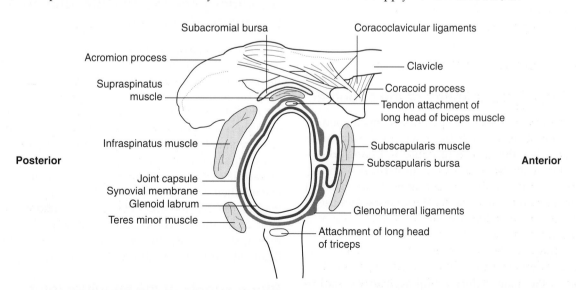

Fig. 12.13 Diagrammatic view of glenoid fossa from the lateral aspect with head of humerus removed. Rotator cuff muscles are shown.

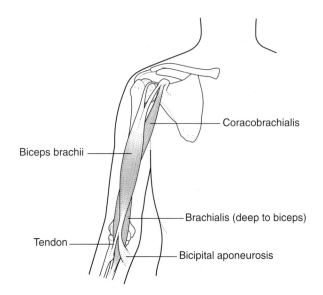

Fig. 12.14 Elbow flexors.

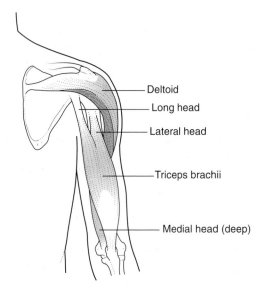

Fig. 12.15 Posterior aspect of arm.

Movements and stability of the shoulder

The articular surfaces of the shoulder are not a good fit. This means that although the range of movement is very extensive, the joint is unstable and liable to disarticulation with the head of the humerus dislocating, usually anteroinferiorly. Compensating to some extent for the lack of bony stability are the rotator cuff muscles and the glenohumeral ligaments.

Abduction

Deltoid is the main abductor. Supraspinatus is said to initiate the movement by holding the head of the humerus on the scapula so that the deltoid can get

some purchase on the movement, but electromyography studies show that both muscles act throughout. When the arm is abducted to about 90°, the greater tuberosity of the humerus comes in contact with the acromion and there is some lateral rotation of the humerus so that more movement is possible.

The accepted wisdom handed down from text to text is that after 90° of abduction the scapula rotates as a result of the action of serratus anterior and trapezius (see above), which allows the arm to be abducted much further. This is wrong, as you will see if you use your eyes: the scapula begins to rotate well before even 45° abduction is reached. Inability to abduct beyond 90°, such as might result from weakness of trapezius and serratus anterior is a nuisance: it would mean that you could not groom your hair, scratch your head, reach for high shelves, and so on.

Nerve supply of abduction:

- deltoid and supraspinatus: axillary, suprascapular nerves (both C5, 6)
- scapular rotation: long thoracic nerve (C5, 6, 7); accessory (eleventh cranial) nerve.

Flexion, extension

See above – pectoralis major, biceps, coracobrachialis, latissimus dorsi.

Rotation

- Lateral rotation: mainly by infraspinatus, teres minor and posterior fibres of deltoid.
- Medial rotation: mainly by pectoralis major, subscapularis and teres major.

Shoulder joint capsule, glenohumeral ligaments, dislocations (Fig. 12.13)

The joint capsule is reinforced by the tendons of the rotator cuff muscles and anteriorly also by three thickenings, the glenohumeral ligaments (Fig. 12.13). With the rotator cuff muscles, these help to compensate for the poor fit of the articular surfaces. Inferior to the joint there is neither rotator cuff muscle nor capsular reinforcement – a potential weakness taken advantage of by shoulder dislocations. Sports players (particularly of racquet sports) and others who habitually hyperextend their shoulder joints may stretch the anterior wall of the capsule and subscapularis tendon so that joint dislocation becomes more common. This can be managed surgically by tightening the glenohumeral ligaments and/or the subscapularis tendon.

Blood supply of the shoulder joint

The blood supply of any joint is profuse. It is necessary

to know only that branches of the anterior and posterior circumflex humerals, axillary and brachial arteries supply the shoulder.

Nerve supply of the shoulder joint

As usual (Hilton's law), sensory fibres from the joint are carried in nerves which supply muscles acting on the joint, particularly the axillary nerve C5, 6.

Clinical box

Synovial cavity and bursas (Fig. 12.13)
The synovial cavity extends inferiorly for some distance, presumably to allow for hyperabduction.

- Subacromial or subdeltoid bursa. This lies between supraspinatus tendon (below) and the acromioclavicular articulation and the attachment of deltoid (above). It has two names because in adduction the bursa is more lateral (subdeltoid), but in abduction it is more medial (subacromial). It is separate from the joint cavity unless supraspinatus tendon is torn.
- Other bursas. There is usually a bursa, an extension of the joint space, deep to subscapularis muscle. Other bursas may also be found.

Nerve injuries
- Axillary nerve: this may be damaged by fractures of the surgical neck of the humerus, or by shoulder dislocations.
- Radial nerve: this may be damaged in the spiral groove by midshaft humeral fractures.

Other conditions
Inflammation of the attachment of supraspinatus to the greater tuberosity is one cause of 'frozen shoulder', rotator cuff syndromes, or impingement sydromes (all meaning much the same). It can be very painful and disabling, substantially limiting movement.

Surface anatomy

Normally the most lateral bony point of the skeleton is the greater tuberosity of the humerus. In shoulder dislocations, the head of the humerus is displaced down and medially, and the most lateral point is then the acromion process.

12.4 Axilla

Overview

The axilla is bounded by the anterior and posterior axillary folds, the humerus and the rib cage. It contains axillary vessels, components of the brachial plexus, and lymph nodes so often involved in breast disease.

Learning Objectives

You should:

- know the boundaries and contents of the axilla
- know the main groups of axillary lymph nodes and the areas and organs, particularly the breast, that drain to them.

Spatial considerations   (Fig. 12.16)

The axilla is like a distorted four-sided pyramid:

- base: skin of the armpit
- anterior wall: anterior axillary fold made up of pectoralis major muscle
- medial wall: chest wall with the long thoracic nerve (to serratus anterior) and the lateral thoracic artery passing down
- posterior wall: posterior axillary fold made up of latissimus dorsi and teres major muscles
- lateral 'wall': the anterior and posterior walls converge on the bicipital groove of the humerus that contains the tendon of the long head of biceps.

Contents

- Vessels: axillary artery and vein with branches and tributaries (see 12.2, p.153).
- Nerves: divisions, cords and branches of the brachial plexus (see 12.2, p. 155).
- Lymph nodes (Fig. 12.17):
  - anterior or pectoral group: lymph from most of the breast
  - posterior or subscapular group: lymph from the upper trunk and axillary tail of the breast

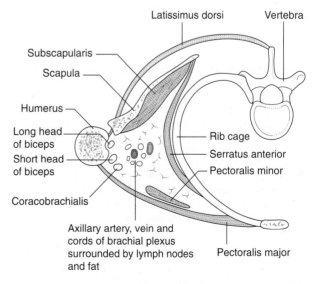

Fig. 12.16   Horizontal section through the axilla.

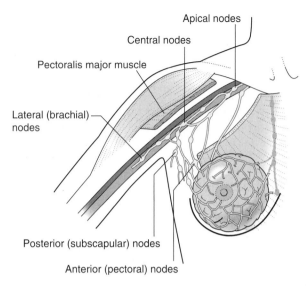

Apical nodes

Central nodes

Pectoralis major muscle

Lateral (brachial) nodes

Posterior (subscapular) nodes

Anterior (pectoral) nodes

Fig. 12.17   Axillary lymph nodes.

- lateral group: lymph from the ulnar side of the upper limb
- central group: lymph from all the above groups
- apical group: lymph from the central group (i.e. all the above) and the deltopectoral (infraclavicular) nodes (lymph from radial side of upper limb, alongside the cephalic vein).
  From the apical group, which gathers all together, lymph passes to the origin of the brachiocephalic veins where it enters the venous system.
- Fascia. The clavipectoral fascia extends from the clavicle down in the floor of the deltopectoral groove (triangle) and splits to enclose pectoralis minor muscle. Below this, it continues as the suspensory ligament of the axilla that attaches to the axillary skin. None of these details is important.

Clinical box

Long thoracic nerve (of Bell)

It is important in axillary surgery (e.g. for breast cancer) not to damage the long thoracic nerve. This would result in winging of the scapula, impaired shoulder abduction and loss of function. The nerve may also be damaged in those poor unfortunates who fall asleep, for whatever reason, with their arms over the back of a chair.

Lymph from the upper limb

Breast surgery in which the lymphatic channels from the upper limb are occluded will result in lymphoedema (lymphatic engorgement) of the upper limb. This is fortunately less common now with improved pharmacological treatments available.

12.5 Arm, elbow, cubital fossa, supination, pronation

Overview

At the elbow, the radiohumeral articulation permits flexion and extension, and the superior radioulnar joint permits pronation and supination. The cubital fossa anterior to the elbow contains the termination of the brachial artery and the median nerve, and is covered by the bicipital aponeurosis. The ulnar nerve passes posterior to the medial epicondyle. Elbow flexion is supplied by C5, 6; extension by C7, 8; pronation and supination by C5, 6.

Learning Objectives

You should:

- know the surface anatomy of the elbow region and the cubital fossa
- understand the mechanism of pronation and supination
- know the innervation of the principal muscles acting at the elbow and superior radioulnar joints.

Bones, joints and ligaments

Mid- and lower humerus   (Fig. 12.9)

- Spiral (radial) groove and triceps attachments: see above.
- Trochlea: rounded articular surface for the ulna.
- Capitulum: rounded articular surface for the radius.
- Coronoid fossa: coronoid process of ulna fits here in flexion.
- Olecranon fossa: olecranon process of ulna fits here in extension.
- Medial epicondyle: the common origin of the forearm superficial flexors is here; the ulnar nerve passes posteriorly to the bone and may be damaged here.
- Lateral epicondyle: the common origin of the forearm extensors is here.

Proximal ulna   (Fig. 12.18)

- Olecranon process: triceps attachment.
- Coronoid process: brachialis is attached to its anterior aspect.

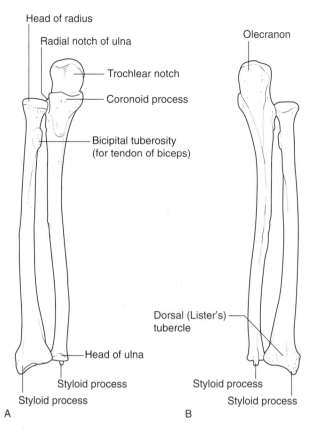

Fig. 12.18   Ulna and radius: (**A**) anterior view; (**B**) posterior view.

- Between the olecranon and coronoid processes is the articular surface for the humerus at which flexion and extension take place.
- Articular surface for radius.
- Interosseous border.

Ulna or ulnar?

Ulna is the name of the bone; ulnar is an adjective that describes other things, as in the ulnar side of the hand.

Proximal radius   (Fig. 12.18)

- Head. This articulates with:
  - the capitulum of the humerus, as part of the elbow flexion–extension mechanism; and
  - the ulna, as part of the pronation–supination mechanism (see below).
- Neck: immediately distal to the head; the deep branch of the radial nerve (posterior interosseous nerve) is vulnerable here. Damage to it (e.g. radial neck fractures, radial head dislocations) would impair function of the wrist and digital extension.
- Bicipital tuberosity. The tendon of biceps attaches here.

Annular ligament: pronation and supination
(Fig. 12.19)

The head of the radius is held against the ulna by the annular ligament attached to the upper and lower margins of the ulnar facet for the superior radioulnar joint. During pronation and supination the head of the radius rotates within this (see below).

Elbow joint   (Fig. 12.19)

Functionally, there are two joints although only one synovial cavity:

- Humerus – ulna: synovial hinge joint for flexion and extension.
- Superior (proximal) radioulnar joint: for pronation and supination. See above.

Injuries

- The ulna can be dislocated posteriorly.
- The head of the radius may be pulled distally, with or without damaging the annular ligament. This is

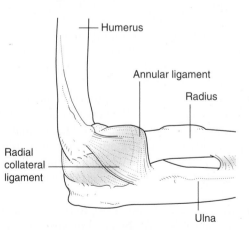

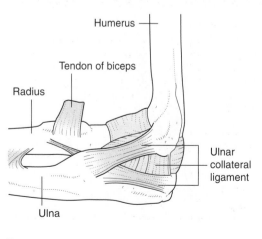

Fig. 12.19   Elbow joint, capsule and ligaments: (**A**) lateral view; (**B**) medial view.

more common in children since the head of the radius is still cartilaginous and the annular ligament is not such a tight fit as in the adult. The deep branch of the radial nerve may be damaged.

Surface anatomy of the elbow region

- The olecranon and the medial and lateral epicondyles are all palpable. Viewed from behind, these should form an almost isosceles triangle with the olecranon at the apex. This arrangement is disrupted in elbow dislocations.
- The head of the radius is also palpable about 2 cm distal to the lateral epicondyle. You can confirm that it is the head of the radius by feeling it rotate during pronation and supination.

Brachial artery   (Fig. 12.20)

- The brachial artery is a continuation of the axillary at the lower border of teres major. It descends in the flexor compartment of the arm. Soon after its origin it gives off:
- The profunda brachii artery, or deep branch (it usually retains its Latin title), which passes laterally with the radial nerve into the spiral groove.

Brachial pulse

The brachial pulse is palpable by pressing the artery from the medial aspect against the humerus. The artery passes anterior to the elbow joint, and bifurcates in the cubital fossa into the radial and ulnar arteries. Occasionally this bifurcation may occur much higher, in the arm itself.

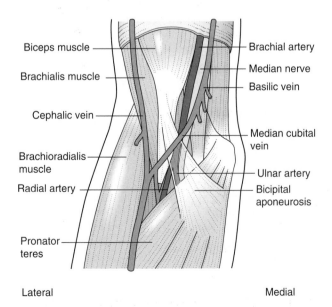

Biceps muscle — Brachial artery
Brachialis muscle — Median nerve
— Basilic vein
Cephalic vein —
— Median cubital vein
Brachioradialis muscle —
— Ulnar artery
Radial artery — Bicipital aponeurosis
Pronator teres —

Lateral   Medial

Fig. 12.20   Cubital fossa and contents.

Cubital fossa   (Fig. 12.20)

The triangular area in front of and slightly distal to the elbow is the cubital, or antecubital, fossa. Cubit means variously ulna, elbow or pertaining to the forearm (the Biblical unit of measurement, the cubit, was the length of the forearm). The fossa is bounded proximally by an imaginary line joining the two humeral epicondyles, and distally by the pronator teres muscle on the ulnar side and the brachioradialis on the radial side.

The cubital fossa is often the site of injections into superficial veins. Its major contents are:

- the biceps tendon (easily palpable), medial (ulnar) to which is
- the brachial artery and its bifurcation, medial (ulnar) to which is
- the median nerve.

Fortunately, from the point of view of inserting needles into superficial veins, these important structures are covered by a sheet of tough fascia extending from the biceps muscle and tendon medially to the deep fascia over the forearm flexor muscles: this is the bicipital aponeurosis and is part of the distal attachment of biceps (see later).

The floor of the fossa is formed by brachialis muscle (lower anterior humerus – coronoid process of ulna) which is an elbow flexor.

Nerves of the elbow region

- Radial nerve. From the spiral groove, the nerve emerges laterally deep between brachialis and brachioradialis. At the elbow it divides into:
  - the superficial branch, usually known simply as the radial nerve, which runs down the radial side of the forearm and supplies overlying skin and that of the back of the hand; and
  - the deep branch (posterior interosseous nerve) which passes through supinator muscle, winds round the neck of the radius and enters the posterior compartment of the forearm to supply extensor muscles.
- Ulnar nerve. From its origin from the medial cord of the brachial plexus, the nerve passes down the medial side of the arm, behind the medial epicondyle of the humerus (where it is vulnerable), through the forearm where it supplies flexor muscles and anterior skin, to the hand (see 12.7, p. 176).
- Median nerve. From its origin from the lateral and medial cords of the brachial plexus, the nerve passes down the arm on brachialis to the cubital fossa where it is medial to the brachial artery. In the forearm it penetrates pronator teres muscle and

continues deep to flexor digitorum superficialis into the forearm and hand flexor muscles and anterior skin.

- Other nerves:
  - Lateral cutaneous nerve of the forearm, the nerve known at its origin as the musculocutaneous, supplying elbow flexors. Its new name indicates its distal function. It is otherwise unimportant.
  - Medial cutaneous nerve of the forearm. Unimportant.

Muscles and movements of the elbow

Flexion   (Figs 12.14, 12.19)

Flexion of the elbow is performed by: brachialis, biceps – musculocutaneous nerve, C5, 6, and brachioradialis – radial nerve, C5, 6.

- Brachialis. Attachments: anterior lower humerus – coronoid process of ulna.
- Biceps. Attachments: scapula – radius. Biceps was considered as a flexor of the shoulder (see 12.3, p. 159). It also flexes the elbow and supinates the forearm. The proximal attachment is to the scapula (long and short heads – see 12.3). The distal attachment has two components:
  - the tendon of biceps, which attaches to the bicipital tuberosity of the radius
  - the bicipital aponeurosis, which passes medially from the lower part of the muscle belly and neighbouring tendon, protecting the contents of the cubital fossa, and blending with the fascia over the forearm flexor muscles.

    There are two bellies that unite inferiorly to attach to the ulna and to the fascia over forearm flexor muscles (see later). The biceps tendon jerk (C5, 6), elicited by tapping the biceps tendon in the cubital fossa, is a commonly used neurological test (see 12.8, p. 177).
- Brachioradialis. Attachments: humerus – radius. This is embryologically an extensor muscle (thus radial nerve) which has strayed from the straight and narrow path. It forms the radial (lateral) edge of the forearm, and the radial border of the cubital fossa. When you are lifting a heavy object held in the hand with the thumb uppermost, this muscle forms the sloping upper edge of the forearm. It is also involved in supination. It is possible to elicit a reflex by tapping the tendon of brachioradialis: this is still often known as the 'supinator' reflex because the old name for the muscle was supinator longus.

Extension   (Fig. 12.15)

The extensor muscle of the elbow is triceps, supplied by the radial nerve (C7, 8). Attachments: scapula, humerus – ulna. Triceps has three heads:

- long, from the infraglenoid tubercle of the scapula
- lateral, from the back of the humerus, above and lateral to the radial groove, more superficial than lateral
- medial, from the back of the humerus, below and medial to the radial groove, more deep than medial.

The radial nerve thus runs through the muscle between the attachments of the lateral and medial heads to the humerus. The triceps tendon jerk (C7, 8), elicited by tapping the attachment of triceps just above the olecranon, is a commonly used neurological test (see 12.8, p. 177).

An accessory extensor of the elbow is anconeus – entirely trivial and unimportant.

Pronation and supination   (Figs 12.19, 12.21)

As described earlier, the head of the radius rotates within the annular ligament. This occurs in pronation and supination as you can demonstrate to yourself. First flex your elbow to about 90° with the palm of your hand facing up and the thumb lateral: this is the supine position. Now turn the palm down, so that the thumb comes to be medial: this is the action of pronation and the forearm is now pronated, or in the prone position. Throughout this movement, the ulna

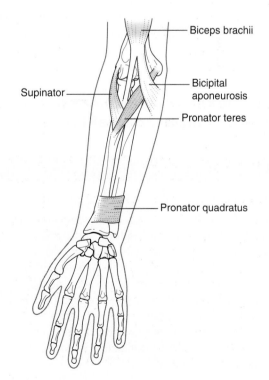

Fig. 12.21   Muscles of pronation and supination: anterior view.

remains almost stationary (as you can feel); it is the radius that moves with its head rotating as above and its distal (inferior) end moving in an arc over the ulna.

- Pronation: pronator teres, pronator quadratus, median nerve, C6.
- Supination: biceps and supinator, musculocutaneous and radial nerves, C5, 6.

Biceps as a supinator: using a screwdriver. With the elbow flexed at 90° the tendon of biceps approaches the bicipital tuberosity of the radius directly from above and is perfectly placed to cause rotation of the radius within the annular ligament. Also, the bicipital aponeurosis aids supination by traction on the fascia over the superficial forearm flexors. Biceps is a very powerful supinator.

Tightening a screw for a right-handed person involves supination against resistance, whereas for a left-handed person it involved pronation against resistance; this is why right-handed people are better screwers and left-handed people are better unscrewers (unless you buy special left-handed screws).

Supinator: humerus, ulna, joint capsule – radius. It is attached to the posterior surface of the proximal ulna, the back of the annular ligament and the adjacent elbow joint capsule and the lateral humeral epicondyle. It sweeps laterally and wraps itself around the lateral aspect of the radius. When it contracts it 'unwraps' the radius so that supination takes place. It is supplied by the radial nerve (C6) which divides into superficial and deep branches on its surface, the deep (posterior interosseous nerve) passing through the substance of the muscle as its approaches the neck of the radius (Fig. 12.3).

12.6 Flexor compartment of the forearm, carpus, carpal tunnel

Overview

The distal radius articulates with the scaphoid and lunate. The radius and scaphoid may be fractured by a fall on the outstretched hand. The radial and ulnar pulses are commonly felt at the wrist, and the surface anatomy of this region is important since it is often injured. Forearm flexor muscles are supplied by the median and ulnar nerves, and extensors by the radial nerve. Flexor tendons pass from the forearm to the hand through the carpal tunnel, which also contains the median nerve, which is therefore vulnerable in carpal tunnel syndrome.

Learning Objectives

You should:

- know the innervation of the principal muscles acting on the wrist
- know the surface markings of the bones, nerves and vessels at the wrist
- know the surface markings of flexor retinaculum and its attachments
- understand the anatomy and the clinical manifestations of carpal tunnel syndrome.

Bones

Revise the cubital fossa, pronation and supination.

Interosseous membrane

This structure is attached to the interosseous borders of the radius and ulna, occupying most of the area between the bones. It separates the flexor compartment anteriorly from the extensor compartment posteriorly and helps to stabilise the two bones, playing a role in weightbearing. Some people regard it as an intermediate radioulnar joint.

Distal radius   (Fig. 12.18)

The distal end of the radius is larger than the proximal end. The head of the radius is the smaller, proximal, end. Note the following:

- interosseous border
- articular surface for ulna
- articular surface for scaphoid and lunate
- dorsal (Lister's) tubercle
- styloid process.

Clinical box

Colles' fracture, Smith's fracture
These are fractures of the lower end of the radius, named after two Dublin surgeons. Colles' fracture involves a dorsal displacement (so-called 'dinner fork' deformity) of the distal radius on the shaft, and Smith's involves an anterior displacement. Colles' fracture is a very common consequence of a fall on the outstretched hand, Smith's after a fall on the back of the flexed wrist.

Distal ulna   (Fig. 12.18)

The distal end of the ulna is smaller than the proximal end. The head of the ulna is the smaller, distal, end. Note the following:

- interosseous border
- articular surface for radius
- styloid process
- distal end.

The ulna does not articulate with the carpal bones at all: between the ulna and the carpal bones is the triangular fibrocartilage of the wrist joint.

Carpal bones (Fig. 12.22)

For most bones it is simply necessary to know only the names. But you must be able to identify them on a skeleton, on a radiograph and know where to palpate the hamate, scaphoid and trapezium.

- Proximal row, radial side to ulnar side:
  - Scaphoid. Articulates with the radius. Palpable in the anatomical snuffbox. The shape and blood supply of the scaphoid are important. It has a narrow waist which is prone to fracture as a result of a fall on the outstretched hand. Since the proximal portion articulates with the radius, blood vessels can enter the proximal portion only through the waist from the distal portion, and if the waist is fractured, the proximal portion may undergo avascular necrosis.
  - Lunate. Articulates with the radius. May dislocate and damage the median nerve.
  - Triquetral.

- Pisiform. This is actually a sesamoid bone in the tendon of flexor carpi ulnaris. It is easily palpable.
- Distal row, ulnar side to radial side:
  - Hamate. This has an anterior projection, the hook, which is palpable on deep palpation in the hypothenar eminence.
  - Capitate. The biggest.
  - Trapezoid.
  - Trapezium. This is immediately distal to the scaphoid and also palpable in the anatomical snuffbox.

The wrist joint

It is not necessary to go into details, but you should know that the radius articulates with the scaphoid and lunate (you can see this on the distal end of the radius), and that movements take place at all the joints between the carpal bones, the radius and the metacarpals. Numerous ligaments connect the bones together: details of these are unnecessary.

Arteries, pulses

The ulnar and radial arteries arise in the cubital fossa and pass down the forearm to the wrist and hand.

- The common interosseous is an early branch of the ulnar artery. It divides into anterior and posterior

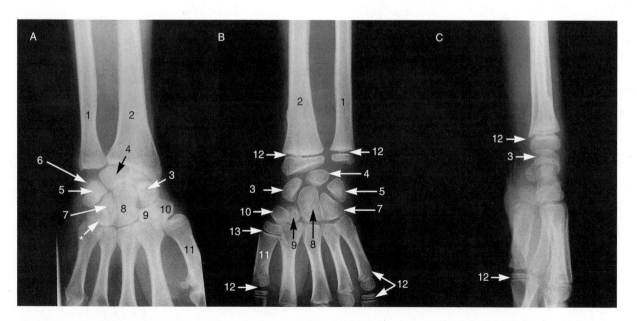

Fig. 12.22 Radiographs of carpus and hand: (**A**) adult; (**B**) child; (**C**) child, lateral view. 1, ulna; 2, radius; 3, scaphoid; 4, lunate; 5, triquetral; 6, pisiform (not present in B or C); 7, hamate, * indicates hook; 8, capitate; 9, trapezoid; 10, trapezium; 11, first metacarpal; 12, epiphyseal lines in B and C – these demonstrate the immaturity of the patient; the lack of a visible pisiform, but the presence of the other carpal bones, means that the child, if normal, is between 7 and 12 years of age; 13, the epiphysis of the first metacarpal is proximal, not distal like those of metacarpals 2–5 – this demonstrates the fact that embryologically, the first metacarpal is a phalanx by another name.

interosseous arteries supplying, respectively, the flexor and extensor compartments of the forearm muscles.

- The radial pulse is palpated just proximal to the wrist joint by pressing the artery on to the anterior surface of the radius, lateral to flexor carpi radialis tendon. It is the most commonly palpated pulse. Distal to this, the radial artery passes laterally to the anatomical snuffbox.
- The ulnar pulse is also easily palpated just proximal to the wrist on the radial side of flexor carpi ulnaris tendon.

Nerves

- The ulnar nerve passes down the ulnar side of the forearm. It is vulnerable to slash wounds in the distal forearm.
- The median nerve passes more or less in the midline of the forearm (hence its name) on the posterior surface of flexor digitorum superficialis muscle. It is less vulnerable, being deep to flexor digitorum superficialis muscle and tendons.
- The radial nerve (the superficial branch: cutaneous only) passes on the radial side of the forearm.

Muscles and movements

Flexor muscles: C6, 7 (Fig. 12.23)

The forearm flexor muscles act upon the wrist joint and fingers. They are for power, unlike the small muscles of the hand (see below) which are for precision. They arise from the common flexor origin (medial epicondyle of the humerus), the proximal radius and ulna and the interosseous membrane. Precise details are not necessary. There are three groups, from superficial to deep:

Superficial flexors (Fig. 12.23A). Four muscles radiate from the common flexor origin. From radial to ulnar sides, these are:

- Pronator teres. Attachments: common flexor origin – mid-shaft of the radius.
- Flexor carpi radialis. Attachments: common flexor origin – first and second metacarpals. This is the large tendon on the radial side of the wrist.
- Palmaris longus. Attachments: common flexor origin – palmar aponeurosis. This is the small tendon more or less in the midline at the wrist. It may be absent on one or both sides.

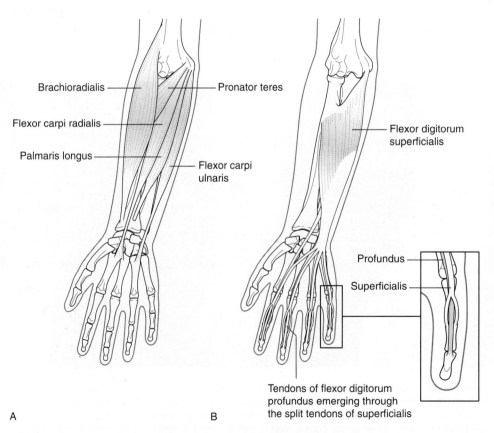

Brachioradialis

Pronator teres

Flexor carpi radialis

Palmaris longus

Flexor carpi ulnaris

Flexor digitorum superficialis

Profundus

Superficialis

Tendons of flexor digitorum profundus emerging through the split tendons of superficialis

A   B

Fig. 12.23   Forearm flexors: (**A**) superficial group; (**B**) intermediate group. Note splitting of tendon of flexor digitorum superficialis to allow tendon of flexor digitorum profundus to pass (see inset).

- Flexor carpi ulnaris. Attachments: common flexor origin – fifth metacarpal by means of the pisiform (sesamoid bone).

Nerve supply: median nerve, except for flexor carpi ulnaris which is supplied by the ulnar nerve.

Intermediate flexors (Fig. 12.23B): flexor digitorum superficialis. Attachments: radius, ulna, interosseous membrane – middle phalanx of each finger (digits 2–5). Nerve supply: median nerve, which passes immediately deep to this muscle.

Deep flexors (Fig. 12.24):

- Flexor digitorum profundus. Attachments: radius, ulna, interosseous membrane – terminal phalanx of each finger (digits 2–5).
- Flexor pollicis longus. Attachments: radius, interosseous membrane – distal phalanx of thumb.
- Pronator quadratus. Attachments: ulna – radius. This is a quadrilateral muscle running from side to side in the distal forearm. It wraps itself over the front of the radius to attach to the lateral side of the radius, so that when it contracts it pulls the distal end of the radius over the ulna in pronation.

Nerve supply: median nerve, except for the two bellies of flexor digitorum profundus to digits 4 and 5 which are supplied by the ulnar nerve.

Do I have to learn all these muscles?

No. These muscles act together and from a functional point of view it is not necessary to be able to recognise or name them individually. They are all supplied by the median and ulnar nerves, C6, 7. Nevertheless, some of them are worth singling out simply as reference points when describing the position of structures or lesions. These are:

- the common flexor origin from the medial humeral epicondyle
- flexor carpi radialis at the wrist
- flexor carpi ulnaris at the wrist.

Extensor muscles   (Fig. 12.25)

These are all supplied by branches of the radial nerve. Details of these are certainly unnecessary. They include: extensor pollicis longus (thumb), extensor pollicis brevis (thumb), abductor pollicis longus (thumb), extensor digitorum (fingers); extensor indicis (the index finger is singled out for special treatment); extensor carpi radialis longus and brevis (to the metacarpals), extensor carpi ulnaris (to the metacarpals). Knowledge of detailed attachments is not necessary. Nerve supply: radial nerve, C6, 7, 8. See wrist drop (12.8, p. 178).

Anatomical snuffbox   (Fig. 12.25)

This is the area at the wrist between the tendons of extensor pollicis longus on the ulnar side (just after it

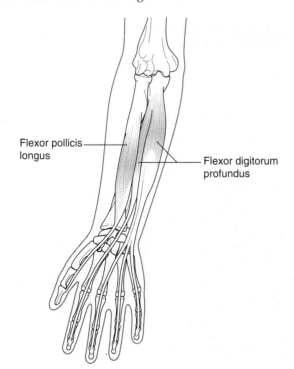

Fig. 12.24   Deep forearm flexors.

Flexor pollicis longus

Flexor digitorum profundus

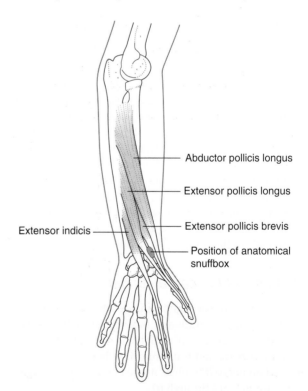

Abductor pollicis longus

Extensor pollicis longus

Extensor pollicis brevis

Position of anatomical snuffbox

Extensor indicis

Fig. 12.25   Superficial forearm extensors and anatomical snuffbox.

has changed direction around the dorsal (Lister's) tubercle of the radius), and extensor pollicis brevis and abductor pollicis longus on the radial side. The radial artery is palpable in the snuffbox together with the scaphoid and the trapezium. Tenderness here is strongly suggestive of a fractured scaphoid.

Other movements

Lateral flexion in both ulnar and radial directions takes place at the radiocarpal joint. Muscles causing these movements are predictable. For example, flexor carpi radialis acts as a radial flexor when used with extensor carpi radialis muscles, but as a flexor when used with flexor carpi ulnaris.

Carpus, carpal tunnel

Wrist creases and surface anatomy

Proximal and distal wrist creases are found on the flexor aspect of the distal forearm. The distal crease marks the approximate level of the radius–scaphoid–lunate articulation. All the carpal bones are distal to the distal wrist crease.

Palpable bones are:

- scaphoid and trapezium on the radial side
- pisiform and hamate on the ulnar side.

Carpal tunnel and flexor retinaculum

(Fig. 12.26)

The proximal and distal rows of carpal bones fit together forming a concavity facing anteriorly (as viewed from the palmar aspect) which is maintained by the flexor retinaculum – attached like a tiebeam to the trapezium and scaphoid laterally and the pisiform and hamate medially. Between the tiebeam and the bones is thus an enclosed space, the carpal tunnel, through which most of the structures pass between hand and forearm.

Surface markings of flexor retinaculum. These are an approximately 2-cm square immediately distal to the middle of the distal wrist crease.

Contents of the carpal tunnel

- Tendons of flexor digitorum superficialis, flexor digitorum profundus and flexor pollicis longus. (The tendon of flexor carpi radialis is in a separate compartment and is unimportant here.)
- Median nerve (the ulnar nerve passes superficial to the tunnel, not through it).

Clinical box

Carpal tunnel syndrome

Swelling in the carpal tunnel (for example caused by fluid retention in pregnancy), or a space-occupying lesion here, may compress the median nerve in the carpal tunnel causing:

- motor loss in the thenar muscles
- sensory changes over the palmar aspect of (usually) the radial three and a half digits.

This is carpal tunnel syndrome. The thenar muscles are involved because the thenar (or recurrent) branch of the median nerve which supplies them does not leave the main trunk of the nerve until after it has passed through the tunnel. The skin over the thenar muscles is not affected because the palmar cutaneous branch is given off by the median nerve proximal to the wrist in the forearm. Carpal tunnel syndrome may require incision of the flexor retinaculum to relieve the pressure.

Ossification of the carpal bones (Fig. 12.22)

It is sometimes useful to know that carpal bones ossify in order of size approximately annually beginning with the capitate (the largest) in year 1. The pisiform, though, does not usually ossify until about year 12. This is relevant to the radiographic appearance of the wrist of a child and may be used to assess chronological age in relation to 'metabolic' age.

12.7 Hand

Overview

The hand is a complex structure permitting great subtlety of digital movement. Power movements are performed by forearm muscles with long tendons, fine movements by intrinsic muscles of the hand. All intrinsic hand muscles are supplied by axons from ventral horn cells of spinal segment T1: thenar muscles principally by the median nerve, hypothenar muscles by the ulnar nerve, and abduction and adduction by both nerves. The radial nerve supplies dorsal skin, the median and ulnar supplying palmar skin. Arterial blood comes from superficial and deep palmar arterial arches formed by branches of the radial and ulnar arteries. Palmar fascial spaces allow infection to collect in the hand and spread to the forearm.

Learning Objectives

You should:

- know the names and surface anatomy of all carpal bones, and be able to recognise them on radiographs
- know the surface markings of the nerves and vessels of the hand
- know the innervation of the thenar and hypothenar muscles
- understand the anatomical basis of dermatome testing in the hand
- understand the anatomical basis of motor nerve testing in the hand.

Digits: names or numbers?

Digit 1 is the thumb or pollux (adjective: pollicis); digit 2 is the index finger; 3 is the middle finger, 4 is the ring finger; 5 is the little finger (pinkie).

Bones   (Fig. 12.22)

Revise carpal bones.

- Metacarpals 1–5
- Phalanges. The thumb (digit 1) has two phalanges, proximal and distal. The fingers (digits 2–5) have three phalanges, proximal, intermediate and distal.

Despite accepted terminology, the first metacarpal is embryologically a phalanx, so the thumb has three phalanges (like the other digits) but no metacarpal. You can see this in a radiograph of an immature hand: the epiphyseal line in the first metacarpal is distal, as for a phalanx, rather than proximal, as for a true metacarpal (Fig. 12.22).

Joints

- Carpometacarpal, metacarpophalangeal and interphalangeal joints are all synovial.
- The first carpometacarpal joint, trapezium – first metacarpal, has reciprocal saddle-shaped articular surfaces to allow for all the movements of which the thumb is capable. Involvement of this joint in a fractured first metacarpal (Bennett's fracture) is potentially serious since poor healing may result in significant loss of mobility.

Movements and muscles

- Flexion, extension, adduction and abduction are defined differently in the thumb as compared with the fingers.

- For the fingers, these movements are as you would expect them to be.
- The thumb, though, is abducted when it is moved forwards from the anatomical position, away from and in a plane at right angles to the palm of the hand, and adducted when it is moved back again. It is extended when it is moved laterally, away from and in the same plane as the palm of the hand, and flexed when this is reversed.
- Digits 2, 4 and 5 are adducted towards the middle finger (3), and abducted away from it. The middle finger can be 'abducted' to both sides.
- Opposition is movement of the thumb across the palm of the hand as in bringing together the thumb and little finger. It is an important component of the precision grip.

Muscles   (Fig. 12.26)

Movements of the digits are brought about by:

- the intrinsic muscles of the hand, which include:
  - thenar muscles
  - hypothenar muscles
  - interosseous muscles
  - lumbricals
- the tendons of the forearm flexors
- the tendons of the forearm extensors.

Thenar muscles   (Fig. 12.26)
The fleshy mound at the base of the thumb is the thenar eminence. It contains:

- Abductor pollicis brevis. Attachments: lateral carpal bones – proximal phalanx of thumb.
- Flexor pollicis brevis. Attachments: lateral carpal bones – proximal phalanx of thumb.
- Opponens pollicis. Attachments: lateral carpal bones – lateral border of first metacarpal, so lying underneath the first two.

Nerve supply of the above three muscles: median nerve (thenar branch, see above), C8, T1.
Deep to these is the:

- Adductor pollicis. Attachments: capitate and metacarpals 2 and 3 – proximal first phalanx. Nerve supply: ulnar nerve, deep branch, C8, T1.

Hypothenar muscles   (Fig. 12.26)
The fleshy mound at the base of the little finger is the hypothenar eminence. It contains three muscles corresponding to the superficial thenar muscles (abductor brevis, flexor brevis, opponens) with digiti minimi substituted for pollicis. Details are not necessary. Nerve supply: ulnar nerve, C8, T1.

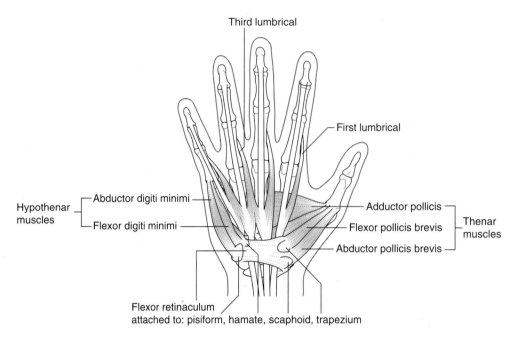

Fig. 12.26 Muscles of the hand: opponens muscles not shown. Opponens muscles (thenar and hypothenar) lie deep to other thenar and hypothenar muscles – see text.

Long flexor tendons   (Figs 12.23, 12.24)
As the tendons of flexor digitorum superficialis approach the phalanges, each splits into two components which pass on either side of the tendon of flexor digitorum profundus to attach to the intermediate phalanx, so superficialis acts at the proximal interphalangeal joint. Profundus tendon attaches to the terminal phalanx, so this muscle acts at the distal interphalangeal joint.

A similar arrangement is found in the thumb: the tendon of flexor pollicis brevis splits to let that of flexor pollicis longus pass through.

Extensor tendons   (Fig. 12.25)
- Extensor carpi radialis and ulnaris tendons are attached to the dorsal surface of the metacarpals.
- Extensor digitorum tendons are attached to the dorsal aspects of all the phalanges by the dorsal extensor expansions. The details are complex and you do not need to know them.

Nerve supply: radial nerve, C6, 7.

Lumbricals: straight finger flexion   (Fig. 12.26)
These four muscles, like short worms (Latin: lumbricus), are attached to the tendons of flexor digitorum profundus in the region of the mid-palm. They pass on the radial side of the bones to the extensor expansion of the same digit in such a way that they flex the metacarpophalangeal joint, but because they attach to the extensor expansion, they extend the interphalangeal joints. The resultant movement is straight finger flexion. You can sometimes see a bulge (or at any rate feel something) caused by the first lumbrical (index finger) when you flex the metacarpophalangeal joint, keeping the finger straight. Nerve supply: ulnar and median nerves, two each, in accordance with the supply of flexor digitorum profundus, of which they are really extensions.

Interosseous muscles: abduction, adduction
(Fig. 12.27)
Three (or four) palmar, four dorsal. Palmar interossei adduct, dorsal interossei abduct (PAD, DAB).

- Palmar: from the palmar surface of metacarpal 2, passing on the ulnar side of the metacarpophalangeal joint, to the dorsal tendon expansion of the same digit, and similarly for digits 4 and 5 except that they pass on the radial side of the metacarpophalangeal joints. Some authorities maintain that there is also a palmar interosseous for the thumb: others say that this is part of flexor pollicis brevis.
- Dorsal: deep to the palmar interossei. Each arises from the sides of adjacent metacarpals and the tendons pass to proximal phalanges and the extensor expansion of digits 2 (radial side), 3 (one muscle radial side, one muscle ulnar side) and 4 (ulnar side). The first dorsal interosseous is the fleshy muscle on the back of the hand between the first and second metacarpals.

Nerve supply: ulnar nerve, deep branch, C8, T1.

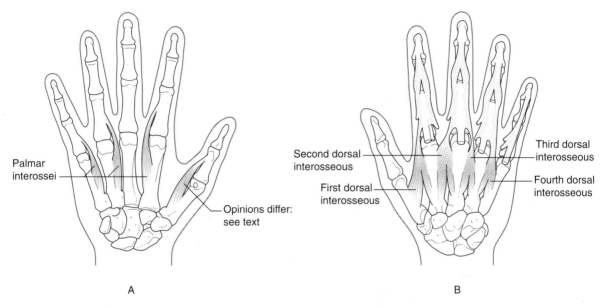

Fig. 12.27 Interossei: (**A**) palmar; (**B**) dorsal.

Clinical box

Functional considerations, nerve injuries
- The hand muscles act in concert. Fine movements, like threading a needle, or writing, depend upon fine movements of all these components.
- If you see a patient with hypothenar muscle weakness, think of ulnar nerve lesion.
- If you see a patient with thenar muscle weakness, think of median nerve lesion.
- If you see a patient with both hypothenar and thenar muscle weakness, think of brachial plexus root lesion, T1. The thenar muscles, hypothenar muscles and interossei, whether supplied by the ulnar nerve or the median nerve, are all supplied by neurons with cell bodies in the ventral grey horn of spinal cord segment T1 (and possibly C8). Damage to T1 ventral horn cells, nerve roots or T1 nerve itself (e.g. Pancoast's tumour; see 10.4, p. 89) may present as a loss of manual dexterity.

Vessels of the hand (Fig. 12.28)

Arteries

- Ulnar artery: passes from forearm to hand superficial to the flexor retinaculum, between the pisiform and hook of the hamate (both of which are palpable). It is usually the main contributor to the superficial palmar arterial arch. The deep branch, to the deep palmar arch, grooves the ulnar aspect of the hook of the hamate.
- Radial artery: passes from forearm to hand, avoiding the flexor retinaculum, by running dorsally deep to the tendons bounding the anatomical snuffbox, then penetrating the first dorsal interosseous muscle and

the adductor pollicis muscle. It is usually the main contributor to the deep palmar arterial arch. Its superficial branch, to the superficial palmar arch, is superficial to the flexor retinaculum.
- Superficial and deep palmar arterial arches. Both radial and ulnar arteries usually contribute to these.
  - Superficial arch: approximately level with the tip of the fully extended thumb.
  - Deep arch: approximately level with the base of the extended thumb.
    Both arches give branches to the distal portions of the hand and the digits.

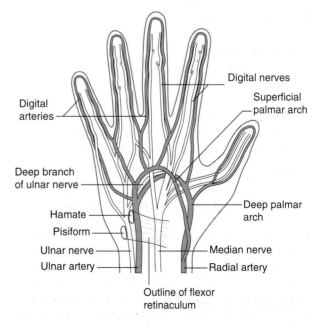

Fig. 12.28 Arteries and nerves in the hand.

Veins

The only important thing to note is that the pattern of superficial veins is, as usual, very variable. There is often a dorsal venous arch on the back of the palm, from either side of which arise the cephalic and basilic veins. Look at your own hand.

Nerves of the hand

Ulnar nerve   (Fig. 12.4)

This passes superficial to the flexor retinaculum with the ulnar artery.

- Palmar and digital branches: these supply hypothenar muscles and palmar skin of the ulnar one and a half digits, and the adjacent palm.
- Dorsal branch: this is given off in the distal forearm and supplies dorsal skin of the ulnar one and a half digits.
- Deep branch: this is given off near the hamate, accompanies the deep branch of the ulnar artery, and supplies interossei and adductor pollicis.

Median nerve   (Fig. 12.4)

After giving off the palmar cutaneous branch in the forearm, which supplies skin over the thenar eminence, the median nerve passes through the carpal tunnel.

- Palmar and digital branches: these supply palmar skin of the radial three and a half digits, and the adjacent palm.
- Thenar, or recurrent, branch: this is given off distal to the flexor retinaculum, and supplies thenar eminence muscles.

Radial nerve   (Fig. 12.3)

In the hand, this is entirely sensory and there are no special points of clinical significance. The territory of the radial nerve is the dorsal skin of the radial three and a half digits (thus mirroring the median nerve).

Cutaneous overlap, variation, clinical considerations

- There is a significant degree of overlap between these cutaneous territories such that:
  - the skin that is supplied *only* by the radial nerve is on the dorsal aspect of the first dorsal interosseous muscle
  - the skin that is supplied *only* by the median nerve is over the thenar eminence
  - the skin that is supplied *only* by the ulnar nerve is on the ulnar edge of the hand.
- Variations in the borders between the territories of the ulnar and median nerves are encountered.
- Weakness and wasting of the thenar muscles means a lesion of the median nerve. Weakness and wasting of the hypothenar muscles means a lesion of the ulnar nerve. Weakness and wasting of both thenar and hypothenar muscles means a lesion of T1 root, probably at the apex of the lung or in the brachial plexus. Make sure you understand this.

12.8 Innervation, nerve testing, surface anatomy

Dupuytren's contracture

A thickening and shortening of part of the palmar aponeurosis may result in flexion of the metacarpophalangeal joints, usually beginning (inexplicably) with that of the ring finger. It occurs more frequently as one gets older and in certain chronic conditions (e.g. liver disease – again inexplicably).

Synovial sheaths   (Fig. 12.29)

Also important clinically, and for similar reasons, are the synovial sheaths or bursas of the palm. In the palm (Fig. 12.29A) the common synovial sheath extends through the carpal tunnel into the forearm, and inflammation of the sheath is a potential cause of carpal tunnel syndrome. Dorsally (Fig. 12.29B), synovial sheaths surround the extensor tendons as they pass deep to the restraining extensor retinaculum (of which you need to know nothing other than that it exists). These sheaths may be inflamed in, for example, racquet players and others who habitually flex and extend their wrists more than most of us. Such inflammation is synovitis.

A fall on the outstretched hand

This may cause:

- fractured clavicle
- Colles' fracture (distal radius)
- fractured scaphoid: tenderness in the anatomical snuffbox
- dislocated lunate: median nerve injury
- Bennett's fracture (first metacarpal)
- mid-shaft humeral fracture: radial nerve damage.

Overview

Principal nerves supplying the upper limb are the axillary, radial, musculocutaneous, median and ulnar. They are vulnerable to injury at certain points close to skin and/or bone.

Learning Objectives

You should:

- know where nerves are vulnerable to injury
- know how to test the axillary, radial, musculocutaneous, median and ulnar nerves for both sensory and motor function
- know how to test specific spinal segments for both sensory and motor function
- know the surface markings of upper limb bones, and principal vessels and nerves.

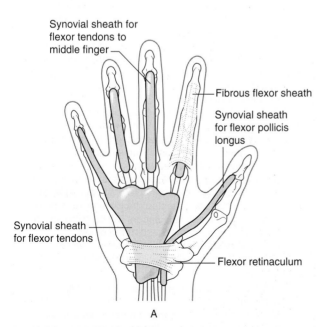

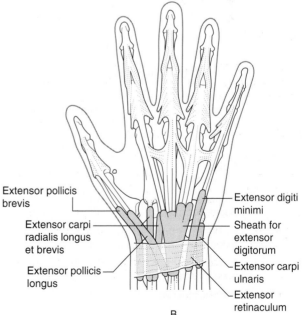

Fig. 12.29   Synovial sheaths of the hand and wrist: (**A**) palmar; (**B**) dorsal. The fibrous flexor sheath is shown only in the index finger.

Nerves: a revision of some important points

Dermatomes (Fig. 6.6, p. 36)

Remember these:

- C5 over deltoid
- C6 over the thumb
- C8 on the medial forearm
- T1, 2 axillary skin.

Sensory nerves

- Over deltoid:
  - axillary nerve.
- Anterior arm:
  - axillary nerve (laterally)
  - medial cutaneous nerve of the arm.
- Anterior forearm:
  - lateral cutaneous nerve of the forearm (continuation of musculocutaneous)
  - medial cutaneous nerve of the forearm.
- Posterior arm and forearm:
  - branches of radial nerve.
- Hand:
  - radial nerve: dorsum of radial three and a half digits
  - ulnar nerve: dorsal and palmar aspects of ulnar one and a half digits
  - median nerve: palmar aspect of radial three and a half digits.

Segmental values for upper limb movements (Table 12.1)

The most frequently tested upper limb reflexes can be remembered thus: biceps jerk C5, 6; triceps jerk C7, 8.

Table 12.1 Segmental values for upper limb movements

Joint	Movement	Segmental value
Shoulder	Abduction, lateral rotation	C5
	Adduction, medial rotation	C6, 7, 8
Elbow	Flexion	C5, 6
	Extension	C7, 8
Forearm	Pronation	C6
	Supination	C5, 6
Wrist	Flexion	C6, 7
	Extension	C6, 7
Fingers	Flexion, extension (long muscles)	C7, 8
Hand	Intrinsic muscles	T1

Clinical box

Sites where injuries may damage upper limb nerves (Figs 12.3, 12.4)

- Shoulder dislocation: axillary nerve.
- Fractured surgical neck of humerus: axillary nerve.
- Fractured mid-shaft of humerus: radial nerve.
- Medial epicondyle of humerus: ulnar nerve.
- Neck of radius, fracture or dislocation: deep branch of radial (posterior interosseous) nerve.
- Slashed wrist: ulnar nerve, palmar cutaneous branch of median nerve.
- Dislocated lunate: median nerve.
- Stabbing in thenar eminence: thenar branch of median nerve (thenar muscles).

Nerve injuries

- Upper trunk of brachial plexus (C5, 6), e.g. from forcible separation of the shoulder (downward) and the neck (as in a motorcycle accident, or during a difficult birth): deltoid, biceps and brachialis are all affected, so the arm is adducted, extended and pronated ('waiter's tip' position). This is Erb's paralysis.
- Lower trunk of brachial plexus (C8, T1), e.g. from forcible separation of the arm (upwards) and the chest (as in a motorcycle accident, or when someone falls from a height and grasps something on the way to arrest the fall): paralysis of the intrinsic muscles of the hand and some forearm muscles. This is Klumpke's paralysis.
- Radial nerve: wrist drop. Since the radial nerve supplies all the extensors including those of the wrist, damage to it causes the forelimb to adopt a characteristic position with a flexed, limp wrist. In this state, grip strength is lost since for maximum power in the digital long flexors, the wrist has to be held in extension. Radial nerve damage may occur:
  - in the arm, e.g. from a mid-shaft fracture of the humerus: wrist drop, elbow extension also affected, inability to extend fingers.
  - at the elbow, e.g. from dislocation of the superior radioulnar joint: wrist drop, inability to extend fingers.
- Ulnar nerve:
  - at the elbow, e.g. from trauma at the medial epicondyle (this is 'banging the funny bone'). Because the median and ulnar nerves both supply forearm muscles, there is no dramatic motor loss except for abduction and adduction of the fingers, though there may be some clumsiness. There is no very characteristic appearance.
  - at the wrist, e.g. from slashed wrist: see above. In this case, though, the finger flexors supplied by the ulnar nerve are not affected (they are in the forearm) and so the ring and little fingers will be more flexed than if the nerve is sectioned at the elbow. Paradoxically, therefore, the hand looks 'worse' although fewer muscles are inactivated.
- Median nerve
  - in the cubital fossa, e.g. from a supracondylar humeral fracture.
  - at the wrist, e.g. from carpal tunnel syndrome. As with ulnar nerve lesions, there is no dramatic motor loss or very characteristic appearance.

- T1 segment or nerve root, e.g. from Pancoast's tumour: paralysis of the intrinsic muscles of the hand with loss of manual dexterity (see 10.4, p. 89).

Testing peripheral nerves
- Musculocutaneous: skin on lateral side of forearm, biceps tendon reflex.
- Axillary: skin over humeral attachment of deltoid, shoulder abduction.
- Radial: skin over first dorsal interosseous muscle, wrist or elbow extension.
- Median: ask the patient to abduct the thumb against resistance.
- Ulnar: finger abduction/adduction – try to stop the patient spreading the fingers (abduction, dorsal interossei), ask the patient to grasp a sheet of paper between the fingers without using the thumb (adduction, palmar interossei).

Testing spinal segments
- C5, 6: biceps tendon jerk; skin over lateral side of arm.
- C7, 8: triceps tendon jerk; skin over centre and medial side of forearm and hand.
- T1: finger abduction/adduction, thumb opposition; skin of medial side of arm, axilla.
  Revise dermatomes: Figure 6.6 (p. 36).

Surface anatomy: a revision of some important points

Shoulder, axilla

- Most lateral bony point: greater tuberosity of humerus except in shoulder dislocations when it is the acromion process.

- Acromioclavicular joint and coracoid process palpable.
- Deltopectoral triangle: cephalic vein passes deep, lymph nodes may be palpable.
- Axillary lymph nodes may be palpable.
- Long thoracic nerve on medial wall of axilla, more or less vertical in the midaxillary line.

Arm, cubital fossa and elbow region

- Brachial pulse medial to belly of biceps.
- Biceps tendon and aponeurosis.
- Brachial pulse: medial to biceps tendon, with median nerve medial to the pulse.
- Ulnar nerve: behind medial epicondyle.
- Head of the radius palpable about 1.5 cm distal to the lateral epicondyle.

Wrist and hand

- Radial pulse: just proximal to the wrist joint lateral to flexor carpi radialis tendon.
- Ulnar pulse: just proximal to the wrist on the radial side of flexor carpi ulnaris tendon.
- Flexor retinaculum: about 2-cm square in the midline just distal to the distal wrist crease – it is in the hand *not* the forearm.
- Anatomical snuffbox: scaphoid, trapezium, radial artery.
- Pisiform and hook of hamate are palpable.
- Superficial palmar arterial arch: level with tip of fully extended thumb.
- Deep palmar arterial arch: level with base of extended thumb.

Self-assessment: questions

Multiple choice questions

1. Concerning the joints and related structures of the pectoral girdle:
   a. The sternoclavicular joint overlies the union of the internal jugular and subclavian veins.
   b. The sternoclavicular joint is cartilaginous.
   c. After fracture of the clavicle, the medial portion is lower than the lateral.
   d. Conoid and trapezoid ligaments are attached to the acromion process.
   e. The subacromial bursa normally communicates with the shoulder joint.

2. In the axilla:
   a. Breast tissue may be present.
   b. Damage to the long thoracic nerve would impair shoulder abduction.
   c. The posterior axillary fold is formed by serratus anterior muscle.
   d. The lateral thoracic artery is a branch of the axillary artery.
   e. Axillary skin is supplied by spinal segment C6.

3. Supraspinatus muscle:
   a. Is involved in the first stages of shoulder abduction.
   b. Is supplied by the axillary nerve.
   c. Is attached to the lesser tuberosity of the humerus.
   d. Is separated from the deltoid muscle by a bursa.
   e. Is on the anterior aspect of the shoulder joint.

4. Serratus anterior muscle:
   a. Is attached to the lateral border of the scapula.
   b. Protracts the scapula.
   c. May be paralysed by pressure on the rib cage in the axilla.
   d. Is supplied from the roots of the brachial plexus.
   e. Is involved in shoulder abduction beyond about 90°.

5. At the shoulder and in the arm:
   a. The rotator cuff is incomplete below.
   b. The brachial pulse may be palpated in the arm just medial to biceps muscle.
   c. Fractures of the surgical neck of the humerus may cause wrist drop.
   d. Mid-shaft humeral fractures may cause wrist drop.
   e. The biceps tendon reflex involves spinal cord segments C7 and C8.

6. In the region of the elbow:
   a. Biceps muscle is attached to the ulna.
   b. The ulnar nerve may be damaged by injuries at the medial humeral epicondyle.
   c. The lateral epicondyle of the humerus gives attachment to forearm flexor muscles.
   d. Brachialis muscle is attached to the ulna and humerus.
   e. The superior radioulnar joint is surrounded by an annular ligament and communicates with the elbow joint.

7. In the cubital fossa:
   a. Brachioradialis forms the lateral border.
   b. The median nerve is medial to the brachial pulse.
   c. The biceps tendon is easily palpable.
   d. The radial nerve is lateral.
   e. The bicipital aponeurosis passes medially.

8. In the forearm and hand:
   a. In the anatomical position, the forearm is supinated.
   b. Sensory loss on the ulnar side of the forearm may be due to C8 lesions.
   c. The radius articulates with the trapezium.
   d. The ulna articulates with the triquetral and pisiform.
   e. Damage to the deep branch of the radial (posterior interosseous nerve) would impair wrist flexion.

9. In the hand:
   a. The radial nerve supplies the dorsal skin over the first dorsal interosseous muscle.
   b. The radial nerve supplies the first dorsal interosseous muscle.
   c. The dermatome over the thumb is usually C6.
   d. The first metacarpal articulates with the trapezium.
   e. The superficial palmar arterial arch is formed mainly by the ulnar artery.

10. In the hand:
    a. The pisiform bone is palpable on the lateral (radial) side of the wrist.
    b. A dislocated lunate may damage the median nerve.
    c. Lumbricals flex the metacarpophalangeal joints.
    d. The capitate is the first carpal bone to ossify.
    e. The deep palmar arch accompanies a nerve containing nerve fibres with cell bodies in ventral horn cells of spinal segment T1.

11. The shoulder joint capsule is strengthened by:
    a. Teres minor muscle anteriorly.
    b. Infraspinatus muscle anteriorly.
    c. Subscapularis muscle posteriorly.
    d. Glenohumeral ligaments anteriorly.
    e. Supraspinatus muscle superiorly.

12. The radial artery:
    a. Is the major contributor to the superficial palmar arch.
    b. Is palpable in the anatomical snuffbox.
    c. Passes through the carpal tunnel.
    d. Penetrates the first dorsal interosseous muscle.
    e. Lies superficial to the tendons bounding the anatomical snuff box.

13. Lumbricals:
    a. Are attached to the tendons of flexor digitorum profundus.
    b. Are supplied by both median and ulnar nerves.
    c. Flex the metacarpophalangeal joints.
    d. Extend the interphalangeal joints.
    e. Are the principal digital abductors.

Matching item questions

Questions 1–10

Match the numbered item to the lettered response. Each lettered response may be used once, more than once, or not at all.

    a. axillary artery
    b. subclavian artery
    c. related to the spiral groove of the humerus
    d. related to the medial humeral epicondyle
    e. related to the surgical neck of the humerus

1. vertebral artery

2. lateral thoracic artery

3. internal thoracic artery

4. profunda brachii artery

5. thoracoacromial artery

6. nerve supplying shoulder abductor muscle

7. nerve supplying hypothenar muscles

8. nerve which when sectioned would give wrist drop

9. nerve supplying skin on the dorsum of the little finger

10. abduction of the fingers

Questions 11–15

Match the numbered item to the lettered response. Each lettered response may be used once, more than once, or not at all.

    a. C5, 6
    b. C7, 8
    c. T1
    d. branch of nerve involved in carpal tunnel syndrome
    e. nerve damaged by dislocated lunate

11. hypothenar muscles

12. biceps tendon reflex.

13. triceps tendon reflex

14. axillary skin

15. upper trunk of brachial plexus

Questions requiring short answers

1. Describe the factors responsible for maintaining stability of the shoulder joint.

2. Describe the axilla and the structures passing through it. Why is it important clinically?

3. How may blood in the subclavian artery reach the axillary artery following occlusion of the third part of the subclavian artery?

4. Name the muscles that are attached to the bicipital groove of the humerus. Give the innervation and function of each.

5. Describe the attachments, function and innervation of biceps brachii muscle.

6. Explain why a left-handed person is likely to find it more difficult to tighten screws with a manual screwdriver than a right-handed person.

7. Explain why, when you forcibly pull a child by the hand, there is more likely to be nerve damage than in an adult. Which nerve is involved, and what would be the consequence?

8. Describe the anatomical basis of carpal tunnel syndrome.

9. How is the hand supplied with arterial blood? Where may peripheral pulses easily be palpated in this region? What is Allen's test?

10. In the hand:
    a. how would you test the sensory function of the ulnar, median and radial nerves?
    b. how would you test the motor function of each nerve?

Self-assessment: answers

Multiple choice answers

1. a. **True.** This is a good surface marking for the introduction of central venous lines, especially on the right.
   b. **False.** It is synovial.
   c. **False.** The lateral portion is pulled down by pectoralis major and the weight of the upper limb.
   d. **False.** They are attached to the coracoid process.
   e. **False.**

2. a. **True.**
   b. **True.** It supplies serratus anterior which is involved in abduction beyond about 90°.
   c. **False.** It is formed by latissimus dorsi.
   d. **True.**
   e. **False.** T1 usually, but not C6.

3. a. **True.**
   b. **False.** It is supplied by the suprascapular nerve, C4, 5.
   c. **False.** It is attached to the greater tuberosity.
   d. **True.** The subacromial or subdeltoid bursa lies between supraspinatus tendon and the attachment of deltoid.
   e. **False.** It is on the superior aspect.

4. a. **False.** It is attached to the medial border of the scapula.
   b. **True.**
   c. **True.** The long thoracic nerve may be involved.
   d. **True.** It is supplied from C5, 6, 7.
   e. **True.**

5. a. **True.**
   b. **True.**
   c. **False.** Wrist drop is caused by damage to the radial nerve, not to the axillary.
   d. **True.**
   e. **False.** It involves segments C5 and C6. The triceps jerk is C7, 8.

6. a. **False.** It is attached to the radius.
   b. **True.** It is immediately behind the epicondyle.
   c. **False.** It gives attachment to forearm extensors. The flexors are attached medially.
   d. **True.**
   e. **True.** Long statements are usually true.

7. a–e. **All true!**

8. a. **True.**
   b. **True.**
   c. **False.** The radius articulates with the scaphoid and lunate.
   d. **False.** It does not articulate with any of the carpal bones.
   e. **False.** It would impair extension.

9. a. **True.**
   b. **False.** The first dorsal interosseous muscle is supplied by the ulnar nerve.
   c. **True.**
   d. **True.**
   e. **True.**

10. a. **False.** It is palpable on the medial (ulnar) side of the wrist.
    b. **True.**
    c. **True.** They bring about straight finger flexion.
    d. **True.** Ossification is usually in the first year after birth.
    e. **True.** It is the deep branch of the ulnar nerve which supplies interossei and adductor pollicis. Anyway, long statements are usually true!

11. a. **False.** Teres minor is posteroinferior.
    b. **False.** Infraspinatus is posterior.
    c. **False.** Subscapularis is anterior.
    d. **True.**
    e. **True.**

12. a. **False.** The ulnar artery is the major contributor to the superficial palmar arch.
    b. **True.**
    c. **False.**
    d. **True.**
    e. **False.**

13. a. **True.**
    b. **True.** The median nerve supplies the two radial lumbricals; the ulnar nerve supplies the two ulnar lumbricals.
    c. **True.**
    d. **True.**
    e. **False.** The principal digital abductors are the dorsal interossei.

Matching item answers

1. b.

2. a.

3. b.

4. c.

5. a.

6. e. The axillary nerve, which passes from medial to lateral behind the surgical neck of the humerus, supplies the deltoid muscle.

7. d. The ulnar nerve passes posterior to the medial epicondyle to supply muscles of the hand.

8. c. The radial nerve is close to the bone in the spiral groove of the humerus, where it may be damaged by midshaft fractures.

9. d. The ulnar nerve supplies skin on the ulnar side of the hand.

10. d.

11. c.

12. a.

13. b.

14. c.

15. a.

Short answers

1. Stability at the shoulder joint is maintained by rotator cuff muscles (supraspinatus, infraspinatus, subscapularis, teres minor) and glenohumeral ligaments. These are important and should be elaborated giving, if you have time, the attachments of the muscles and their nerve supply. The glenoid labrum has a minor role.

2. Describe the distorted pyramidal shape, the anterior and posterior axillary folds and the floor. The important contents are the brachial plexus, axillary artery and branches, and lymph nodes, which you could describe in some detail. No account of the axilla should omit its relevance to the spread of breast cancer. See 12.4 (p. 163).

3. The scapular anastomosis may be involved in bypassing a blocked distal subclavian artery. Blood from the subclavian passes into branches which communicate with the anastomosis round the scapula, e.g. dorsal scapular artery, internal thoracic artery (via intercostals and connections).

Blood passes the 'wrong way' up the subscapular artery and reaches the third part of the axillary artery. See also Figure 10.25 (p. 86).

4. Latissimus dorsi and teres major are attached to the floor and medial edge of the bicipital groove of the humerus; pectoralis major is attached to its lateral edge. The nerve supply of latissimus dorsi and teres major is through branches of the posterior cord of the brachial plexus. Their functions are shoulder adduction, extension, and medial rotation. Pectoralis major, supplied by medial and lateral pectoral nerves, flexes and adducts the shoulder.

5. The long head of biceps brachii is attached to the supraglenoid tubercle, and the tendon passes inside the capsule of the shoulder joint to the bicipital groove of the humerus. The short head is attached to the coracoid process of the scapula. Distally the attachment is to the bicipital tuberosity of the radius. The muscle functions as a flexor and supinator at the elbow, and as a flexor at the shoulder. Nerve supply is by the musculocutaneous nerve, C5, 6.

6. See Biceps as a supinator: using a screwdriver (12.5, p. 168).

7. The head of the radius is kept in place by the annular ligament. The bone is not completely ossified in a child and therefore the head may more easily slip out if the arm is pulled distally. This may occur, for example, when you are trying to cross the road with your child and you misjudge the speed of an oncoming vehicle, or, regrettably, in cases of child abuse. The posterior interosseous nerve may be damaged as it winds round the neck of the radius with resultant paralysis or weakness of digital extension.

8. The median nerve passes through the carpal tunnel and may be compressed within it. This would result in altered sensation (e.g. tingling, numbness) in the cutaneous distribution of the nerve (palmar aspect of hand and radial three and a half digits, but not over the thenar eminence because the branch that supplies this comes off in the forearm, before the nerve reaches the carpal tunnel), and weakness or paralysis of the muscles supplied distal to the carpal tunnel (thenar muscles). This is most easily tested by opposition of the thumb.

9. Blood supply to the hand is via the radial and ulnar arteries, which form deep and superficial arches. See Allen's test in 12.7 (p. 176).

10. a. Sensory function is tested as follows:
    - median nerve – skin over thenar eminence
    - ulnar nerve – skin over medial edge of palm
    - radial nerve – skin on dorsal aspect of first dorsal interosseous.
    b. Motor function is tested as follows:
    - median nerve – abduction of the thumb against resistance
    - ulnar nerve – abduction and adduction of the fingers
    - radial nerve – extension of the wrist or fingers.

13 Lower limb

13.1 The big picture

First, some words of caution

Parts of this chapter assume that you have already studied the upper limb. When comparing the lower limb with the upper, there are some potentially confusing issues that you need to keep in mind:

- Thigh, leg. "Thigh' means lower limb from groin to knee. 'Leg' means knee to ankle, not the entire lower limb.
- Lateral, medial, tibial, fibular. In the lower limb, unlike the upper limb, lateral and medial are unambiguous. Nevertheless, in the leg, the terms tibial (medial) and fibular or peroneal (lateral) are also used.
- Anterior, posterior, flexors, extensors. During development, the lower limb rotates medially so that muscles and skin supplied by anterior divisions of ventral rami become medial (above the knee) or posterior (below the knee), and muscles and skin supplied by posterior divisions come round to be lateral and in front. So, extensors are at the front, flexors at the back, the knee points forwards (not backwards like the elbow) and the dorsum of the foot is at the front, not the back.
- Peroneal (from Greek) and fibular (from Latin) are synonymous. Peroneus and peroneal are used by many older books but are increasingly being replaced by fibularis and fibular. If you use peroneal, spell it correctly: perineal means something else altogether.

Arteries   (Fig. 7.1, p. 44; Fig. 13.1)

Arterial blood to the lower limb comes from the femoral artery and its branches, with the gluteal arteries (from the internal iliac) supplying the gluteal region.

- Femoral. This is the principal artery to the lower limb. It enters the thigh behind the midpoint of the inguinal ligament and descends into the popliteal fossa where it becomes the popliteal.
- Profunda femoris. The profunda femoris is an early branch of the femoral. It supplies the thigh and gives a series of branches which encircle the femur and contribute to the supply of the hip joint.
- Popliteal. At the lower border of the popliteal fossa the popliteal artery divides into anterior and posterior tibial arteries.
- Anterior tibial. This descends in the anterior (extensor) compartment becoming the:
- Dorsalis pedis artery of the foot.
- Posterior tibial. This descends in the posterior (flexor) compartment, entering the foot posteromedial to the ankle and dividing into:
- Medial and lateral plantar arteries. The lateral plantar anastomoses with the continuation of the dorsalis pedis that passes into the sole between the first (big toe) and second metatarsals.
  Palpable pulses. These are the femoral, popliteal, dorsalis pedis, and posterior tibial.

Veins, deep fascia, fascia lata

(Fig. 7.2, p. 45)

Venous blood drains to the femoral vein, thence to the external iliac and inferior vena cava. As in the upper limb there are deep and superficial systems.

- Superficial veins are immediately subcutaneous, superficial to the deep fascia. Although the pattern of superficial veins is variable, one is particularly important: the great (or long) saphenous vein (saphenous: from Greek, meaning visible), which empties into the femoral vein by passing through a defect in the deep fascia at the top of the thigh, the saphenous opening. Note that the deep fascia of the thigh is called the fascia lata.
- Deep veins accompanying the arteries (venae comitantes) converge to form the popliteal vein,

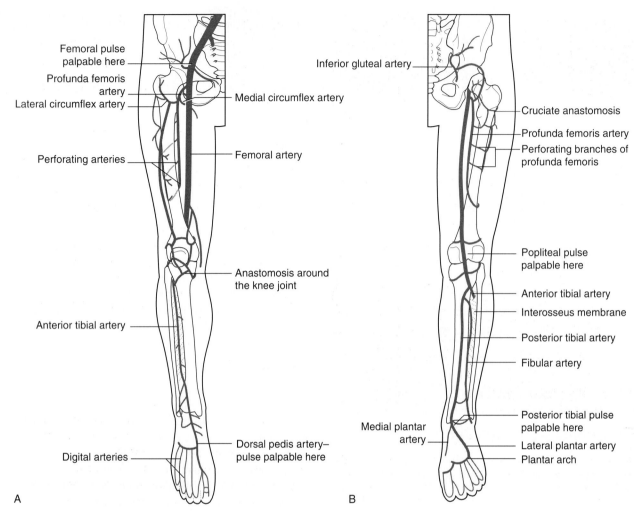

Fig. 13.1 Arteries of the lower limb: (**A**) anterior view; (**B**) posterior view.

which in turn becomes the femoral. They receive blood from superficial veins through connections which, since they penetrate the deep fascia, are known as perforating veins, or simply perforators.

Since we stand on our feet, venous return from the lower limb is often against gravity. Venous disease of the lower limb is common and the mechanism of venous return is important. It is dealt with in 13.6 (p. 206).

Lymph   (Fig. 7.4, p. 46; Fig. 13.2)

All lymph drains to inguinal nodes.

- From the medial side, lymph drains directly to inguinal nodes.
- From the lateral side, lymph drains to the popliteal nodes behind the knee, thence to inguinal nodes.

- From inguinal nodes, lymph passes to external iliac nodes, thence to para-aortic nodes, the cisterna chyli and thoracic duct to the venous system at the origin of the left brachiocephalic vein.

Nerves

- From the lumbar plexus (L1–5): to the anterior and medial thigh – hip flexion and adduction and knee extension. Revise the lumbar plexus (Fig. 11.26, p. 127).
- From the sacral plexus (L4–S4): to the rest of the lower limb – hip extension and abduction, knee flexion and all ankle and foot movements. Revise the sacral plexus (Fig. 11.31, p. 132).
- Dermatomes and myotomes. As in the upper limb, the muscles and skin supplied by one segmental nerve are not adjacent as in the trunk. The dermatomes (sensory) are shown in Figure 6.6 (p. 36).

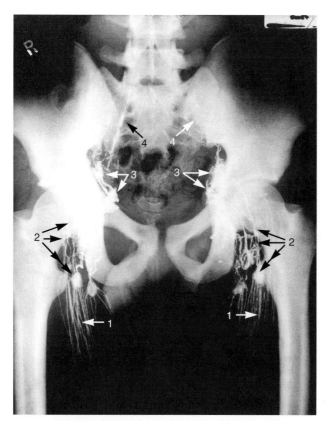

Fig. 13.2 Lymphangiogram. Radio-opaque dye was injected into the superficial tissues of both feet: this image was taken some time later after the dye had been taken up into the lymphatics. 1, lymphatic channels leading to: 2, inguinal nodes, leading to: 3, external iliac nodes, leading to: 4, common iliac nodes, from where lymph passes to para-aortic nodes.

Is this patient male or female?

13.2 Hip joint, gluteal region and upper thigh

Overview

The head of the femur articulates with the acetabulum of the hip bone. The hip joint is surrounded by large muscles, bones, joint and ligaments reflecting the forces imposed as a result of our bipedal gait. The blood supply of the joint and the head of the femur is an important consideration in patients with fractured femoral necks. Hip flexion and medial rotation are performed by muscles in and around the femoral region; extension and lateral rotation by posterior muscles (gluteal and hamstrings). The principal nerves in this region are the femoral anteriorly, vulnerable to injury in the femoral triangle, and the sciatic posteriorly, at risk in ill-judged injections and posterior dislocations of the hip.

Learning Objectives

You should:

- know the structure of the hip joint and how it may be injured
- know the blood supply of the joint and head of the femur
- know the principal muscle groups acting on the joint, and their innervation
- know the structures in the femoral triangle, and the anatomy of femoral hernia
- know the surface markings of the sciatic and femoral nerves, and the femoral artery in the femoral triangle
- understand the effects of damage to the femoral and sciatic nerves.

Bones

Sacrum (Fig. 11.29, p. 130)

- Posterior surface: provides attachment for gluteus maximus, and foramina for dorsal rami of sacral nerves are evident (not important).
- Anterior surface: provides attachment for piriformis, and foramina for ventral rami of sacral nerves are evident.

Hip bone (Fig. 11.29, p. 130; Fig. 13.3)

- Anterior surface of ilium: provides attachment for iliacus which, with psoas from the vertebral column, forms the main hip flexor, iliopsoas.
- Posterior (gluteal) surface of ilium: provides attachment for gluteus medius and gluteus minimus.
- Ischial tuberosity: provides attachment for posterior muscles of the thigh (hamstrings); these extend the hip and flex the knee.
- Pubic symphysis: a midline secondary cartilaginous joint.
- Pubic crest and pecten: provide attachment for pectineus (not important).
- Obturator foramen: this is a large defect closed by membrane in which is a small hole allowing the obturator neurovascular bundle to pass between pelvis and medial thigh.
- Ischiopubic ramus (lower border of obturator foramen formed by ramus of ischium and inferior ramus of pubis): provides attachment for adductor muscles.

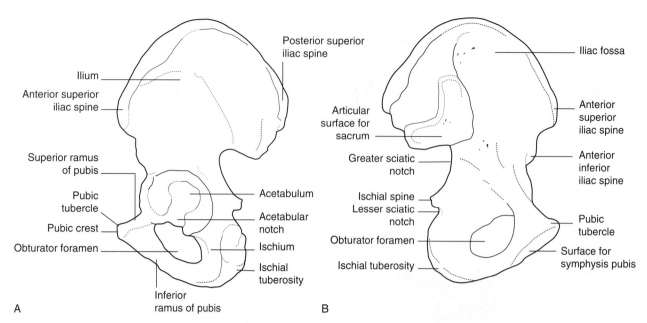

Fig. 13.3 Hip bone: (**A**) lateral view; (**B**) medial view.

- Acetabulum: articular surface for the head of the femur. The acetabular notch allows a branch of the obturator artery to enter the round ligament (ligamentum teres) of the head of the femur, which attaches the femur to the hip bone. The components of the hip bone, the ilium, ischium and pubis, meet in the centre of the acetabulum, the three parts fusing at about 16 years of age.

Femur   (Fig. 13.4)

- Head: this articulates with the acetabulum. A small pit, the fovea capitis, marks the attachment of the round ligament.
- Neck: note the many small foramina which allow blood vessels to enter the bone.
- Lesser trochanter: for the distal attachment of iliopsoas.
- Greater trochanter: provides attachment for gluteus medius and gluteus minimus.
- Trochanteric line, the ridge on the anterior surface of the femur connecting the two trochanters: the iliofemoral ligament of the hip joint capsule is attached here.
- Trochanteric fossa, between the greater trochanter and the femoral neck: provides attachment for piriformis, obturator externus and obturator internus.
- Gluteal tuberosity, on the posterior aspect of femur: provides attachment for part of gluteus maximus.
- Linea aspera: provides attachment for adductors, vastus muscles and the short head of biceps femoris.
- Adductor tubercle: provides attachment for adductor and vastus muscles.

- Shaft: this is smooth, except for the linea aspera posteriorly.

Hip joint   (Figs 13.5–13.7)

This is a ball and socket synovial joint. The acetabulum is deepened by the acetabular labrum, a rim of hyaline cartilage which, with the transverse acetabular ligament, closes the acetabular notch.

Joint capsule: iliofemoral, pubofemoral and ischiofemoral ligaments   (Figs 13.6, 13.7)

The fibrous capsule is attached proximally to the acetabular margin and distally to the intertrochanteric line on the anterior surface of the femur and about half-way up the femoral neck above and behind. Inferiorly, it extends some way down the medial border of the femur to provide sufficient slack capsule which can be taken up on abduction. The fibres of the capsule form three strong ligaments:

- Iliofemoral ligament. Attachments: anterior inferior iliac spine and acetabular margin (proximally) – intertrochanteric line (distally). This strengthens the front of the joint capsule.
- Pubofemoral and ischiofemoral ligaments. Attachments: pubic and ischial margins of the acetabulum (proximally) – upper end of intertrochanteric line (distally), but passing *behind* the femoral neck and head through the trochanteric fossa. They reinforce the back of the joint capsule.

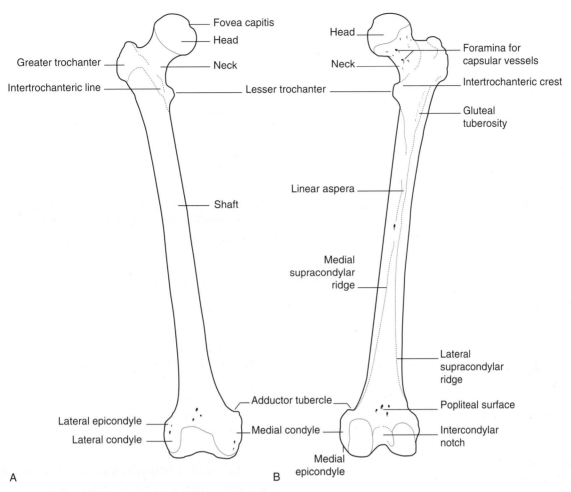

Fovea capitis

Head

Greater trochanter

Neck

Intertrochanteric line

Lesser trochanter

Shaft

Adductor tubercle

Lateral epicondyle

Medial condyle

Lateral condyle

Medial epicondyle

A

Head

Neck

Foramina for capsular vessels

Intertrochanteric crest

Gluteal tuberosity

Linear aspera

Medial supracondylar ridge

Lateral supracondylar ridge

Popliteal surface

Intercondylar notch

B

Fig. 13.4 Femur: (**A**) anterior view; (**B**) posterior view.

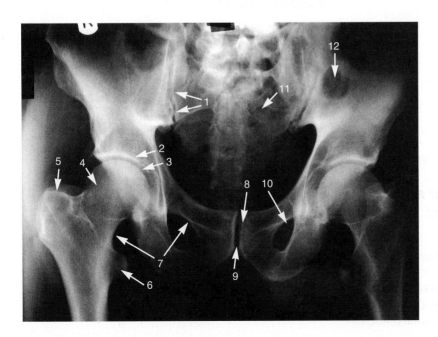

Fig. 13.5 Radiograph of pelvis and hip joints: 1, sacroiliac joint; 2, articular surface of acetabulum; 3, articular surface of head of femur; 4, neck of femur; 5, greater trochanter; 6, lesser trochanter; 7, Shenton's line; 8, pubic symphysis; 9, subpubic angle (narrower in males, wider in females); 10, bony obturator foramen; 11, margin of anterior sacral foramen; 12, (black area) air in the descending colon.

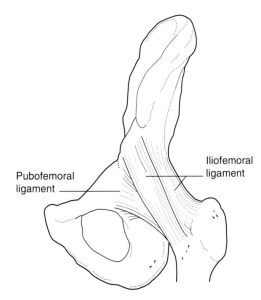

Fig. 13.6 Iliofemoral and pubofemoral ligaments.

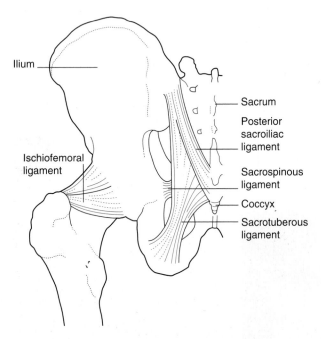

Fig. 13.7 Posterior ligaments of hip and sacrum.

Blood supply of head of femur and hip joint: cruciate and trochanteric anastomoses

- Capsular (retinacular) vessels arise from the cruciate and trochanteric anastomoses posterior to the hip joint and neck of the femur. These receive blood from the gluteal and obturator arteries (from the internal iliac), and from circumflex femoral branches of the profunda femoris artery.
- Terminal branches of the nutrient artery from the shaft. In children these do not reach the femoral

head, since vessels never cross the epiphyseal plate of developing bone.
- Artery of the round ligament (from the obturator). This is never sufficient to keep the femoral head viable if the other sources of blood are compromised (e.g. in fractures of the femoral neck).

Avascular necrosis of the femoral head may occur after a fracture of the femoral neck. It may also occur in children for reasons that are not entirely clear: this is Perthes' disease.

Flexion and adduction at the hip, femoral triangle, adductor compartment

Flexion   (Fig. 13.8)

Nerve supply: femoral nerve (L2–4) and direct branches from the lumbar plexus.

- Iliopsoas. Attachments: anterior surface of iliac crest (iliacus) and lumbar vertebral column and discs (psoas) – lesser trochanter. It is the principal flexor supplied directly from the lumbar plexus. It passes deep to the inguinal ligament.
- Sartorius. Attachments: anterior superior iliac spine – medial side of upper end of tibia.
- Pectineus. Attachments: superior border (pecten) of pubis – lesser trochanter with iliopsoas. It also has an adductor role and receives fibres from the obturator nerve as well as the femoral.
- Rectus femoris. Attachments: anterior inferior iliac spine – patella, tibia. It is part of quadriceps, the extensor of the knee, but since it is attached to the pelvis, it has a minor additional role as a hip flexor.

Adduction   (Fig. 13.8)

Nerve supply: obturator nerve, L2, 3, 4.

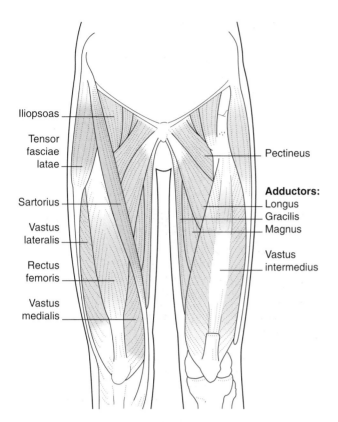

Fig. 13.8 Anterior thigh.

Labels in Fig. 13.8:
Iliopsoas
Tensor fasciae latae
Sartorius
Vastus lateralis
Rectus femoris
Vastus medialis
Pectineus
Adductors:
Longus
Gracilis
Magnus
Vastus intermedius

- Adductor longus. Attachments: below pubic tubercle – linea aspera of femur.
- Gracilis (strictly speaking, adductor gracilis). Attachments: inferior ramus of pubis – medial side of tibia.
- Adductor brevis. Attachments: inferior ramus of pubis – linea aspera of femur.
- Adductor magnus. Attachments: ischiopubic ramus – linea aspera and adductor tubercle of femur. Just above the attachment to the adductor tubercle the muscle fibres part to allow the femoral artery and vein to pass between the anterior and posterior compartments: the femoral/popliteal boundary.

Femoral region (Fig. 13.9)

- At the midpoint of the inguinal ligament, the femoral artery passes from abdomen to thigh. Lateral to it is the femoral nerve and medial the femoral vein. Medial to the vein is:
- The femoral canal – a short extension of the abdominal cavity beneath the inguinal ligament into the thigh. It contains nothing in particular other than a few lymph nodes. Medial to it is:
- The lacunar ligament, an extension of the inguinal ligament which passes on to the superior pubic ramus.
- The femoral ring is the opening of the femoral canal to the abdominal cavity.

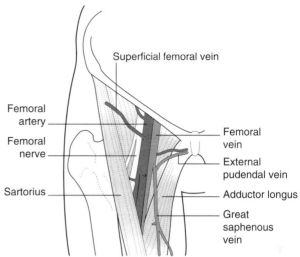

Fig. 13.9 Femoral triangle. Note the termination of the great saphenous vein.

Labels in Fig. 13.9:
Femoral artery
Femoral nerve
Sartorius
Superficial femoral vein
Femoral vein
External pudendal vein
Adductor longus
Great saphenous vein

- The femoral sheath encloses the canal, the vein and the artery, but not the nerve.

Femoral triangle and vessels
(Figs 13.9, 13.10)

- The base of the triangle is the inguinal ligament, the

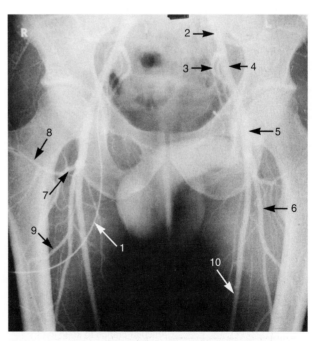

Fig. 13.10 Femoral arteries displayed after radio-opaque dye was injected into the aorta. 1, catheter; 2, common iliac artery; 3, internal iliac artery and branches (can you identify any of them?); 4, external iliac artery; 5, femoral artery; 6, profunda femoris artery; 7, branch of profunda femoris artery giving; 8, circumflex femoral artery; 9, perforating branch of profunda femoris artery; 10, femoral artery becomes popliteal about here.

medial border of sartorius laterally, and the medial border of adductor longus medially. Its floor is formed by (from above down) iliopsoas, pectineus and adductor longus.

- The femoral artery passes to the apex of the femoral triangle and then runs for a short distance under sartorius to the gap in adductor magnus where it enters the popliteal fossa. The subsartorial 'canal' is also called the adductor or Hunter's canal.
- The profunda femoris artery arises in the upper part of the femoral triangle and is large, its size reflecting the importance of the thigh muscles and hip joint. It provides a series of arteries that encircle the femur, the uppermost of which, the circumflex femorals, contribute to the cruciate and trochanteric anastomoses supplying the hip joint. The lower branches perforate the fascia between the anterior and posterior thigh muscles and are known as perforating arteries (not to be confused with perforating veins joining the deep and superficial venous systems).

Femoral and obturator nerves

(Figs 13.11, 13.12)

- The femoral nerve enters the thigh immediately

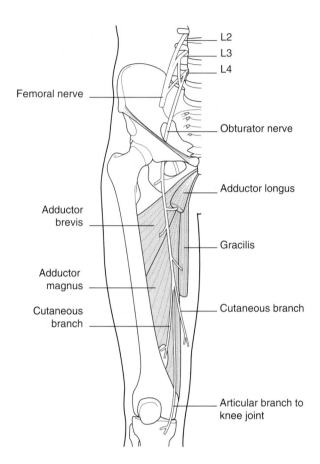

Fig. 13.12 Obturator nerve.

lateral to the femoral pulse at the inguinal ligament. It divides into numerous branches:
  - to knee extensors
  - medial and intermediate cutaneous nerves of the thigh (the lateral cutaneous is a separate nerve, see Fig. 11.26, p. 127)
  - saphenous nerve (sensory), which continues through the subsartorial canal and then becomes superficial, running down the medial side of the lower thigh and leg with the great saphenous vein to the foot. It supplies a strip of medial skin over and around it and thus a branch of the femoral nerve carries L4 fibres all the way to the foot.
- The obturator nerve enters the thigh through the obturator foramen and supplies:
  - hip adductor muscles
  - skin of the upper medial thigh
  - sensory fibres to the knee joint.
- Both femoral and obturator nerves are formed from ventral rami of L2, 3, 4, the obturator from anterior divisions, and the femoral from posterior divisions. Posterior divisions at the front? Yes: remember the embryonic medial rotation: see the beginning of this chapter.

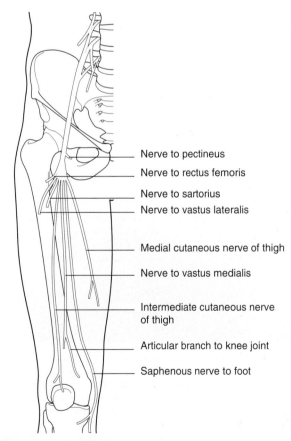

Fig. 13.11 Femoral nerve.

Hip abduction, rotation, extension; gluteal region

Abduction and medial rotation   (Fig. 13.13)

Nerve supply: superior gluteal nerve, L4, 5, S1.

- Gluteus medius. Attachments: posterior ilium – greater trochanter. This is deep to gluteus maximus.
- Gluteus minimus. Attachments: posterior ilium – greater trochanter. This is deep to gluteus medius.

These muscles are hip abductors: if you contract them whilst seated, this is what they do. But if you are standing with, say, your right foot on the ground and you contract them on the right, they will raise the opposite side of the pelvis, allowing you to lift your left foot. This is their principal function: the hip abductors contract on the weightbearing side during locomotion to allow body weight to be supported on the ipsilateral lower limb. If they are weakened or paralysed (e.g. poliomyelitis affecting L4, 5, S1), the pelvis will dip to the non-weightbearing side resulting in a waddling gait, the Trendelenburg gait (not to be confused with the waddling gait that workers in the fashion industry, and others, try hard to acquire).

- Tensor fasciae latae. Attachments: lateral iliac crest – lateral longitudinal thickening of fascia lata, the iliotibial tract, which passes between the ilium and

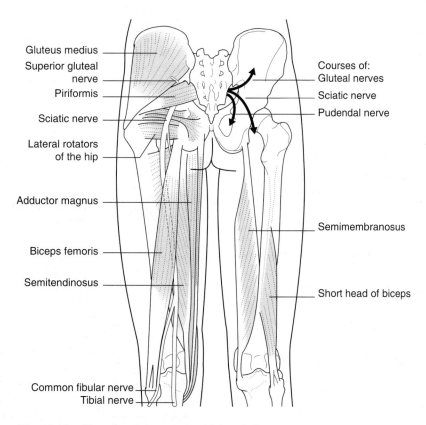

Fig. 13.13   Gluteal region, posterior thigh, sciatic nerve.

the lateral condyle of the tibia. Many authorities regard this muscle as an extensor, but my eyes and hands tell me it is an abductor, and it is supplied by the superior gluteal nerve.

Extension (Fig. 13.13)

- Gluteus maximus. Attachments: posterior surface of iliac crest, sacrum, coccyx, sacrotuberous ligament – femur and tibia via iliotibial tract (see below).

  Nerve supply: inferior gluteal nerve, L5 S1, 2.

  Gluteus maximus is the big superficial muscle of the backside. Less than one quarter of its fibres are attached to the femur, to the gluteal tuberosity just below the greater trochanter. Most fibres pass to the iliotibial tract of the fascia lata (see above). Gluteus maximus is a powerful extensor of the hip, used particularly for antigravity movements such as rising from the kneeling or sitting position, or climbing stairs.

- Hamstrings (semitendinosus, semimembranosus, biceps femoris). Attachments: ischial tuberosity – femur, tibia and fibula.

  Nerve supply: tibial and common fibular nerves, L5, S1, 2, 3.

These hip extensors are also important knee flexors and are considered in detail in that section.

Lateral rotation: direct branches of L4–S2
(Fig. 13.13)

None of these muscles is particularly important.

- Piriformis. Attachments: anterior aspect of sacrum – greater trochanter (through greater sciatic foramen).
- Obturator externus. Attachments: outer margins of obturator foramen and membrane – trochanteric fossa.
- Obturator internus. Attachments: inner margins of obturator foramen and membrane – trochanteric fossa. This muscle turns a right angle through the lesser sciatic foramen. As it emerges it is joined above and below by fibres attached to the margins of the foramen, the superior gemellus and inferior gemellus (definitely not important).
- Quadratus femoris: ischial tuberosity – greater trochanter.

Other features of gluteal region and the hip

Greater and lesser sciatic foramina

The greater sciatic foramen transmits:

- the superior gluteal nerve and vessels above piriformis
- the inferior gluteal nerve and vessels, the pudendal nerve and vessels, and (usually) the sciatic nerve below piriformis. The pudendal nerve immediately then dives into the lesser sciatic foramen to pass in the ischioanal fossa of the perineum.

Sciatic nerve (Fig. 13.13)

- The nerve roots of L4–S3 form two large nerves, the tibial (anterior divisions supplying flexors) and the common fibular or fibular (posterior divisions supplying extensors). These nerves, although separate entities, are usually bound together as the sciatic nerve, the two components separating in the popliteal fossa. However, they may be separate throughout their length, with the common fibular nerve passing above or through piriformis and the tibial through or below piriformis.
- The sciatic nerve in the gluteal region is immediately posterior to the hip joint capsule and may be damaged by posterior hip dislocations.

> **Clinical box**
>
> **Sciatic nerve surface markings: injections**
> Surface markings of sciatic nerve:
> - halfway between posterior superior iliac spine and ischial tuberosity, to
> - halfway between ischial tuberosity and greater trochanter.
>
>   To be sure to avoid the nerve, intramuscular injections must be given in the upper outer quadrant of the backside.

13.3 Knee joint, movements, muscles, posterior thigh, popliteal fossa

Overview

At the knee, the femur articulates with the tibia. Ligaments of the joint include cruciate ligaments that limit flexion and extension and which have a role in weighbearing. Extension is performed by the quadriceps muscle (femoral nerve) and flexion by the hamstrings (tibial nerve). In addition, at the end of extension, a small degree of rotation permits 'locking'. There are numerous bursas round the joint, some of which may become inflamed and enlarged. Posteriorly, the popliteal pulse may be palpated in the popliteal fossa, and laterally the common fibular nerve is vulnerable at the neck of the fibula.

Learning Objectives

You should:

- know the surface anatomy of the knee joint
- know the structure of the knee joint and how it may be injured
- know how to test the ligaments of the knee joint
- know the principal muscle groups acting on the joint, and their innervation
- know the position of bursas around the knee joint
- understand why the popliteal artery is at risk in supracondylar femoral fractures.

Bones

Distal femur   (Fig. 13.14)

- Articular condyles: articulate with the tibia, the medial is bigger than the lateral. The patella articulates anteriorly.
- Linea aspera: this provides attachment for vastus muscles and the short head of biceps femoris. The linea aspera widens to form the:
- Popliteal surface, immediately related to the popliteal artery.
- Intercondylar notch: provides attachment for cruciate ligaments.

Proximal tibia   (Fig. 13.14)

- Articular surfaces: receive the femoral condyles, the medial is bigger than the lateral.
- Intercondylar eminence: provides attachments for cruciate ligaments and menisci.
- Tibial tuberosity: provides attachment for the patellar ligament.
- Facet for articulation of fibula (superior tibiofibular joint).

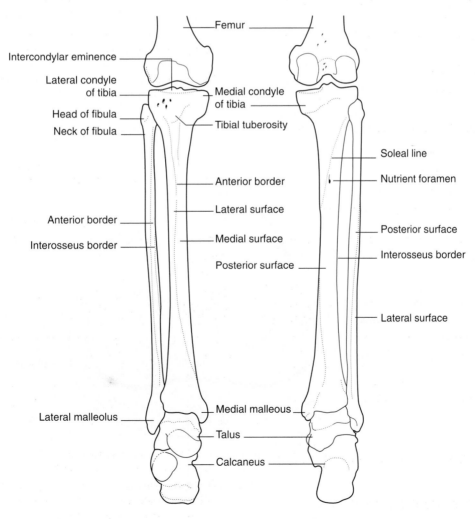

Fig. 13.14   Distal femur, tibia, fibula, talus: (**A**) anterior view; (**B**) posterior view.

Proximal fibula (Fig. 13.14)

- Head: this articulates with the tibia.
- Neck: this is related to the common fibular nerve.

Patella

- This is a sesamoid bone in the tendon of quadriceps femoris.

Knee joint

Synovial cavity

The synovial cavity has medial and lateral compartments that communicate anteriorly behind an infrapatellar fat pad. It extends superiorly for about a handsbreadth above the upper margin of the patella – the suprapatellar bursa (see below). There are two articulations between the tibia and femur, right and left, and one between the anterior femur and the patella.

Menisci (semilunar cartilages) and collateral ligaments (Figs 13.15, 13.16)

- Medial and lateral menisci form partial cushions between tibia and femur and are attached to the intercondylar eminence of the tibia.
- The medial collateral ligament, a broad and flat band, is a thickening of the knee joint capsule and is attached to the medial meniscus. It is taut in knee extension and prevents knee abduction.

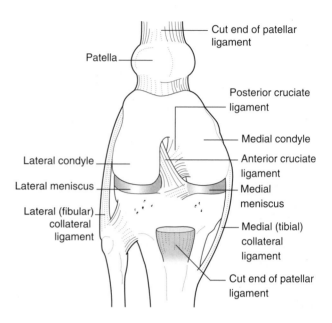

Fig. 13.15 Knee joint, anterior view with patella lifted upwards.

- The lateral collateral ligament is a cord-like structure, attached neither to the lateral meniscus nor the knee joint capsule. It is taut in knee extension and prevents knee adduction.
- The medial meniscus is more commonly injured in twisting ('cartilage') injuries than the lateral, partly because it is less mobile than the lateral and can not move out of the way.

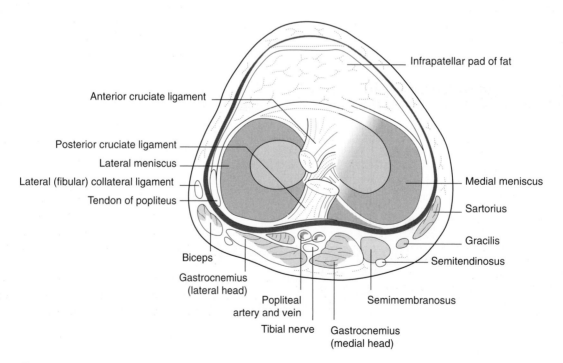

Fig. 13.16 Knee joint, articular surface of tibia viewed from above.

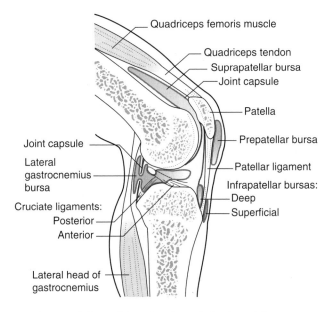

Fig. 13.17   Schematic section through the knee joint.

Labels on figure:
- Quadriceps femoris muscle
- Quadriceps tendon
- Suprapatellar bursa
- Joint capsule
- Patella
- Prepatellar bursa
- Patellar ligament
- Infrapatellar bursas:
  - Deep
  - Superficial
- Joint capsule
- Lateral gastrocnemius bursa
- Cruciate ligaments:
  - Posterior
  - Anterior
- Lateral head of gastrocnemius

Cruciate ligaments   (Figs 13.16, 13.17)

- The anterior cruciate ligament is attached to the anterior intercondylar area of the tibia and passes upwards, backwards and laterally to the lateral side of the intercondylar notch of the femur. It limits anterior movement of the tibia on the femur (or posterior movement of the femur on the tibia). We can manage without it if it is torn.
- The posterior cruciate ligament is attached to the posterior intercondylar area of the tibia and the lateral meniscus. It passes upwards, forwards and medially (the two ligaments thus making a cross – hence the name) to the medial side of the

intercondylar notch of the femur. It limits posterior movement of the tibia on the femur (or anterior movement of the femur on the tibia). It takes the weight of the body when we are standing with our knees bent, or when we descend stairs or a slope. We can not easily manage without it.

Movements and muscles

Extension   (Figs 13.8, 13.17)

Nerve supply: femoral nerve, L3, 4.
- Quadriceps femoris. Attachments: ilium and femur – patella and tibia. There are four parts, all converging on the patellar tendon.
  - Rectus femoris: from anterior inferior iliac spine and neighbouring ilium.
  - Vastus lateralis: from lateral side of linea aspera.
  - Vastus medialis: from medial side of linea aspera. Muscle fibres extend more distally than for the other components, attaching directly to the upper medial aspect of the patella. The patella has a tendency to dislocate laterally since, because of the angle between the thigh and the leg, quadriceps as a whole pulls it somewhat laterally. These fibres of vastus medialis counteract this tendency.
  - Vastus intermedius: from upper two-thirds of femoral shaft.

Note: the tendon between the muscle and the patella is the quadriceps tendon; that from patella to tibia is the patellar ligament or tendon.

Knee jerk (patellar tendon reflex). Tapping the patellar tendon to elicit the knee jerk tests the femoral nerve and spinal segments L3, 4. It is an important part of a general neurological examination.

Flexion   (Fig. 13.13)

Nerve supply: tibial nerve, L5–S3.
  The hamstrings are attached to the ischial tuberosity above.

- Biceps femoris. This passes laterally to the head of the fibula. Its tendon is easily palpated as it approaches the fibula. Its long head comes from the ischial tuberosity, and its short head (supplied by the common fibular nerve) from the lower part of the linea aspera.
- Semitendinosus. This passes medially and ends in a long tendon attached to the medial side of the upper tibia, in company with sartorius and gracilis.

Clinical box

Testing the ligaments
- Collateral ligaments. Take the leg in your hands and, keeping the knee straight, try (gently!) to abduct and adduct the knee. There should be little if any movement.
- Cruciates. Ask the patient to sit with the knees flexed to about a right angle. Sit on the foot of the side you are testing. Grasp the upper tibia in your hands and try to pull it forwards. If it comes forwards more than it should, the anterior cruciate is torn. Now push backwards. If the tibia goes back more than it should, the posterior cruciate is torn. Since someone (who?) imagined this to be similar to pulling and pushing a drawer open and closed, it is called the drawer test.

- Semimembranosus. This passes medially ending in a wide membrane-like aponeurosis, deep to semitendinosus, attached to the medial side of the upper tibia and knee joint capsule.
- Both semi- muscles are palpable.

Locking, unlocking: tibial nerve, L4, 5, S1

Imagine you are sitting with your knee flexed. Now extend it. The lateral articular surfaces (smaller) reach the end of available movement before the medial, and the tibia rotates to allow more extension on the medial side. This is locking, and the rotation is passive. This happens when you stand from a sitting position, and the locking mechanism means that the knee is reasonably stable in extension without muscular activity maintaining it in this position.

At the beginning of flexion, unlocking must occur. This is not passive: popliteus muscle exists for this purpose. It arises from the posterior surface of the tibia and passes upwards and laterally to the lateral joint capsule and, by a part that penetrates the joint capsule, to the lateral meniscus and lateral condyle of the femur. It is having to cope with this unlocking mechanism that makes good artificial knees tricky to develop.

Clinical box

Bursitis
There are many bursas associated with the knee joint. Some of them are shown in Figure 13.17.
- Suprapatellar: an extension of the cavity of the knee joint. If the patella bounces when tapped, there is probably a knee joint effusion. An enlarged suprapatellar bursa may be palpable.
- Prepatellar. In the days when housemaids scrubbed floors, the superficial prepatellar bursa often became inflamed: housemaid's knee.
- Infrapatellar, superficial and deep, on either side of the patellar tendon: separate from the joint. In the days when clergymen knelt on hard wooden surfaces to pray, this bursa often became inflamed: clergyman's knee.
- Semimembranosus: between membrane and joint, may communicate with the joint.
- Popliteus: between popliteus tendon and the back of the joint, communicating with the joint and the lateral gastrocnemius bursa.

Popliteal fossa, neck of fibula, superior tibiofibular joint

This is a diamond-shaped area behind the knee. It is bounded above by the diverging hamstrings (biceps laterally, semi- muscles medially) and below by the lateral and medial heads of gastrocnemius. It contains the popliteal vessels and the two divisions of the sciatic nerve.

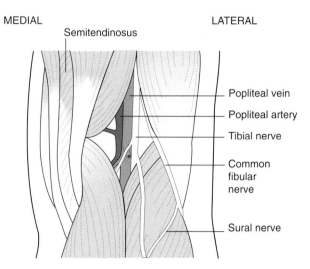

Fig. 13.18   Popliteal fossa.

The popliteal artery and pulse   (Fig. 13.18)

The artery is deep (= anterior) in the fossa, immediately adjacent to the posterior surface of the femur. It is vulnerable here: in a supracondylar femoral fracture, the distal portion of the femur may be pulled posteriorly by the gastrocnemius with the sharp edge of the fracture severing the artery.

The popliteal pulse is palpated by pressing from behind against the back of the femur. The leg muscles must be relaxed, so ask the patient to sit with feet and backside on the same surface.

The popliteal artery divides at the lower margin in the popliteal fossa to give:

- the posterior tibial artery, which descends in the posterior compartment of the leg
- the anterior tibial artery, which descends in the anterior compartment of the leg.

The fibular artery, running close to the fibula in the posterior compartment, is usually a branch of the posterior tibial, but the pattern varies.

Nerves

- The tibial and common fibular nerves diverge in the upper part of the popliteal fossa, the tibial continuing more or less vertically and the common fibular passing laterally to the neck of the fibula. Both nerves are vulnerable to trauma in the fossa. Both nerves give branches to form the sural nerve supplying skin over the posterior calf.
- The common fibular is also vulnerable at the neck of the fibula, at just the right height to take the maximum impact from a car bumper (fender) injury. This nerve here is equivalent to the radial nerve at

the radial neck: damage to the one may cause wrist drop; to the other foot drop.

- At the neck of the fibula, the common fibular nerve divides into:
  - deep fibular: supplies muscles that extend (dorsiflex) the ankle
  - superficial fibular: supplies muscles that evert the ankle.

Again, compare the common fibular nerve with the radial in the upper limb.

Superior tibiofibular joint

It is synovial, separate from the knee joint, and unimportant.

13.4 Ankle joint and movements: posterior, anterior and lateral compartments of leg

Overview

The ankle joint is formed by the talus, tibia and fibula. Dorsiflexion is performed by muscles supplied by the deep fibular nerve, and plantarflexion by muscles supplied by the tibial nerve. Stability is provided by muscles and ligaments, the lateral ligament being frequently injured. Palpable pulses around the ankle include the posterior tibial and anterior tibial. Tendons passing from the leg to the foot are surrounded in the ankle region by synovial sheaths and restrained by retinacula.

Learning Objectives

You should:

- know the surface anatomy of the ankle joint and principal ligaments
- know the principal muscle groups acting on the joint, and their innervation
- know the position of the peripheral pulses around the ankle.

Bones

Distal tibia (Fig. 13.14)

- Medial aspect. This is directly subcutaneous: feel your own. Because of this it is painful when it is kicked. The lack of muscular attachments also

means it has a relatively poor blood supply, and fractures are sometimes slow to heal.

- Soleal line. An obvious ridge running upwards and laterally on the posterior of the bone. It is caused by the attachments of soleus (below) and popliteus (above).
- Interosseous border: to which is attached the interosseous membrane.
- Medial malleolus: the large bony prominence palpable medially at the ankle.

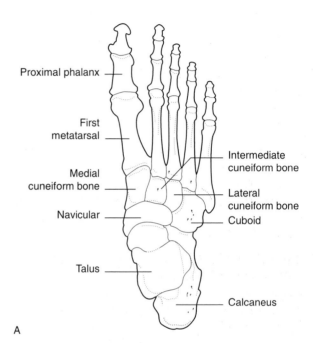

A

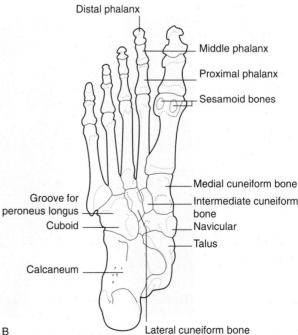

B

Fig. 13.19 Foot bones: (**A**) view from above; (**B**) view from below.

- Articular surface: the internal aspect of the medial malleolus and the distal surface of the shaft. It forms about two-thirds of the proximal articular surface of the ankle joint.

Distal fibula (Fig. 13.14)

- Interosseous border: to which is attached the interosseous membrane.
- Lateral malleolus: the large bony prominence palpable laterally at the ankle.
- Articular surface: the internal aspect of the lateral malleolus forms about one-third of the proximal articular surface of the ankle joint.
- There is nothing else below the neck of the fibula that is important.

Talus (Figs 13.14, 13.19)

- Body (proximal). This articulates with the tibia and fibula, the lateral articular surface being larger than the medial (tibial). There is a separate articular surface for the posterior part of the calcaneus: this is considered in 13.5 (p. 204).
- Neck. Like the scaphoid, to which it is equivalent, the talus has a narrow central section which may be fractured. It is liable to avascular necrosis, since in twisting it may tear its blood supply.
- Head (distal). This is palpable. It articulates with the anterior part of the calcaneus and navicular and is considered in 13.5.

Calcaneus (calcaneum) (Figs 13.19, 13.20)

This is considered in more detail in 13.5, but at this stage note the sustentaculum tali (Latin: support of the talus), which extends medially from the bone and is palpable inferior to the head of the talus.

Other foot bones (Figs 13.19, 13.20)

These are not directly relevant to the ankle joint although some of them provide attachments for muscles that act on the ankle. They are considered in 13.5.

Ankle joint (Fig. 13.20)

- The distal ends of the tibia and fibula are united by fibrous tissue (inferior tibiofibular joint) and form a mortise into which the body of the talus fits.
- The dorsum of the foot is at the front (see p. 185).
- Moving the distal foot down is plantarflexion, the equivalent of flexion at the wrist.
- Moving the distal foot up is dorsiflexion, the equivalent of extension at the wrist.
- Turning the sole of the foot medially (inwards) is inversion.
- Turning the sole of the foot laterally (outwards) is eversion.

Inferior tibiofibular joint and ankle ligaments
(Fig. 13.21)

- Inferior tibiofibular ligaments: the fibres are oblique rather than horizontal, so there is some 'give' at this

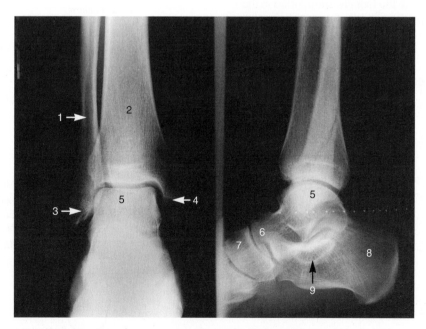

Fig. 13.20 Radiographs of ankle joint, posterior and lateral views: 1, fibula; 2, tibia; 3, lateral malleolus; 4, medial malleolus; 5, body of talus; 6, head of talus; 7, navicular; 8, calcaneus; 9, sustentaculum tali of calcaneus.

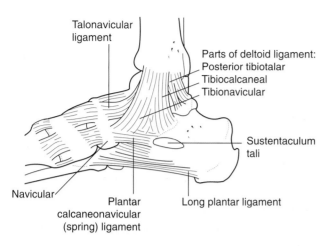

Fig. 13.21 Medial ankle ligaments.

joint, but otherwise there is no significant movement of the tibia and fibula.

- Lateral ligaments: calcaneofibular, anterior talofibular and posterior talofibular. The anterior talofibular ligament is most often the site of an ankle 'sprain'. Tenderness just below and in front of the lateral malleolus is indicative of a torn anterior talofibular ligament.
- Deltoid (medial) ligament. From the medial malleolus, the medial ligament spreads out as a triangle (hence the name). There are two parts:

  - superficial: down and back to the sustentaculum tali of the calcaneus
  - deep: backwards and downwards to the entire length of the sustentaculum tali, down to the spring ligament (see 13.5) and down and forwards to the navicular. It is a very strong ligament – so strong that the sustentaculum may be fractured rather than the ligament torn.

Stability

The articular surface of the talus is wider in front than behind so that when the ankle is dorsiflexed, the wider part of the articular surface of the talus is in the mortise formed by the tibia and fibula and the joint is stable. In plantarflexion, though, the narrower part of the talus is in the mortise and the joint is therefore somewhat unstable. Fortunately, we do not walk with the ankle in plantarflexion, but ballet dancers need to be very careful.

Movements and muscles

Plantarflexion, toe flexion, inversion
(Fig. 13.22)

Muscles which plantarflex the ankle and invert the foot occupy the posterior compartment of the leg.

Nerve supply: tibial nerve, L4, 5, S1, 2.

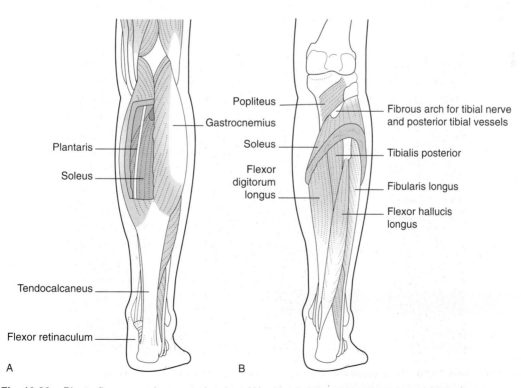

Fig. 13.22 Plantarflexor muscles, posterior view: (**A**) with window cut in gastrocnemius; (**B**) with gastrocnemius and most of soleus removed.

Superficial flexors. Attached to the calcaneus by the Achilles tendon (tendo calcaneus): gastrocnemius (from femur) and soleus (from tibia, fibula):

- Gastrocnemius: medial and lateral heads attached to medial and lateral condyles of the femur. They form obvious bulges at the back of the leg and unite on the Achilles tendon (tendo calcaneus), which is attached to the lower part of the posterior surface of the calcaneus.
- Soleus. This is attached to the soleal line on the posterior surface of the tibia and the upper third of the back of the fibula. Between these two bones is a fibrous arch, deep to which pass the tibial nerve and the posterior tibial artery and veins. It is a very bulky muscle and contains the soleal venous plexus, so important in the soleal muscle pump (see p. 207). It is attached by the Achilles tendon to the calcaneus.
- Plantaris. This very small muscle from the lateral condyle of the femur has a very long tendon that joins the Achilles tendon. It is very unimportant, so everyone remembers it.

Deep flexors. Attached to the bones of the sole of the foot: tibialis posterior, flexor digitorum longus, flexor hallucis longus:

- Tibialis posterior. Attachments: posterior tibia, fibula, interosseous membrane – navicular, inferior surface. Its tendon grooves the posterior surface of the medial malleolus and is palpable at the ankle. The tendon sends slips to every tarsal and metatarsal bone except the talus and first metatarsal.
- Flexor digitorum longus. Attachments: posterior tibia – distal phalanges of digits 2–5. Its tendon grooves the medial malleolus and is palpable at the ankle.
- Flexor hallucis longus. Attachments: posterior fibula – distal phalanx of first (big) toe (with part of flexor digitorum longus). Its tendon grooves the back of the tibia and passes immediately deep to the sustentaculum tali of the calcaneus. Its tendon is not easily palpable, being deeply situated. Note that in the leg the long flexor of the big toe is lateral to that of the other toes, whereas in the foot the big toe is medial. The tendons cross in the foot.

Ankle jerk. Tapping the Achilles tendon to elicit the ankle jerk tests the tibial nerve and spinal segments S1, 2. It is an important part of a general neurological examination.

Clinical box

Achilles tendon rupture
This occasionally happens, either when the tendon is under tension, or sometimes for no very good reason. A sharp pain at the back of the ankle, coupled with tenderness on gentle squeezing of the tendon – the squeeze test – is usually indicative.

Dorsiflexion, eversion   (Fig. 13.23)

Nerve supply: common fibular nerve, L4, 5, S1.

Ankle dorsiflexion and toe extension: deep fibular nerve. These muscles occupy the anterior compartment of the leg:

- Tibialis anterior. Attachments: tibia, interosseous membrane – medial cuneiform and first metatarsal. This fleshy muscle and its tendon anterior to the medial side of the ankle are palpable.
- Extensor digitorum longus. Attachments: fibula, interosseous membrane – extensor expansion of digits 2–5. These tendons are palpable. On the dorsum of the foot they are joined by tendons of extensor digitorum brevis. The tendon passing to the fifth toe may be reinforced by a slip from the fibula – fibularis tertius. Forget about it.
- Extensor hallucis longus. Attachments: fibula, interosseous membrane – base of distal phalanx of first (big) toe. The tendon is palpable.

Ankle eversion: superficial fibular nerve (Fig. 13.28). Muscles that evert the foot occupy the lateral compartment of the leg:

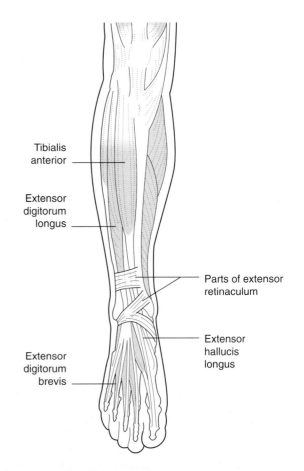

Tibialis anterior

Extensor digitorum longus

Parts of extensor retinaculum

Extensor hallucis longus

Extensor digitorum brevis

Fig. 13.23   Dorsiflexor muscles.

- Fibularis longus. Attachments: fibula – inferior surface of medial cuneiform and first metatarsal. The tendon enters the foot laterally but then crosses under the bones to the medial side, grooving the under surface of the cuboid. Both muscle and tendon are palpable.
- Fibularis brevis. Attachments: fibula – base of fifth metatarsal.

Arrangements to help tendons turn corners

- Flexor retinaculum (Fig. 13.24). The tendons of tibialis posterior (superficial), flexor digitorum longus and flexor hallucis longus (deep) enter the foot behind the medial malleolus deep to the flexor retinaculum. Other structures which accompany them are the tibial nerve, the posterior tibial artery and its venae comitantes.
- Extensor retinaculum (Figs 13.23, 13.24). Extensor tendons (extensor hallucis, extensor digitorum, fibularis tertius) pass from leg to foot behind the extensor retinaculum, which is in two parts: an upper transverse band, and a lower Y-shaped band. Other structures that accompany them are the deep fibular nerve, the anterior tibial artery and its venae comitantes.
- Fibular retinaculum (Fig. 13.25). The tendons of fibularis longus and brevis pass between ankle and foot deep to the superior and inferior fibular retinacula.
- Synovial sheaths. As the tendons pass deep to the retinacula at the ankle, they are enclosed in synovial

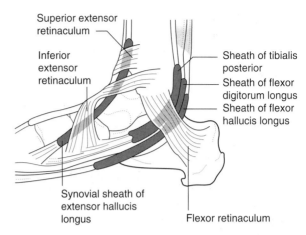

Fig. 13.25   Lateral leg muscles.

sheaths. As at the wrist, it is more important that you know that they exist rather than details of them. Athletes (jumpers, gymnasts, basketball players, etc.) and others may suffer from tenosynovitis of these tendons and sheaths – a condition which can be painful and disabling. Pain fibres are conveyed in the nearest local cutaneous nerve.

Pulses at the ankle   (Fig. 13.1)

Posterior tibial

The posterior tibial pulse is easily palpable just behind the medial malleolus, deep to the flexor retinaculum. Feel your own.

Anterior tibial and dorsalis pedis

The anterior tibial pulse is easily palpable between the tendons of extensor hallucis longus and digitorum longus. At the level of the malleoli, the anterior tibial artery becomes the dorsalis pedis artery, another important palpable pulse. Feel your own.

13.5 Foot

Overview

Because the foot is less often injured than the hand, you do not require such detailed knowledge of it. Revise the hand before proceeding. The small muscles of the foot are equivalent to those of the hand, and, together with foot bones and ligaments, constitute a dynamic structure that adapts to posture, stance and terrain. Inversion and eversion take place at several joints in the foot, inversion being supplied by the tibial nerve and eversion by the superficial fibular. The dorsalis pedis pulse is usually palpable on the dorsum of the foot.

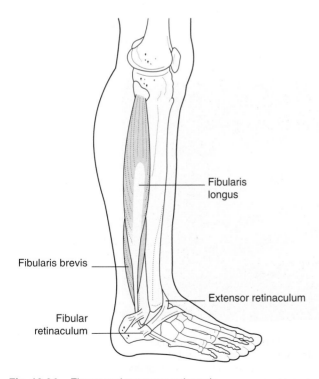

Fig. 13.24   Flexor and extensor retinacula.

Learning Objectives

You should:

- know the names and surface anatomy of all foot bones, and be able to recognise them on radiographs

- understand the subtalar and talocalcaneonavicular joints

- know where to palpate for the dorsalis pedis pulse.

Bones (Figs 13.19, 13.26)

- Tarsal bones: learn the names, be able to recognise the bones on radiographs, and point out the following surface features:
  - head of the talus
  - sustentaculum tali of the calcaneus
  - tuberosity of the navicular
  - cuboid.
- Metatarsals 1–5, and phalanges, as in the hand.

Otherwise, you do not need to learn details of the bones.

Joints

Talus – calcaneus – cuboid – navicular

There are two separate talocalcaneal articulations and one also includes the navicular. There is disagreement concerning the nomenclature of these joints and the version that follows is as good as any.

- Subtalar joint. This is directly underneath the talus, in line with the tibia.
- Talocalcaneonavicular joint. This is anterior to the head of the talus and involves the sustentaculum tali, the head of the talus, the spring ligament and the navicular.
- Calcaneocuboid joint. This is a separate joint cavity, but is a functional unit with the talocalcaneonavicular joint, the two together being called by some the midtarsal joint. However, this term is used differently by different authorities.

Other joints, foot movements

There is no need to bother with the details of other tarsal joints.

Inversion and eversion are composite movements that involve several joints. Disease of any one synovial cavity will result in limitation of foot function. This involves all the small movements that must take place during locomotion, not only the obvious ones concerned with taking a step, but also the small adjustments concerned with adapting foot position to an uneven or sloping surface. You do not need to learn details, but try to appreciate that joint diseases in the foot will affect our stance and our ability to get about.

Ligaments

There are numerous tarsal ligaments: some are worth reading about.

- Medially in the sole: spring (plantar calcaneonavicular) ligament: sustentaculum tali of

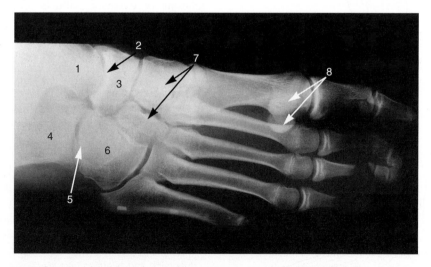

Fig. 13.26 Radiograph of foot: 1, head of talus; 2, talonavicular articulation of talocalcaneonavicular joint; 3, navicular; 4, calcaneus; 5, calcaneocuboid articulation; 6, cuboid; 7, cuneiform bones; 8, sesamoid bones in the tendons of the long flexors (hallucis usually, digitorum sometimes).

calcaneus – navicular. This forms part of the articular surface for the talocalcaneonavicular joint: its upper surface is covered by articular cartilage. It is continuous with the deltoid ligament (see 13.4, p. 201). Note that the bones to which the spring ligament is attached are palpable.

- Laterally in the sole: long and short plantar (calcaneocuboid) ligaments. The long plantar also sends slips to the middle three metatarsals. The short plantar is deep (superior) to the long plantar and the tendon of fibularis longus runs between them on its way from the lateral side of the foot to the medial cuneiform.
- On the dorsum: bifurcate ligament: calcaneus – cuboid, navicular.

Muscles and arches of the foot

Muscles of the sole

Nerve supply: medial and lateral plantar nerves, L5–S3.

Muscles of the sole are equivalent to the thenar, hypothenar, lumbricals and interosseous muscles of the hand except that:

- hallucis replaces pollicis
- there are no opponens muscles.

As in the hand, the first toe has no lumbrical. There is no need to learn details of actions or attachments: for most practitioners these are superfluous. The muscles are innervated as in the hand: regard the medial plantar nerve as the equivalent of the median nerve and the lateral plantar as the equivalent of the ulnar, except that the medial plantar (median equivalent) supplies only one lumbrical, that of the second toe.

Muscle actions

Although we can train our toes to wield paintbrushes etc., it is sufficient to regard the small muscles of the foot as dynamic ligaments, constantly contracting and relaxing in response to subtle changes in posture, activity and orientation of the supporting surface.

Long flexor tendons

- Flexor hallucis longus, flexor digitorum longus:
  - After passing behind the medial malleolus, these tendons cross.
  - An additional muscle, flexor accessorius (quadratus plantae) connects the tendon of flexor digitorum longus to the lower surface of the calcaneus and converts the oblique pull of the long tendon to one in line with the axis of the foot itself.

- Sesamoid bones are found in these tendons - we walk on them.
- Fibularis longus, from the lateral side; tibialis posterior, from the medial side (see above).

Arches of the foot

The foot is described as having a medial longitudinal arch, a lateral longitudinal arch, and a transverse half-arch, the two of which, when the feet are together, presumably constitute a whole arch. These arches are maintained by the numerous ligaments and small muscles of the foot, and the pull of the long tendons (see above) must also be an important load-bearing factor.

Plantar fascia

This is tougher than the palmar fascia in the hand. The skin is so tightly attached to it that infiltration of local anaesthetics, for instance in order to deal with something as simple as a plantar wart, may be difficult and painful.

Dorsum of the foot

- Extensor digitorum brevis: deep fibular nerve. It is unimportant except that its fleshy belly may be mistaken for a tumour.
- The superficial dorsal venous arch gives rise medially to the great saphenous vein, and laterally to the small saphenous vein.

Arteries of the foot   (Fig. 13.1)

- Branches of the posterior tibial artery (see above): medial and lateral plantar arteries. The lateral plantar curves medially under the metatarsals to anastomose with a branch of the dorsalis pedis artery that has passed between the first and second metatarsals.
- Dorsalis pedis artery, a continuation of the anterior tibial artery. See above.

Nerves of the foot

- Branches of the tibial nerve (Fig. 13.27):
  - medial plantar: fewer muscles, more skin (like the median in the hand): plantar skin of the medial three and a half digits
  - lateral plantar: more muscles, less skin (like the ulnar in the hand): plantar skin of the lateral one and a half digits.
- Branches of the common fibular nerve (Fig. 13.28):
  - deep fibular: only a tiny area of skin at the base of the first and second toes
  - superficial fibular: most of the skin of the dorsum.

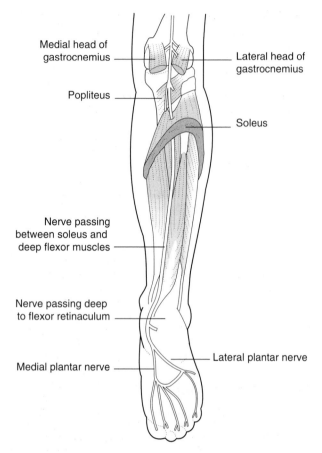

Medial head of gastrocnemius

Lateral head of gastrocnemius

Popliteus

Soleus

Nerve passing between soleus and deep flexor muscles

Nerve passing deep to flexor retinaculum

Medial plantar nerve

Lateral plantar nerve

Fig. 13.27 Tibial nerve.

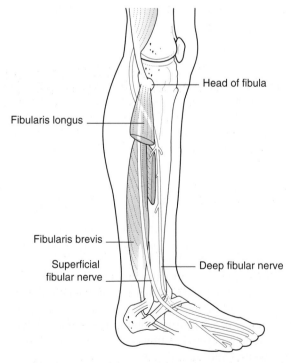

Head of fibula

Fibularis longus

Fibularis brevis

Superficial fibular nerve

Deep fibular nerve

Fig. 13.28 Common fibular nerve and branches.

13.6 Venous drainage of the lower limb (Figs 13.9, 13.29)

Overview

Venous return from the lower limb is driven by the soleal muscle pump enclosed within the tough deep fascia. As blood in deep veins is squeezed upwards, it is replaced by blood drawn in from the superficial veins through perforating veins. When this process is disrupted, venous disease results.

Learning Objectives

You should:

- know the surface markings of the great saphenous vein
- understand the effect of the muscle pump
- understand the function of the perforating veins
- know how the great saphenous vein terminates
- understand the basis of venous disease.

Mechanism of venous return

- Superficial veins:
  - Great saphenous vein. This is formed medially from the dorsal venous arch of the foot and ascends in front of the medial malleolus and behind the knee, continuing up the thigh to penetrate the fascia lata below and lateral to the pubic tubercle at the saphenous opening. It drains into the femoral vein. Below the knee it is accompanied by the saphenous nerve.
  - Small saphenous vein. This is formed laterally from the dorsal venous arch of the foot and ascends on the back of the calf accompanied by the sural nerve. It penetrates the deep fascia in the popliteal fossa, and joins the popliteal vein.

There are several tributaries in the calf and thigh (details not necessary).

- Deep veins: venae comitantes of the deep arteries unite to form the popliteal vein, which becomes the femoral.
- Perforators, permitting blood to flow from superficial to deep.

The effective venous return from the lower limb depends upon a pumping mechanism within the deep fascia.

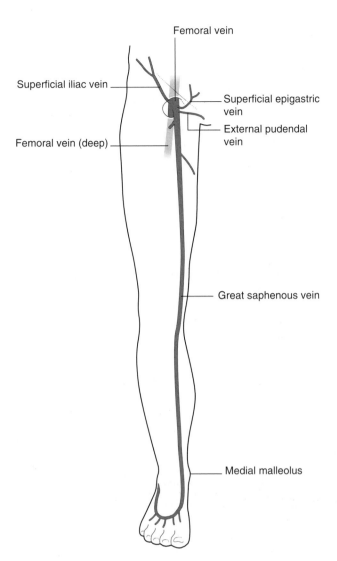

Fig. 13.29   Great saphenous vein.

Femoral vein

Superficial iliac vein

Superficial epigastric vein

External pudendal vein

Femoral vein (deep)

Great saphenous vein

Medial malleolus

13.7 Innervation, nerve testing, surface anatomy

Overview

Principal nerves supplying the lower limb are the femoral, obturator, tibial and common fibular. They are vulnerable to injury at certain points close to skin and/or bone.

Learning Objectives

You should:

- know where nerves are vulnerable to injury
- know how to test the femoral, obturator, tibial and common fibular nerves for both sensory and motor function
- know how to test specific spinal segments for both sensory and motor function
- know the surface markings of lower limb bones, and principal vessels and nerves.

- The deep fascia, in the thigh called fascia lata, is a tough fibrous layer, in no way elastic. The valves in the deep veins permit blood to flow only towards the heart so when muscles within the deep fascial sleeve contract, deep veins are compressed and blood flows upwards (because of the valves). When the muscles relax, blood is sucked into the deep veins through the perforators from the superficial system, the perforators also containing valves allowing blood to flow only in this direction.
- Below the knee, one of the largest muscles surrounding the deep veins is the soleus, and this mechanism is known as the soleal muscle pump.
- The chances of a blood cell passing from foot to femoral vein through the length of the great saphenous vein are very small – it is likely to be sucked into the deep system through a perforator.

Nerves: a revision of some important points

Dermatomes (Fig. 6.6, p. 36)

Remember these:
- L3 at the knee (over the patella)
- S2 over the popliteal fossa
- L5 under the first toe
- S1 under the fifth toe.

Sensory nerves (Fig. 13.30)

- Gluteal region:
  - posterior cutaneous branches of sacral plexus.
- Anterior thigh:
  - branches of genitofemoral and ilioinguinal
  - lateral cutaneous nerve of the thigh
  - intermediate and medial cutaneous nerves of the thigh (branches of the femoral).

- Posterior thigh and popliteal fossa: sacral plexus:
  - posterior cutaneous nerve of the thigh (sacral plexus).
- Leg:
  - saphenous nerve (from femoral): medial skin; since it accompanies the great saphenous vein it may be damaged by surgical procedures on the vein.
  - sural nerve (from tibial and common fibular in the popliteal fossa): posterolateral skin
  - superficial fibular nerve: lower anterior skin; it may be affected by trauma at the fibular neck.
  - lateral cutaneous nerve (from common fibular nerve); it may be affected by trauma at the fibular neck.
- Foot:
  - superficial fibular nerve: dorsum
  - saphenous nerve: medial skin
  - sural nerve: lateral skin
  - medial and lateral plantar nerves (branches of tibial nerve).

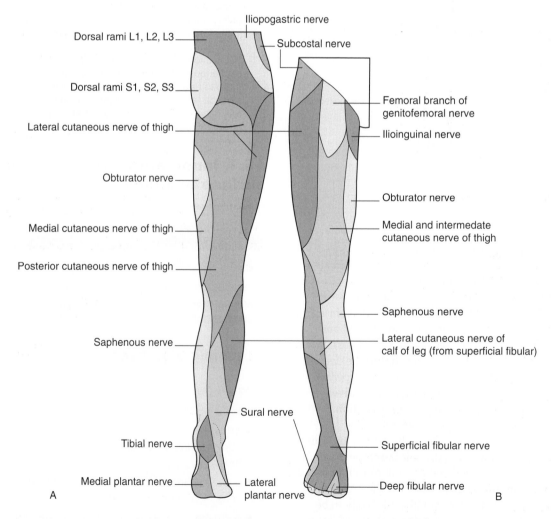

Fig. 13.30 Cutaneous nerves of lower limb: (**A**) posterior view; (**B**) anterior view.

Segmental values for movements and reflexes

Hip
Flexion, adduction, medial rotation   L2, 3
Extension, abduction, lateral rotation L4, 5, S1

Knee
Extension   L3, 4
Flexion   L5, S1

Ankle
Dorsiflexion   L4, 5
Plantarflexion S1, 2

Foot
Inversion L4
Eversion   L5, S1

The most frequently tested reflexes of both limbs can be remembered thus: ankle jerk, knee jerk, biceps jerk, triceps jerk: *1 2, 3 4, 5 6, 7 8* (plus S, L or C as appropriate).

Clinical box

Sites where injuries may damage lower limb nerves
- Anterior superior iliac spine: lateral cutaneous nerve of the thigh (neuralgia paraesthetica).
- Posterior dislocation of the hip: sciatic nerve.
- Popliteal fossa trauma: tibial and/or common fibular nerves.
- Neck of fibula, fracture or trauma: common fibular nerve.
- Foot drop. Damage to common fibular nerve at the neck of the fibula would result in paralysis or weakness of dorsiflexion and eversion: the foot would be plantarflexed and inverted. This is foot drop. Sensory changes would be present in the skin of the anterior leg and dorsum of the foot.
- Great saphenous vein procedures: saphenous nerve.

Testing peripheral nerves
- Femoral: skin over anterior thigh, knee jerk.
- Obturator: skin over medial thigh, hip adduction.
- Tibial: ankle jerk.
- Deep fibular: ankle dorsiflexion.
- Superficial fibular: skin of dorsum of foot, ankle eversion.

Testing spinal segments
- L1, 2: skin over front of upper thigh.
- L3, 4: knee jerk, skin over patella and medial side of leg.
- L5: skin over lateral side of leg.
- S1, 2: ankle jerk, skin over lateral side of foot and back of thigh.
- S3, 4: skin over medial gluteal region.

Revise dermatomes: Figure 6.6 (p. 36).

Surface anatomy: a revision of some important points

Gluteal region

- Sciatic nerve: halfway between posterior superior iliac spine and ischial tuberosity, curving to about halfway between ischial tuberosity and greater trochanter.

Thigh

- Femoral pulse: midpoint of inguinal ligament.
- Femoral vein: medial to femoral pulse.
- Femoral nerve: lateral to femoral pulse.
- Saphenous opening in fascia lata, femoral hernia: about 2 cm below and lateral to pubic tubercle.

Knee

- Popliteal pulse: press deep in popliteal fossa against popliteal surface of femur.
- Suprapatellar bursa: extends about one handsbreadth above upper margin of patella.
- Prepatellar bursa: directly over patella.
- Head of fibula: tendon of biceps femoris.
- Common fibular nerve: neck of fibula.

Ankle region and foot

- Posterior tibial pulse: immediately posterior to medial malleolus.
- Dorsalis pedis pulse: between tendons of extensors hallucis and digitorum longus.
- Great saphenous vein: anterior to medial malleolus.
- Lateral ligaments of ankle: below and in front of lateral malleolus.
- Sustentaculum tali of calcaneus: attachment of deltoid ligament.

Self-assessment: questions

Multiple choice questions

1. At the hip joint:
   a. Quadriceps femoris is the principal flexor.
   b. The profunda femoris artery contributes little to the cruciate anastomosis.
   c. The capsule is directly related to the sciatic nerve posteriorly.
   d. Blood supply to the head of the femur may be impaired if the joint capsule is torn.
   e. Disease in the hip may present as pain in the knee.

2. In the gluteal region and at the back of the thigh:
   a. It is safe to give intramuscular injections in the inferomedial quadrant.
   b. The hamstrings flex both hip and knee joints.
   c. Gluteus maximus is an abductor of the hip joint.
   d. Paralysis of gluteus maximus and medius causes the Trendelenburg gait.
   e. The pudendal nerve is directly related to the ischial spine.

3. In the thigh:
   a. Sartorius is attached to the anterior inferior iliac spine.
   b. Ovarian pain may be referred to medial skin of the thigh.
   c. The saphenous opening transmits the great saphenous vein.
   d. At the inguinal ligament the femoral vein is lateral to the femoral artery.
   e. Semitendinosus is on the lateral side.

4. At the knee joint:
   a. The anterior cruciate ligament is tested by pushing the tibia posteriorly on the femur.
   b. The lateral (fibular) collateral ligament is firmly attached to the lateral meniscus.
   c. The medial meniscus is more likely to be torn than the lateral.
   d. Popliteus tendon penetrates the joint capsule.
   e. The suprapatellar bursa does not communicate with the joint.

5. The tibial nerve supplies:
   a. Hip flexors.
   b. Knee flexors.
   c. Anterior femoral skin.
   d. Skin of the sole of the foot.
   e. Plantarflexors.

6. The posterior tibial artery:
   a. Is a branch of the femoral artery.
   b. Is related to the medial malleolus.
   c. Divides into medial and lateral plantar arteries.
   d. Supplies dorsiflexors.
   e. Is accompanied by the sural nerve.

7. At the ankle and in the foot:
   a. The great saphenous vein is posterior to the medial malleolus.
   b. Tibialis posterior tendon passes deep to the flexor retinaculum.
   c. Eversion and inversion mainly take place at the ankle joint.
   d. The Achilles tendon is attached to the talus.
   e. The spring ligament is attached to the sustentaculum tali.

8. The capsule of the hip joint:
   a. Is attached along the intertrochanteric crest posteriorly.
   b. Carries blood vessels to the head of the femur.
   c. Limits flexion of the hip.
   d. Is directly related to the sciatic nerve posteriorly.
   e. Has the psoas bursa as an immediate anterior relation.

9. The sartorius muscle:
   a. Is inserted onto the lateral side of the tibia.
   b. Crosses the thigh deep to the quadriceps femoris muscle.
   c. Forms the anterior wall of the adductor canal.
   d. Forms the medial boundary of the femoral triangle.
   e. Extends the hip joint.

10. The sural nerve:
    a. Is a branch of the femoral nerve.
    b. Passes down the leg with the short saphenous vein.
    c. Supplies muscles of the foot.
    d. Is related to the neck of the fibula.
    e. Supplies skin over the anterior aspect of the leg.

11. At the knee, the following bursas usually or always communicate with the joint space:
    a. Suprapatellar.
    b. Semimembranosus.
    c. Popliteus.
    d. Deep infrapatellar.
    e. Prepatellar.

12. The anterior tibial artery:
    a. Is a branch of the femoral artery.
    b. Is related to the medial malleolus.
    c. Divides into medial and lateral plantar arteries.
    d. Supplies the dorsiflexor muscles.
    e. Is palpable in the foot.

13. Concerning the foot:
    a. Fracture of the neck of the talus may cause avascular necrosis of the body.
    b. The talus has two separate articulations with the calcaneus.
    c. The deltoid (medial) ligament is stronger than the lateral ligament of the ankle.
    d. A laceration in the femoral triangle may cause sensory loss on the medial side of the foot.
    e. The great saphenous vein is medial.

Matching item questions

Questions 1–5

Match the numbered item to the lettered response. Each lettered response may be used once, more than once, or not at all.
    a. femoral nerve
    b. tibial nerve
    c. nerve related to the neck of the fibula
    d. obturator nerve
    e. genitofemoral nerve

1. supplies knee extensors

2. damage to this nerve may result in foot drop

3. is related to the ovarian fossa in the pelvis

4. a branch of this supplies skin on the medial side of the foot

5. cutaneous sensation of the medial thigh

Questions 6-12

Match the numbered item to the lettered response. Each lettered response may be used once, more than once, or not at all.
    a. profunda femoris artery
    b. popliteal artery
    c. L3, 4
    d. S1, 2
    e. anterior superior iliac spine

6. blood supply to the hip joint

7. sartorius muscle

8. branch of artery palpable deep to the inguinal ligament

9. may be damaged by supracondylar femoral fracture

10. contributes to obturator nerve

11. patellar tendon reflex

12. Achilles tendon reflex

Questions requiring short answers

1. A patient is stabbed in the thigh just below the middle of the inguinal ligament. What structures are in danger? What will be the effect of section of the major nerve here?

2. Describe or draw the main arterial tree of the lower limb. Name three sites where peripheral pulses may be palpated. Where are these vessels liable to injury?

3. Describe the venous drainage of the lower limb, indicating the normal direction of blood flow between the superficial and deep veins.

4. Describe the blood supply of the head of the femur in the adult. How is this relevant to femoral neck fractures?

5. Describe the knee joint cartilages and ligaments. How would you test the ligaments? List the muscle groups that perform flexion and extension and the segmental innervation of these muscle groups. Names of individual muscles are *not* required.

6. What is foot drop? How may it be caused?

7. A 20-year-old student twists his ankle playing basketball. There is marked tenderness anterior to the lateral malleolus. Name the bones constituting the ankle joint and state the injury that has occurred. List the muscle groups acting on the joint and give their nerve supply and segmental innervation.

8. List the structures attached to and/or related to the sustentaculum tali of the calcaneus.

Self-assessment: answers

Multiple choice questions

1. a. **False.** Psoas is the principal flexor.
   b. **False.** It is very important.
   c. **True.** Posterior dislocations of the hip joint may damage the nerve.
   d. **True.** The important capsular (retinacular) vessels may be damaged.
   e. **True.** Sensory information from both joints passes in the same nerves, so referred pain from hip to knee is not unusual.

2. a. **False.** This is the most unsafe area.
   b. **False.** They flex the knee and extend the hip.
   c. **True.**
   d. **True.**
   e. **True.**

3. a. **True.**
   b. **True.** Ovarian pain may be referred to the territory of the obturator nerve. Revise the pelvis.
   c. **True.**
   d. **False.** The vein is medial to the artery at the inguinal ligament.
   e. **False.** Biceps is lateral.

4. a. **False.** Pull the tibia anteriorly on the femur.
   b. **False.** It is not attached (unlike the medial).
   c. **True.**
   d. **True.** (Why does this matter?)
   e. **False.** It is part of the joint.

5. a. **False.** The femoral nerve supplies these.
   b. **True.**
   c. **False.** Anterior femoral skin is supplied by the femoral nerve and its branches.
   d. **True.** Plantar branches of the tibial nerve supply skin on the sole of the foot.
   e. **True.**

6. a. **False.** It is a branch of the popliteal artery.
   b. **True.**
   c. **True.**
   d. **False.** Dorsiflexors are supplied by the anterior tibial artery.
   e. **False.** It is nowhere near the sural nerve.

7. a. **False.** It is anterior. Anyone who gets this wrong is foolish: they have only to look down at their ankles.
   b. **True.**
   c. **False.** Eversion and inversion take place at joints in the foot.
   d. **False.** It is attached to the calcaneus
   e. **True.**

8. a. **False.** It is attached to the intertrochanteric line anteriorly, but posteriorly it is well up the neck.
   b. **True.**
   c. **False.** It limits extension.
   d. **True.**
   e. **True.**

9. a. **False.** The sartorius muscle is inserted on the medial side of the tibia.
   b. **False.** Sartorius is superficial to quadriceps femoris.
   c. **True.**
   d. **False.** It forms the lateral boundary of the femoral triangle.
   e. **False.** It flexes the hip joint (but only weakly).

10. a. **False.** It is a branch of the tibial and common fibular nerves (the saphenous nerve is a branch of the femoral).
    b. **True.**
    c. **False.** It is a cutaneous nerve.
    d. **False.** The common fibular nerve is so related.
    e. **False.** It supplies skin over the posterior aspect of the leg.

11. a. **True.**
    b. **True.**
    c. **True.**
    d. **False.**
    e. **False.**

12. a. **False.** It is a branch of the popliteal.
    b. **False.** The posterior tibial is so related.
    c. **False.** The posterior tibial does so.
    d. **True.**
    e. **False.** In the foot, by definition, it is called the dorsalis pedis artery. (Sorry! I agree that this is a nit-picking question, but it does illustrate that names can make all the difference.)

13. a. **True.** Compare it with the scaphoid in the upper limb.
    b. **True.** It has an articulation posteriorly at the subtalar joint, and another anteriorly at the talocalcaneonavicular joint.
    c. **True.**
    d. **True.** Saphenous nerve function would be lost if the laceration severed the femoral nerve.
    e. **True.**

Matching items answers

1. a. Quadriceps femoris, the extensor of the knee, is supplied by the femoral nerve.

2. c. The common fibular nerve may be damaged at the neck of the fibula, causing foot drop.

3. d.

4. a. The saphenous nerve is a branch of the femoral nerve.

5. e.

6. a.

7. e.

8. a. Profunda femoris is a branch of the femoral artery, whose pulse is palpable at the inguinal ligament.

9. b.

10. c.

11. c.

12. d.

Short answers

1. The femoral nerve, artery, and vein, with branches and tributaries, may be damaged. Section of the femoral nerve will cause functional loss of knee extensors (quadriceps), reduced or absent knee jerk, and loss of skin sensation over the anterior thigh.

2. Figure 13.1 shows the main arteries of the lower limb and the sites of palpable pulses. The femoral artery is liable to injury in the anterior thigh; the popliteal artery is vulnerable in supracondylar femoral fracture. See page 198.

3. The main points are as follows. There are superficial (name the long and short saphenous veins) and deep systems; perforators have valves to allow blood to go from superficial to deep; the soleal pump draws blood into the deep system; if the valves in the perforators are destroyed, blood will go from deep to superficial and cause venous disease of the saphenous veins.

4. The most important vessels supplying the head of the femur are the capsular (retinacular) vessels. Next in importance are branches of the nutrient artery (not in the child because these do not cross the epiphyseal plates) and least important is the artery of the round ligament of the head. Femoral neck fractures will damage the capsular vessels and/or the branches of the nutrient artery. (You could give information about the trochanteric and cruciate anastomoses if you like.)

5. See 13.3, page 196. The important ligaments you should mention are the menisci, the cruciates and the collaterals. Test the cruciates by the drawer test, and the collaterals by passive abduction/adduction: there should be very little. Flexion: hamstrings, L5, S1. Extension: quadriceps femoris, L3, 4.

6. Foot drop is paralysis or weakness of dorsiflexion and eversion. It is caused by damage to the common fibular (peroneal) nerve at the neck of the fibula, often as a result of direct trauma from, for example, a road traffic accident.

7. The ankle joint consists of the tibia, fibula and talus. The lateral collateral ligaments have been torn. Ankle dorsiflexion is performed by the muscle groups of the anterior compartment, supplied by the deep fibular nerve, L4, 5. Ankle plantarflexion is performed by the muscle groups of the posterior compartment, supplied by the tibial nerve, S1, 2.

8. The following structures are attached to the sustentaculum tali of the calcaneus: deltoid ligament, spring ligament.
   Related structures are:
   - superficial: tendons of flexor digitorum longus, tibialis posterior
   - inferior (a smooth groove is visible on the bone): tendon of flexor hallucis longus.

14 Head and neck

14.1 The big picture

Overview

The head houses the brain, main sense organs and the upper end of the respiratory and alimentary systems. 12 pairs of cranial nerves arise from the brain. Arterial blood comes from the common carotid and vertebral arteries. Veins drain principally to the internal jugular vein, and lymph to the deep cervical chain.

Learning Objectives

You should:

- understand the main components of the skull and cervical vertebral column
- know that cranial nerves arise from the brain and supply structures mainly in the head and neck
- know that arterial blood comes from the common carotid and vertebral arteries.

Skeleton

The skeleton of the head and neck serves several functions. Some of its components, the neurocranium, protect the brain and organs of the special senses. Some components, the viscerocranium, provide structural support for the cranial end of the gut tube and attachments for its muscles. Cervical vertebrae provide structural support for the head and muscle attachments for head and neck movements, and cartilages in the anterior neck provide a structural framework for the upper end of the respiratory system and attachments for muscles of phonation.

Nerves

- Cranial nerves. The 12 pairs of nerves that pass through or into the skull bones are probably the most important aspects of head and neck anatomy as far as the general physician is concerned. They serve various functions:
    - special senses: olfaction, vision, balance, hearing
    - sustenance: ingestion, digestion
    - communication: facial expression, speaking.
    A survey and analysis of the cranial nerves follows (14.4, p. 225) to provide a foundation for their various aspects that appear and reappear as the several regions and functions of the head and neck are considered. Cranial nerves are referred to by Roman numerals, I, II, III, etc.
- Cervical spinal nerves 1–8 supply structures in the neck and contribute to the innervation of the upper limb, upper thoracic skin and diaphragm. They are similar in form and function to other spinal nerves.

The brain attempts to integrate, coordinate and control these neural functions.

Arteries

- Carotid system. The right and left common carotid arteries bifurcate to give the internal and external carotid arteries of each side.
    - Internal carotid arteries enter the cranium to supply the brain. Within the cranium they supply the eye and orbit and terminate by contributing to the arterial circle of Willis with the vertebrobasilar system.

- External carotid arteries give branches in the neck to supply the neck, scalp, skull bones and cranial dura mater.
  - Branches of the two carotid systems communicate, particularly in the scalp and around the orbit.
- Vertebrobasilar system. The vertebral arteries supply the cervical vertebrae and spinal cord. They enter the cranial cavity through the foramen magnum, uniting to form the basilar artery, which supplies the brain stem. It terminates by contributing to the arterial circle of Willis with the internal carotids.
- The arterial circle of Willis supplies the brain.

Veins

- Dural venous sinuses within the cranium: these form an intracranial network of veins that receive blood from the brain and drain to the:
- Internal jugular veins: deep veins in the neck, with tributaries from the face and neck.
- External and anterior jugular veins: superficial veins from the skull, face and superficial tissues.
- There are many communicating channels between the internal and external systems.
- Venous blood from the cranial cavity also drains through the foramen magnum to the internal vertebral venous plexus of the vertebral column.

Lymph nodes

- Groups of lymph nodes, many palpable, are shown in Figure 14.1. In the head, lymph from a particular organ or region passes, in general, to whichever

group of nodes is nearest. These then drain to the deep cervical chain and thence to the venous system at the union of the internal jugular and subclavian veins. The palpable lymph node at the top of the deep cervical chain, just behind the angle of the mandible, is the tonsillar or jugulodigastric node. If you suffered as a child from frequent attacks of tonsillitis, you may have a permanently enlarged tonsillar node.

- The entrance to the gut tube is surrounded by Waldeyer's ring of lymphoid tissue: tonsils, adenoids, and lingual tonsils. This is continuous with the upper end of the deep cervical chain and drains to it.
- Retropharyngeal nodes. Involvement of nodes between the vertebral column and the pharynx is dangerous. The nodes are deep and therefore impalpable, so if disease spreads to this group of nodes, it is likely to go undetected until it has also spread elsewhere, by which time it is likely to be too late for effective treatment. Retropharyngeal nodes are connected to the deep cervical nodes of both sides and so provide a pathway for lymphatic spread across the midline.

14.2 Skull bones and joints, cranial cavity

Overview

The skull is made up of several separate bones united by fibrous sutures. The only synovial joint in the skull is the temporomandibular joint at which the movements of chewing occur. The internal aspect of the cranium is divided into three cranial fossas. There are numerous named foramina to allow structures to pass through the cranium. The fetal skull is different from the adult skull in a number of ways apart from size.

Learning Objectives

You should:

- know the names of the skull bones and the principal features of the mandible, occipital bone, sphenoid bone, temporal bone, and the position of the pterion
- know the names and boundaries of the three cranial fossas
- know the principal skull foramina as listed
- understand how the skull grows and how the fetal skull differs from the adult skull.

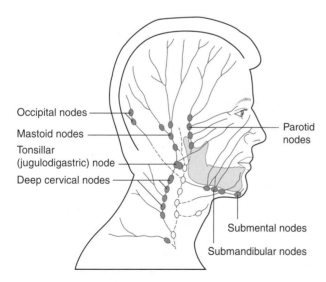

Occipital nodes
Mastoid nodes
Tonsillar (jugulodigastric) node
Deep cervical nodes
Parotid nodes
Submental nodes
Submandibular nodes

Fig. 14.1 Head and neck lymph nodes. The submental nodes are in the midline, connecting the two groups of submandibular nodes.

Bones

There are two types of skull bones:

- Neurocranium: flat bones of the vault of the skull. These consist of two plates of cortical bone, inner and outer tables or diploë, between which is the diploic cavity containing marrow. This is a site of haemopoiesis and so has a rich blood supply.
- Viscerocranium: these are bones of the base of the skull surrounding the nasal cavity and sinuses, oral cavity, pharynx and larynx.

Study the bones of the skull (Figs 14.2–14.6). Most of them reach the external surface of the skull, so identify and palpate them on yourself. Four of them (see below) are worth studying in some detail.

Mandible (Fig. 14.6)

The right and left mandibles fuse in the second year after birth.

- Body and ramus, lateral aspect:
  - mental foramen
  - angle.

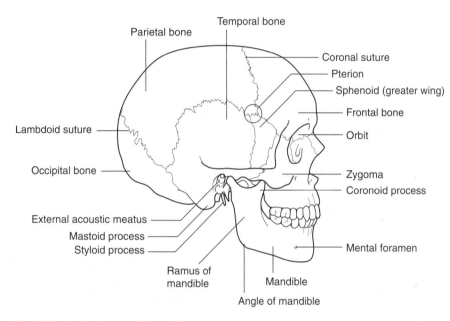

Fig. 14.2 Lateral view of the skull.

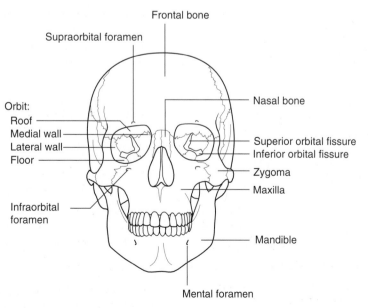

Fig. 14.3 Anterior view of the skull.

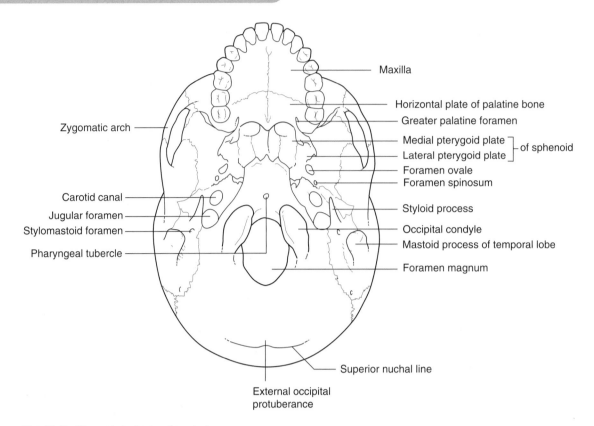

Fig. 14.4 Base of skull, view from below.

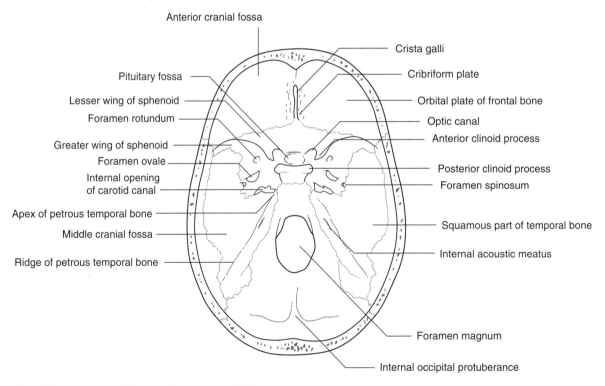

Fig. 14.5 Base of skull, internal aspect, cranial fossas.

A Lateral aspect

B Medial (internal) aspect

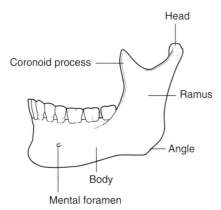
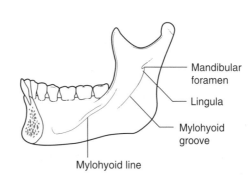

Fig. 14.6   Mandible: (**A**) lateral (external) aspect; (**B**) medial (internal) aspect.

- Body and ramus, medial (internal) aspect:
  - angle
  - mandibular foramen, lingula
  - mylohyoid line and groove.
- Alveolar (teeth) sockets.
- Coronoid process.
- Neck, head (condyle), articular surface.

Occipital bone   (Figs 14.4, 14.5)

- Basi-occiput: equivalent to the vertebral bodies below:
  - foramen magnum
  - condyles: convex, for the reciprocal surface of the atlas
  - hypoglossal (condylar) canal
  - pharyngeal tubercle.
- Squamous part, external aspect:
  - external occipital protuberance
  - superior nuchal lines.
- Squamous part, internal aspect:
  - internal occipital protuberance, ridges for meningeal attachments.

Sphenoid bone   (Fig. 14.5)

- Body, articulating with the basi-occiput.
- Sphenoid air sinus.
- Pituitary fossa (sella turcica), dorsum sellae, clinoid processes.
- Greater wing, lesser wing, optic foramen, superior orbital fissure, foramen rotundum, foramen ovale, foramen spinosum, spine (inferior aspect).
- Lateral and medial pterygoid plates, hamulus (palpable in the mouth behind and medial to the third upper molar).

Temporal bone   (Figs 14.2, 14.4, 14.5)

- Petrous temporal: ridge and apex.

- Internal acoustic (internal auditory) meatus.
- Mastoid process, mastoid antrum and air cells, middle ear cavity, orifice for Eustachian tube.
- Squamous temporal.
- Tympanic part.
- External acoustic (external auditory) meatus.
- Articular (condylar) surface for the head of the mandible.
- Zygomatic process forming the zygomatic arch with the zygoma.
- Carotid canal, foramen lacerum.
- Styloid process.
- Stylomastoid foramen.

Pterion (Fig. 14.2).   This is an area on the lateral side of the skull where the frontal, parietal, temporal and sphenoid bones meet. Its surface marking is about 4 cm above a point one-third of the way from ear to eye. Its importance will be pointed out later (p. 270).

Bones worth only a brief survey

- Parietal: diploë, grooves for meningeal vessels.
- Frontal: supraorbital margin and notch, frontal sinus.
- Zygoma: zygomatic arch formed by zygoma and temporal bone.
- Ethmoid: crista galli, perpendicular plate, cribriform plate, ethmoid sinuses, superior and middle turbinates.
- Maxilla: infraorbital margin and foramen, maxillary sinus, palatal shelf and alveolar sockets.

Bones you need only to have heard of

- Vomer: a midline, unpaired, bone forming the posterior part of the nasal septum.
- Lacrimal bone: on the anteromedial aspect of the orbit, near the opening of the nasolacrimal duct.

- Inferior turbinate: the lowest of the three bones projecting into the nasal cavity from the lateral wall (the other two are parts of the ethmoid).
- Palatine: deep in the skull, forming the posterolateral palate and part of the lateral side of the nasal cavity.
- Nasal bone: the bony part of the nasal bridge, sometimes fractured.

Internal aspect of the cranium, cranial fossas   (Fig. 14.5)

- The floor of the internal aspect of the cranial cavity is divided into three cranial fossas:
  - Anterior cranial fossa: anterior to the lesser wing of the sphenoid, related to the frontal lobes of the brain and the olfactory bulbs. Its features include the cribriform plate and crista galli of the ethmoid.
  - Middle cranial fossa: between the lesser wings of the sphenoid and the ridge of the petrous temporal bones, related to the temporal lobes and cavernous (venous) sinus. Its features include the pituitary fossa, foramina for cranial nerves II–VI, the carotid canal, and foramen spinosum.
  - Posterior cranial fossa: posterior to the ridge of the petrous temporal bone, related to the medulla, pons and cerebellum. It is covered by the tentorium cerebelli. Its features include foramina for cranial nerves VII–XII and the foramen magnum.
- The vault of the skull is formed by frontal, parietal, squamous temporal and squamous occipital bones.

The internal aspect of the vault displays grooves for meningeal vessels supplying bones and dura, and ridges for dural attachments forming intracranial partitions and the edges of the dural venous sinuses.

- Cranial meninges, meningeal vessels and venous sinuses are described in 14.12 (p. 270).

Skull foramina

Although not all these are important clinically, they are given here for the sake of completeness (Table 14.1). The list is not exhaustive.

Most other foramina transmit emissary veins draining the diploic cavities, some of which (e.g. those emerging from the occipital and temporal bones) are large.

Joints and growth of the skull

Sutures   (Fig. 14.2)

Sutures are fibrous joints (see 4.2, p. 21), the most important being:

- coronal – between the frontal bone and the two parietal bones
- sagittal – between the two parietal bones
- lambdoid – between the parietal bones and the occipital bone.

Suture lines are irregular and sometimes contain islands of bone (sutural bones, of no significance). Once sutures have fused no movement is possible, but before that there may be a little and the edges of the sutures may overlap. This is particularly so during childbirth

Table 14.1   Foramina in skull bones

Bone	Name	Contents	Effect of damage at the foramen
Ethmoid	Cribriform plate	I	Post-traumatic anosmia and CSF rhinorrhoea
Sphenoid	Optic foramen	II, ophthalmic artery	Not likely, eye blindness
	Superior orbital fissure	III, IV, Va, VI	Fractures may cause squints
	Foramen rotundum	Vb	Not likely
	Foramen ovale	Vc	Not likely
	Foramen spinosum	Middle meningeal artery	Not likely
Sphenoid/temporal	Carotid canal	Internal carotid artery	Not likely
Mandible	Inferior alveolar	Inferior alveolar nerve and vessels	Mandibular fractures may damage this nerve (mental anaesthesia)
	Mental	Mental nerve	Mental anaesthesia
Temporal bone	Stylomastoid foramen	VII	Facial palsy, weakness
	Internal acoustic meatus	VII, VIII	Deafness, balance disorders
Occipital/temporal	Jugular foramen	IX, X, XI, internal jugular vein	Not likely
Occipital	Hypoglossal canal	XII	Not likely
	Foramen magnum	Lower brain stem, vertebral arteries, XI, meninges	Trunk and limbs paralysis, death

when the fetal skull is deformed as it passes through the mother's pelvis. Growth at the sutures stops at about puberty, after which they are gradually obliterated from inside out. The metopic suture between the two frontal bones fuses during childhood (but may persist for longer), the sagittal suture fuses in the third decade, and those around the temporal bone may be present until old age.

Primary cartilaginous joints

The joint between the occipital and sphenoid bones is a primary cartilaginous joint (see 4.2, p. 21). Fusion of these bones occurs when anteroposterior growth ceases after puberty, usually in the mid-20s.

Synovial joints

There is only one on each side, the temporomandibular joint (see p. 245).

Fetal and neonatal skull

Fontanelles

Until the bones are completely ossified, the defects between them are occupied by fibrous connective tissue. Two such areas are large at birth:

- posterior fontanelle, in the midline between the occipital and parietal bones; it closes in the first 6 months of postnatal life
- anterior fontanelle, in the midline between the frontal and parietal bones; it closes between 18 months and 2 years after birth. It is clinically useful:
  - It can be used to assess intracranial pressure and the state of hydration. In a healthy baby it should be slightly convex and 'give' only a little to the touch, but if the child is dehydrated the fontanelle will be concave and feel 'floppy'. In raised intracranial pressure it may bulge markedly.
  - Through it, drugs can be injected into the subarachnoid space and samples of cerebrospinal fluid can be withdrawn more easily than by performing a lumbar puncture. Beware: a needle inserted in the midline will yield blood, not cerebrospinal fluid, because of the superior sagittal sinus: see Figure 14.37.

Cephalhaematoma

A cephalhaematoma is a subperiosteal haemorrhage: the blood collects between the bone itself and the over-lying periosteum. It may occur during birth, possibly as a result of the inept use during delivery of forceps or some other mechanical extraction device. The haema-toma is limited to the shape of the underlying bone, since the periosteum is attached to the bone at the sutures.

Other differences between the neonatal skull and a mature skull

Three of the more obvious are:

- Size: always state the obvious.
- Several protuberances of the skull bones form as a result of muscular attachments, of which a good example is the mastoid process, which develops postnatally as a result of the action of sternocleidomastoid. The lack of a mastoid process means that the facial nerve emerging from the stylomastoid foramen is superficial and vulnerable.
- As a proportion of the skull as a whole, the face is much smaller in the newborn, reflecting the fact that the child has not yet had to use its gut tube for sustenance.

14.3 Cervical vertebrae, joints and muscles of the neck

Overview

There are seven cervical vertebrae with special functional adaptations in C1 and C2 to allow for nodding and rotation. Elsewhere, features of cervical vertebrae are similar to those of other vertebrae. The cervical spine is more mobile than other regions of the vertebral column.

Learning Objectives

You should:

- know the principal features of C1 and C2 vertebrae
- understand the anatomy of nodding and rotation
- know the movements of the cervical spine, the muscles that produce them and their innervation
- understand the relationship of cervical spinal nerves to cervical vertebrae, and some of the causes of neck pain.

Vertebrae (Fig. 14.7)

Vertebrae C3–C7

Revise the features of a typical vertebra (Fig. 5.1, p. 26). Vertebrae C3–7 are typical cervical vertebrae (see 5.4, p. 26), the particular features of which are:

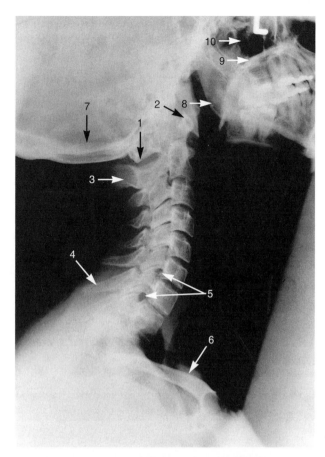

Fig. 14.7 Radiograph of cervical spine, lateral view: 1, posterior arch of atlas; 2, anterior arch of atlas; 3, posterior tubercle of axis; 4, spinous process of C7 (vertebra prominens); 5, intervertebral foramina for nerves C7 and C8; 6, clavicle; 7, occipital bone; 8, angle of mandible; 9, palate; 10, maxillary sinus.

- triangular vertebral canal
- foramen in the transverse process (foramen transversarium) for vertebral vessels
- anterior and posterior tubercles on the transverse processes
- bifid posterior spinous process for the attachment of a tough nuchal ligament (ligamentum nuchae).

Vertebra C2, the axis   (Fig. 14.8)

- Vertebra C2 can be thought of as a typical cervical vertebra with its body extended upwards to form the dens (tooth) or odontoid (tooth-like) process. This is a pivot around which vertebra C1 rotates. Embryologically, the dens is the body of C1, which has fused with C2, so there is no intervertebral disc between C1 and C2.
- There are large articular facets on the upper surface of the lateral sides of the body: these are the articulations for gliding movements with the atlas. Unlike facet joints elsewhere in the vertebral

column, these are anterior to the emerging spinal nerves.

Vertebra C1, the atlas   (Fig. 14.8)

Noteworthy features of the atlas are:

- it has no body (see above)
- anterior arch, the posterior surface of which has a facet for articulation with the dens
- posterior arch
- lateral masses where the anterior and posterior arches meet, palpable immediately behind the angle of the mandible (the atlas is surprisingly wide)
- inferior articular facets for reciprocal surfaces on the axis (see above)
- superior articular facets, concave, for the convex occipital condyles, for nodding movements
- groove for the vertebral artery (see below) on the superior surface.

The atlas is higher than you might think: it lies behind the mouth, so radiographs of the dens and atlas are taken through the open mouth (if the mouth were closed, teeth would obscure the radiographic view).

Joints of the cervical vertebral column

Joints below C2

These are as described in Chapter 5 (5.5, p. 27). There are symphyses with intervertebral discs in the midline and the facet joints laterally. The mobility of the cervical vertebral column means that there is considerable wear and tear on the facet joints and disease of them can cause cervical nerve root irritation and neck pain.

C2–C1: atlanto-axial joints and ligaments
(Fig. 14.8)

- In the midline. There is a synovial joint between the dens and the back of the anterior arch of the atlas (where facets may be seen), and a synovial bursa between the dens and the cruciate ligament behind it. The dens is kept in place by the cruciate ligament.
- Laterally. The lateral articular surfaces are flat to allow for gliding movements during rotation.

Cruciate ligament (Fig. 14.8).   This cross-shaped ligament separates the dens from the spinal meninges. The horizontal component of the ligament is attached to the sides of the spinal canal, and the vertical component runs from the lower part of the body of C2 to the occipital bone above. There is a synovial bursa between the ligament and the posterior aspect of the dens.

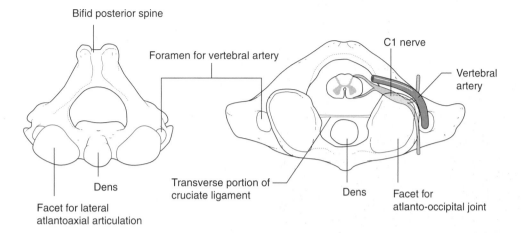

A Axis (C2) from above

Bifid posterior spine

Foramen for vertebral artery

Dens

Facet for lateral
atlantoaxial articulation

Transverse portion of
cruciate ligament

B Atlas (C1) from above

C1 nerve

Vertebral
artery

Dens

Facet for
atlanto-occipital joint

C Atlas, axis viewed from the side

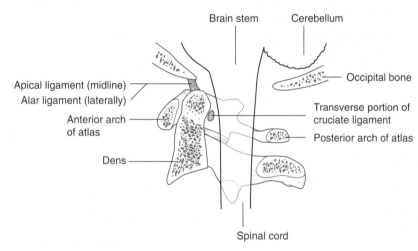

Brain stem   Cerebellum

Apical ligament (midline)
Alar ligament (laterally)

Anterior arch
of atlas

Dens

Occipital bone

Transverse portion of
cruciate ligament

Posterior arch of atlas

Spinal cord

Fig. 14.8 Atlas and axis: (**A**) axis (C2) from above; (**B**) atlas (C1) from above; (**C**) atlas and axis viewed from the side.

Atlanto-occipital joints

These are synovial joints with reciprocally curved surfaces for nodding. They are anterior to the spinal nerves as they emerge from the intervertebral foramen.

Clinical box

Pithing
Pithing takes place when the cruciate ligament ruptures and the dens is forced back into the central nervous system, resulting in death. This is thought to occur in judicial hanging. It may also occur in sudden neck movements if, for example, rheumatoid disease of the synovial bursa between the dens and the cruciate ligament causes degeneration of the ligament. An anaesthetist, or anyone who manipulates the neck, for example for tracheal intubation, needs to be careful when dealing with an aged rheumatic patient. On a lateral

Clinical box (*cont'd*)

radiograph of the cervical spine, if there is more than about 3 mm between the anterior arch of the atlas and the dens, it is likely that the dens is in danger of damaging the low medulla.

Notochordal remnants
Midline structures in this region (dens, apical ligament) are derived from the notochord, and tumours of notochordal remnants, chordomas, occasionally develop here.

Movements of the cervical spine

Flexion and extension occur, as in the rest of the vertebral column. Lateral flexion and rotation are not limited by ribs, as they are in the thorax. The cumulative result

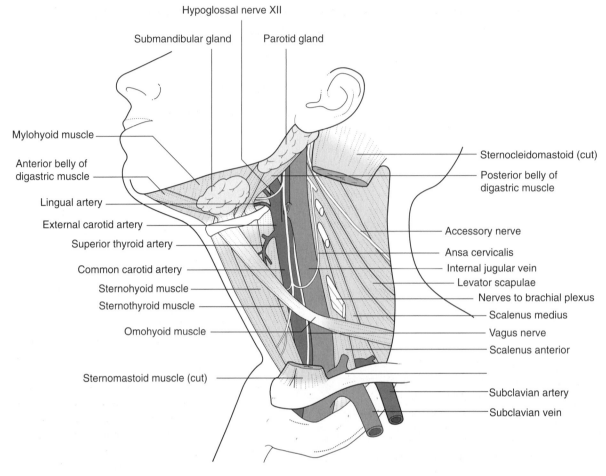

Hypoglossal nerve XII

Submandibular gland

Parotid gland

Mylohyoid muscle

Anterior belly of digastric muscle

Lingual artery

External carotid artery

Superior thyroid artery

Common carotid artery

Sternohyoid muscle

Sternothyroid muscle

Omohyoid muscle

Sternomastoid muscle (cut)

Sternocleidomastoid (cut)

Posterior belly of digastric muscle

Accessory nerve

Ansa cervicalis

Internal jugular vein

Levator scapulae

Nerves to brachial plexus

Scalenus medius

Vagus nerve

Scalenus anterior

Subclavian artery

Subclavian vein

Fig. 14.9 Side of neck: muscles and nerves.

of smaller movements between adjacent vertebrae adds up to great flexibility.

Muscles (Fig. 14.9)

Flexion, lateral flexion

- Sternocleidomastoid. Attachments: sternum, clavicle – mastoid process. Nerve supply: accessory nerve (cranial XI). Sternocleidomastoid flexes the cervical spine and moves the chin upwards and away from the muscle. It is a good test of accessory nerve function: to test the right accessory nerve, ask the patient to rotate his head to the left against the resistance of your hand on his chin.
- Scalene muscles: lateral flexion. Nerve supply: branches from cervical nerves. These muscles arise from the transverse processes of C3–6, scalenus anterior passing to the first rib between the subclavian vein and artery, and scalenus medius passing to the first rib behind the subclavian artery (see 10.4, p. 85).
- Prevertebral (longus) muscles run between anterior

aspects of upper thoracic and cervical vertebrae and the skull. You need only know that they exist.

Extension

- Trapezius. Attachments: external occipital protuberance and nuchal ligament – spine and acromion of scapula. Nerve supply: accessory nerve (cranial XI). Trapezius extends the head and cervical spine and its role in shoulder abduction has been considered (12.3, p. 162). Shrugging the shoulders against resistance is a test of accessory nerve function.
- Postvertebral muscles ('erector spinae') muscles (see 5.5, p. 27). Nerve supply: dorsal rami of spinal nerves.
- Small suboccipital muscles run between the atlas, the spinous process of the axis and the occipital bone and are supplied by branches of C1 and C2 nerves. They are responsible for movements that take place from minute to minute as we move our heads for listening, expressing emotion, talking, viewing and listening. You need know nothing of their detailed anatomy.

Clinical box

Greater occipital nerve, C2
The greater occipital nerve is the dorsal ramus of C2. It is a large sensory nerve which emerges posteriorly between vertebrae C1 and C2, and passes backwards between the suboccipital muscles before turning upwards to supply the skin of the back of the head and scalp as far forwards as the vertex. It has been suggested that compression of the nerve in the suboccipital region, perhaps by muscular tension, may be the cause of many headaches – a theory which has not been disproved – so perhaps there is something in the postural exercises advocated by adherents of the Alexander technique who maintain that certain relaxation exercises involving the cervical spine and skull can improve posture, lessen neck pain and generally promote a feeling of well-being.

14.4 Cranial nerves

You will need to return to this section repeatedly as you come across cranial nerves in other parts of the text.

Overview

Cranial nerves arise from the brain. They are numbered I–XII *roughly* in the order from top (rostral) to bottom (caudal) that they arise. Some are simple, either motor nerves or sensory nerves; some are complex: mixed motor and sensory, with parasympathetic and other impulses travelling with them and their branches on what appears at first sight to be a haphazard basis. Despite their complexity, cranial nerves have one or two functions that matter more than the others. In the clinical situation cranial nerves are often referred to by number alone (I, II, III, etc.).

Learning Objectives

You should:

- know the names and numbers of all 12 cranial nerves
- be able to refer to cranial nerves by number only
- know the most important function of each cranial nerve
- know how to test each cranial nerve (this will not be possible until you have completed your study of the head and neck)
- know the principal features of the course of each cranial nerve (this will not be possible until you have completed your study of the head and neck).

Functions, attachments and skull foramina of cranial nerves (Table 14.2)

A brief analysis

- Sensory nerves: I, II, VIII. These are nerves of the special senses.
- Motor nerves: III, IV, VI, XI, XII:
  - III, IV and VI innervate muscles that move the eyeball.
  - XI innervates sternocleidomastoid and trapezius.
  - XII innervates tongue muscle.
- Mixed nerves: V, VII, IX, X. These nerves supply structures derived from embryonic branchial arches at the cranial end of the gut tube.
  - Motor fibres are called branchiomotor: they are responsible for movements of the mandible, face, pharynx and larynx.
  - Sensory components convey a mixture of cutaneous sensation (e.g. tactile, pain, temperature) and visceral sensation (e.g. taste) from the face, mouth, nose, pharynx and larynx, and in the case of X, visceral sensation from the thorax and abdomen.
- Preganglionic parasympathetic fibres leave the brain stem in III, VII, IX and X but in order to reach their destinations those in III, VII and IX leave these nerves and hitch a lift with branches of V, with the ganglion (synapse) somewhere on the way. Parasympathetic fibres in X pass to the thorax and abdomen. See page 235 and Figure 14.14.
- Sensory fibres in cranial nerves:
  - Cutaneous and oral sensation (tactile, pain, temperature): most impulses reach the brain stem in V, with a few in X. In the brain stem they pass to the trigeminal sensory nuclei, so called (presumably) because the trigeminal nerve contributes most.
  - Visceral sensation (e.g. taste, impulses from chemoreceptors): impulses reach the brain stem in VII, IX and X. In the brain stem the impulses pass to the nucleus of the solitary tract (tractus solitarius) in the medulla. See page 235 and Figure 14.15.

Cranial nerve attachments and skull foramina (Table 14.3)

Cranial nerves I and II are attached to the cerebral hemispheres, and nerves III to XII to the brain stem (midbrain, pons and medulla). All nerves except IV arise from the ventral aspect.

Olfactory nerve: I

The olfactory nerve is the nerve of smell. It transmits impulses from the olfactory epithelium of the nose to the brain and is described in 14.9 (p. 256).

Table 14.2 Cranial nerve types and functions

Nerve	Type	Main function (less important functions in brackets)	Typical symptoms of damaged nerve
I Olfactory	Sensory	Smell	Anosmia
II Optic	Sensory	Vision	Visual impairment
III Oculomotor	Motor	Movements of eyeball, upper eyelid Parasympathetic: pupilloconstriction, accommodation	Squints, ptosis Dilated pupil, poor accommodation
IV Trochlear	Motor	Superior oblique (only)	Squint
V Trigerinal	Mixed		
Va Ophthalmic	Sensory	Eyeball, anterior scalp, upper face	Sensory loss in affected area
Vb Maxillary	Sensory	Nasal cavity and sinuses, palate, upper teeth, mid-face	Sensory loss in affected area
Vc Mandibular	Motor	Muscles of mastication	Impaired chewing
	Sensory	Chin, temple, oral cavity, tongue, temporomandibular joint, lower teeth, ear	Sensory loss in affected area
VI Abducens	Motor	Lateral rectus (only)	Medial squint
VII Facial	Mixed		
	Motor (Motor)	Muscles of facial expression (Parasympathetic: lacrimal, nasal, palatine, submandibular, sublingual glands)	Facial palsy, weakness (Dry mouth)
	(Sensory)	(Taste, anterior tongue)	(Loss of taste)
VIII Vestibulocochlear	Sensory	Balance and position in space, hearing	Disturbance of balance and/or deafness
IX Glossopharyngeal	Mixed		
	Sensory	Oropharynx, posterior tongue, carotid body and sinus	Not often involved in disease
	(Sensory)	(Taste, posterior tongue)	Loss of taste
	(Motor)	(Stylopharyngeus)	
	(Motor)	(Parasympathetic, parotid gland)	Dry mouth
X Vagus	Mixed		
	Motor	Muscles of pharynx, larynx for swallowing, phonation	Impaired swallowing, hoarseness of voice (depends upon site of lesion)
	(Motor)	(Parasympathetic: cardiac muscle; muscles and glands of foregut and midgut)	Not much
	Sensory (Sensory)	Sensation from ear, pharynx, larynx (Sensation from heart, lungs, abdominal viscera)	Abolition of cough reflex
	(Sensory)	(Taste: epiglottic region)	Loss of taste, abolition of cough reflex
XI Accessory	Motor	Sternocleidomastoid, trapezius	Limited head and neck movements and shoulder abduction beyond 90°
XII Hypoglossal	Motor	Tongue muscles	Impaired chewing and speaking

Optic nerve: II

The visual pathways are described in 14.11 (p. 266).

Oculomotor nerve: III

The oculomotor nerve innervates muscles that move the eyeball and is described with the orbit and eyeball (14.11, p. 264).

Trochlear nerve: IV

The trochlear nerve innervates one of the muscles that move the eyeball and is described with the orbit and eyeball (14.11, p. 264).

Trigeminal nerve: V   (Fig. 14.10)

The trigeminal nerve conveys sensation from the face and anterior scalp, the oral and nasal cavities, the teeth and the meninges, and its mandibular division is motor to the eight muscles of the first branchial arch, known as the muscles of mastication.

It arises from the pons and passes forwards over the apex of the petrous temporal bone to the trigeminal

Table 14.3 Cranial nerve attachments and foramina

Brain attachment	Nerve	Foramen or canal (cranial bone in brackets)
Forebrain		
Cerebral cortex, frontal lobes	I	Cribriform plate (ethmoid)
Diencephalon	II	Optic canal (sphenoid)
Midbrain		
Upper, ventral aspect	III	Superior orbital fissure (sphenoid)
Lower, dorsal aspect	IV	Superior orbital fissure (sphenoid)
Hindbrain		
Pons	V	
	Va	Superior orbital fissure (sphenoid)
	Vb	Foramen rotundum (sphenoid)
	Vc	Foramen ovale (sphenoid)
Pontomedullary junction, medial	VI	Superior orbital fissure (sphenoid)
Cerebellopontine angle	VII	Internal acoustic meatus, facial canal, stylomastoid foramen (temporal)
Cerebellopontine angle	VIII	Internal acoustic meatus (temporal)
Medulla	IX, X	Jugular foramen (between occipital and temporal)
Medulla, spinal cord	XI	Jugular foramen (between occipital and temporal): see text
Medulla	XII	Hypoglossal canal (occipital)

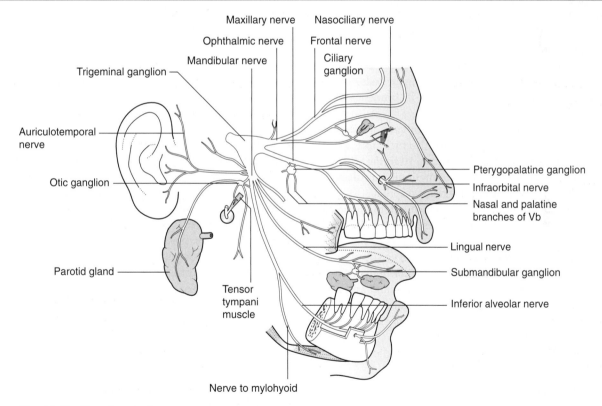

Fig. 14.10 The trigeminal nerve.

(sensory) ganglion in a slight depression on the bone. It then divides into the ophthalmic (Va), maxillary (Vb) and mandibular (Vc) nerves, each described separately below.

Clinical notes

- Shingles. The trigeminal ganglion, like all sensory ganglia, may harbour the herpes zoster virus causing shingles, a painful vesicular eruption in the sensory distribution of the nerve. The virus may have been latent for years following an attack of chickenpox.
- Trigeminal neuralgia. This is severe pain in the distribution of one or more branches of V. Its cause is frequently unknown but it may require partial destruction of the trigeminal ganglion to inactivate pain fibres.

Ophthalmic nerve: Va

The ophthalmic nerve conveys sensation from the eyeball, the skin of the upper face and anterior scalp, the lining of the upper part of the nasal cavity and sinuses, and the meninges of the anterior cranial fossa.

Some peripheral branches pick up parasympathetic fibres from elsewhere on their way to the ciliary and iris muscles, and the lacrimal gland.

Origin, course and branches

From the trigeminal ganglion, Va passes forwards in the lateral wall of the cavernous sinus and divides into the frontal (the largest), nasociliary and lacrimal (the smallest) branches, which pass through the superior orbital fissure into the orbit.

- Frontal nerve: supplies skin of forehead and scalp, and the frontal sinus. The nerve passes directly beneath the frontal bone and divides into supraorbital (larger, lateral) and supratrochlear (smaller, medial) nerves, which turn upwards at the supraorbital margin to supply the skin of the forehead and scalp.
- Nasociliary nerve: supplies the eyeball, upper part of the nasal cavity and neighbouring air cells, anterior nasal skin, and meninges. Its branches include:
  - Long and short ciliary nerves conveying sensory fibres from the eyeball. They also pick up parasympathetic impulses from III to the ciliary ganglion, and deliver postganglionic impulses to the ciliary body and constrictor pupillae.
  - Anterior ethmoidal nerve, which enters the nasal cavity to supply the upper part and associated sinuses. At the bridge of the nose it becomes superficial as the external nasal nerve supplying cutaneous sensation down to the nasal tip.
- Lacrimal nerve: supplies the lacrimal gland and a small area of adjacent skin and conjunctiva. It is unimportant, supplying a small area of skin laterally. It picks up postganglionic parasympathetic impulses from the pterygopalatine ganglion for the lacrimal gland.

The nerve contains

- Somatic sensory fibres: to the trigeminal sensory nuclei.
- In peripheral branches only, parasympathetic impulses from the Edinger–Westphal nucleus and III: to the ciliary ganglion (synapse) and eyeball (see p. 235).
- In peripheral branches only, parasympathetic impulses from the superior salivatory nucleus and pterygopalatine ganglion (synapse): to the lacrimal gland (see p. 235).

Clinical testing

- Test the cutaneous sensation of the forehead and anterior scalp.
- Corneal reflex. When the cornea is touched, usually with a wisp of cotton wool, the subject blinks. This tests Va and VII. The nerve impulses pass thus: cornea → nasociliary nerve → Va → principal sensory nucleus of V → brain stem interneurons → facial motor nucleus → VII → orbicularis oculi muscle. It does *not* test II, III, IV or VI.

Maxillary nerve: Vb

The maxillary nerve conveys sensation from the malar skin (skin between lower eyelid and mouth), from the nasal cavity and sinuses, and from maxillary teeth. Some of its branches pick up postganglionic fibres from the pterygopalatine ganglion to lacrimal, nasal and palatine glands.

Origin, course and branches

From the trigeminal ganglion, Va passes through the foramen rotundum into the pterygopalatine fossa where it divides into:

- Infraorbital nerve: to infraorbital skin, upper lip, maxillary sinus. This runs forwards between the orbit and the maxillary sinus and emerges at the infraorbital foramen.
- Zygomatic nerve: enters the orbit through the inferior orbital fissure and divides into nerves that penetrate the zygoma to supply overlying skin. It also conveys postganglionic parasympathetic impulses from the pterygopalatine ganglion on their way to the lacrimal nerve and gland.
- Nasal branches: pass to the nasal cavity and sinuses. Branches also convey postganglionic impulses from the pterygopalatine ganglion to nasal glands.
- Greater and lesser palatine nerves: descend in similarly named canals to the palate. Branches also convey postganglionic impulses from the pterygopalatine ganglion to palatal glands.
- Superior alveolar (dental) nerves: pass directly through the maxilla to the maxillary teeth and sinus.
- Pharyngeal branch: passes posteriorly to the nasopharynx.

The nerve contains

- Somatic sensory fibres: to the trigeminal sensory nuclei.
- In peripheral branches only, parasympathetic impulses from the superior salivatory nucleus and VII: to lacrimal, nasal and palatal glands (see p. 235).

Clinical testing

Test the cutaneous sensation of the lower eyelid, cheek and upper lip.

Mandibular nerve: Vc

The mandibular nerve is a mixed sensory and motor nerve. It conveys sensation from:

- skin over the mandible, side of the cheek and temple
- oral cavity and contents including the anterior tongue
- external ear, tympanic membrane and temporomandibular joint
- meninges of the cranial vault.

It conveys motor fibres to the eight muscles derived from the first branchial arch:

- temporalis, masseter
- medial, lateral pterygoids
- mylohyoid, anterior belly of digastric
- tensor tympani, tensor palati.

As an aid to memory, note the four groups of two: 2 tensors, 2 pterygoids, 2 big chewing muscles, 2 in the floor of the mouth. These muscles are sometimes known as the muscles of mastication, but this is misleading since effective mastication also requires muscles supplied by other nerves: buccinator (VII) and tongue (XII) – muscles which are *never* called muscles of mastication.

Some of the peripheral branches of Vc also convey parasympathetic impulses to the salivary glands, and taste fibres from the anterior portion of the tongue.

Origin, course and branches

- From the trigeminal ganglion, the mandibular nerve passes through the foramen ovale into the infratemporal fossa where it gives:
  - four main branches: inferior alveolar, lingual, auriculotemporal, buccal
  - branches to the muscles listed above.
- Inferior alveolar nerve: lower teeth, skin, mylohyoid, digastric. The inferior alveolar nerve descends between medial and lateral pterygoids and enters the mandibular foramen. It continues as the mental nerve emerging from the mental foramen of the mandible and supplies skin. Immediately before the mandibular foramen it gives the nerve to mylohyoid and anterior belly of digastric.
- Lingual nerve: tongue sensation. The lingual nerve descends between medial and lateral pterygoids and is joined by the chorda tympani, a nerve connecting the lingual nerve with VII. The lingual nerve is immediately below and medial to the third lower molar (wisdom) tooth and passes forwards in the floor of the mouth, crosses medially beneath the submandibular duct and supplies the anterior tongue and gums. Fibres it exchanges with the chorda tympani are taste fibres from the anterior tongue, and parasympathetic fibres to the submandibular ganglion.
- Auriculotemporal nerve: skin of temple, temporomandibular joint, external ear. The auriculotemporal nerve arises immediately beneath the foramen ovale by two rootlets on either side of the middle meningeal artery. It passes above (or through) the parotid gland, between the temporomandibular joint and the external acoustic meatus, and ascends on the side of the head close to the superficial temporal artery. For a short distance between its origin and the parotid gland it conveys parasympathetic impulses from the inferior salivatory nucleus to the otic ganglion for innervation of the parotid gland.
- Buccal nerve: skin and mucosa of cheek. The buccal nerve passes between the two heads of lateral pterygoid to the cheek. (It does *not* supply buccinator).
- Muscular branches: deep temporal nerves to temporalis, and twigs to other muscles.
- Meningeal branches: branches in the infratemporal fossa re-enter the middle cranial fossa through the foramen ovale, and other foramina.

The nerve contains

- Sensory fibres: to the trigeminal sensory nuclei.
- Branchiomotor fibres: from the trigeminal motor nucleus (pons).
- In peripheral branches only, taste fibres to the nucleus of the solitary tract: from the anterior portion of tongue via the lingual nerve, chorda tympani, VII.
- In peripheral branches only, parasympathetic impulses:
  - from the superior salivatory nucleus and VII to the submandibular and sublingual glands (see p. 235)
  - from the inferior salivatory nucleus and IX to the parotid gland (see p. 235).

First branchial arch

The mandibular nerve is the main nerve of the first branchial arch, which gives rise to a precursor of the mandible (Meckel's cartilage), the spine of the sphenoid, the sphenomandibular ligament, the malleus and incus, and the eight muscles listed above. All these structures are related to mandibular nerve function in some way.

Clinical testing

- Sensory: test the cutaneous sensation of the chin and lower lip.
- Motor: feel the contractions of masseter and temporalis. Ask your patient to open the jaw against

resistance (pterygoids, mylohyoid, anterior digastric).

Abducens nerve: VI

The abducens nerve innervates one of the muscles that move the eyeball and is described with the orbit and eyeball (14.11, p. 265).

Facial nerve: VII   (Fig. 14.11)

The facial nerve supplies the muscles of facial expression.

Its intracranial portion also conveys:

- taste sensation from the anterior portion of the tongue and oral cavity, which is conveyed to the facial nerve by the chorda tympani
- parasympathetic fibres for the first part of their journey to the submandibular, sublingual, lacrimal, nasal and palatine glands.

Origin, course and branches

VII arises from the cerebellopontine angle by two adjacent roots, the motor root (larger, more medial) and the nervus intermedius (smaller, more lateral; sensory and parasympathetic fibres), so named because it is found between two larger nerves (the motor root of VII and VIII).

Intracranial course, within the cranial cavity and temporal bone.

- The roots of VII enter the internal acoustic meatus (with VIII) and merge.
- At the lateral extremity of the meatus is the geniculum where the nerve turns posteriorly into the facial (Fallopian) canal. The greater petrosal nerve arises here. The geniculate ganglion at this site houses the cell bodies of sensory fibres in the facial nerve.
- The facial canal runs posteriorly along the medial wall of the tympanic (middle ear) cavity, and a branch passes to stapedius (attached to the stapes). The nerve turns downwards and laterally, and just before it emerges from the temporal bone it gives off the chorda tympani, which passes anteriorly across the tympanic membrane to the lingual nerve (Vc) in the infratemporal fossa.
- VII emerges at the stylomastoid foramen.

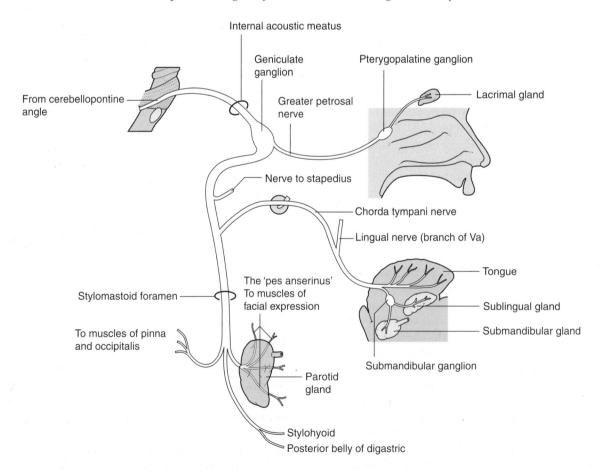

Fig. 14.11   The facial nerve.

Extracranial course and branches.

- Outside the stylomastoid foramen, small branches arise to supply the occipital belly of occipitofrontalis, stylohyoid and the posterior belly of digastric.
- VII enters the parotid gland in which it forms an intricate plexus. Branches of VII are the most superficial structures passing through the gland.
- Five groups (usually) of branches emerge from the anterior border of the gland: temporal, zygomatic, buccal, mandibular and cervical. These supply the muscles of facial expression, including orbicularis oculi, orbicularis oris and buccinator.

The nerve contains

- Branchiomotor fibres: from the facial motor nucleus. Fibres pass dorsally, then loop ventrally around the abducens (VI) nucleus causing an elevation (facial colliculus) on the floor of the fourth ventricle.
- In the intracranial portion only, taste fibres to the solitary tract and nucleus: reach the intracranial portion of VII through the chorda tympani from the lingual nerve. They carry taste sensation from the anterior portion of the tongue.
- In the intracranial portion only, preganglionic parasympathetic impulses from the superior salivatory nucleus: to lacrimal, nasal and palatine glands, and to the submandibular and sublingual glands (see p. 235).
- Somatic sensory fibres: to the trigeminal sensory nuclei from a small and variable area of skin near or in the ear.

Second branchial arch, otic vesicle and facial nerve

The facial nerve is the nerve of the second branchial arch that gives rise to part of the hyoid bone, the styloid process, the stylohyoid ligament, the stapes, and the muscles listed above. Muscles of facial expression migrate into the superficial tissues.

Clinical notes

- The most important thing about the intracranial course of VII is its relationship to the temporal bone and middle ear. It can be affected in ear disease (see p. 260).
- The most important thing about the extracranial course of VII is its relationship to the parotid gland. It can be affected in parotid disease (see p. 242).
- Geniculate herpes. The herpes zoster virus may lie dormant in the geniculate ganglion (after an attack of chickenpox) and at some later stage cause a vesicular eruption in the small area of skin around the external acoustic meatus supplied by the facial nerve. There may also be signs on the anterior portion of the tongue as a result of taste fibres with cell bodies in the geniculate ganglion. The

inflammation may spread to involve the motor fibres in VII and a lower motor neuron lesion arising thus is known as Ramsay Hunt's syndrome.

Clinical testing

- Observe the face. Normal facial movements (lips, eyelids, emotions) and the presence of normal facial skin creases indicate an intact nerve.
- Test strength by trying to force apart the tightly closed eyelids; this should be difficult.
- Test the corneal reflex; see Va above.

Vestibulocochlear nerve: VIII

The vestibulocochlear nerve is the nerve of equilibration (vestibular) and hearing (cochlear) and is described in 14.10 (pp. 261–262).

Glossopharyngeal nerve: IX

The main function of the glossopharyngeal nerve is the sensory supply of the oropharynx, posterior third of the tongue, Eustachian tube and middle ear.

Its other functions are:

- motor to stylopharyngeus
- sensory from the middle ear, carotid sinus and carotid body
- conveying parasympathetic fibres part of the way to the parotid gland.

Origin, course and branches

- IX arises from the medulla by rootlets lateral to the olive, above those of X.
- It leaves the posterior cranial fossa through the jugular foramen. Superior and inferior sensory ganglia for the cell bodies of sensory fibres in the nerve are situated in and near the jugular foramen.
- The tympanic branch is given off in the jugular foramen. This contains parasympathetic impulses from the inferior salivatory nucleus (for the parotid gland) and sensory fibres from the ear.
- It descends in the neck, emerging lateral to stylopharyngeus, and gives a branch to the carotid body, then enters the pharynx between the superior and middle constrictors. Branches contribute sensory fibres to the pharyngeal plexus.

The nerve contains

- Visceral sensory fibres: to the nucleus of the solitary tract.
- Branchiomotor fibres: from the nucleus ambiguus to stylopharyngeus.
- In the proximal part of the nerve only, parasympathetic impulses from the inferior salivatory nucleus: to the parotid gland (see p. 235).

Third branchial arch

The glossopharyngeal nerve is the nerve of the third branchial arch that gives rise to part of the hyoid bone and the stylopharyngeus muscle. Arterial components of the third arch form part of the common and internal carotid arteries, thus explaining the carotid sinus innervation.

Clinical testing

Gag reflex. Sensation supplied by the glosso-pharyngeal nerve is different in quality to that supplied by the trigeminal. Put your finger on the anterior part of your tongue (Vc) and then on the posterior part (IX) to demonstrate this. The gag reflex is mediated by IX (afferent limb) and X (efferent limb), so it tests both nerves.

Vagus nerve: X   (Fig. 14.12)

The vagus is a mixed motor and sensory nerve supplying the gut tube as far as the splenic flexure of the transverse colon. This includes the pharynx and larynx for swallowing and phonation, and these are its most important functions.

It also supplies parasympathetic and sensory fibres to the heart, tracheobronchial tree and abdominal viscera and conveys a few cutaneous sensory fibres from the posterior part of the external acoustic meatus and the tympanic membrane.

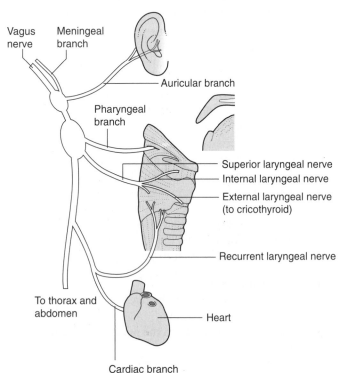

Vagus nerve
Meningeal branch
Auricular branch
Pharyngeal branch
Superior laryngeal nerve
Internal laryngeal nerve
External laryngeal nerve (to cricothyroid)
Recurrent laryngeal nerve
To thorax and abdomen
Heart
Cardiac branch

Fig. 14.12   The vagus nerve.

Origin, course and branches

The vagus is the most extensively distributed cranial nerve, its name reflecting both the distribution and the type of sensation it conveys (Latin: *vagus* = vague, indefinite, wandering).

- X arises from the medulla by rootlets lateral to the olive, below those of IX.
- It leaves the posterior cranial fossa through the jugular foramen. Superior and inferior sensory ganglia for the cell bodies of sensory fibres in the nerve are situated in and near the jugular foramen.
- The auricular branch passes through a canal in the temporal bone and conveys sensory fibres from the posterior part of the external acoustic meatus and tympanic membrane.
- It descends in the carotid sheath between the internal jugular vein and the carotid arteries. It gives pharyngeal branches, and the superior laryngeal nerve.
- Cardiac (slowing the heart rate) and tracheal (sensory) branches arise in the root of neck and upper thorax. It enters the thorax and, on the left side, crosses the arch of the aorta.
- Recurrent laryngeal nerves arise in the mediastinum: that on the left is related to the ligamentum arteriosum, that on the right to the subclavian artery. Both recurrent nerves re-ascend between the trachea and oesophagus to supply laryngeal muscles and give sensory fibres to the larynx below the vocal cords, the trachea and the oesophagus.
- The vagus forms the oesophageal plexus and enters the abdomen through the oesophageal hiatus in the diaphragm. See Chapters 10 and 11.

The nerve contains

The motor function of the vagus in the neck is branchiomotor: in the thorax and abdomen it is parasympathetic.

- Branchiomotor fibres: from the nucleus ambiguus to pharyngeal and laryngeal muscles.
- Parasympathetic fibres: from the dorsal motor nucleus of vagus to the heart and thoracoabdominal viscera (foregut and midgut, see p. 235).
- Somatic sensory fibres: to the trigeminal sensory nuclei. From the posterior wall of the external acoustic meatus and the posterior portion of the external surface of the tympanic membrane, fibres pass in the auricular branch of X to the main trunk in the jugular foramen.
- Visceral sensory fibres: to the nucleus of the solitary tract from taste buds in the epiglottic area, visceral sensory fibres from gut tube derivatives and aortic baro- and chemoreceptors.

Fourth and sixth branchial arches
The vagus is the nerve of the fourth and sixth branchial arches. Structures derived from these include the pharyngeal and laryngeal cartilages and muscles. The sixth arch artery on the left gives rise to the ductus arteriosus (ligamentum after birth) around which the left sixth arch nerve, the recurrent laryngeal, is trapped in embryonic life. The sixth arch artery on the right degenerates, so the right recurrent laryngeal nerve is related to the most caudal persisting branchial arch artery, the fourth, which becomes the right subclavian.

An alternative view of the vagus
The vagus controls the entry into the gut tube (swallowing), and mediates sensation of most of the gut tube. This includes the bronchial tree, another gut tube derivative. What about the heart? This develops from cells initially found in the wall of the yolk sac, from which the gut tube develops. Sustenance is a common theme here, whether the absorption of nutrients from the yolk sac (gut tube) or their propulsion round the body by the force of cardiac contractions. Perhaps the 'big picture' is that the vagus is the nerve of sustenance – the yolk sac nerve.

Clinical testing
- If speech is normal, there is no need to test X at all since it supplies the muscles that move the vocal cords causing phonation.
- Say 'aah'. Observing the elevation of the palate when a subject says 'aah' tests motor function in fibres from the nucleus ambiguus in X.
- Gag reflex – see IX above.

Accessory nerve: XI

The accessory nerve has two parts: cranial and spinal. Oddly enough, when clinicians refer to the eleventh cranial nerve, or accessory nerve, they mean the spinal accessory.

- Cranial accessory. This arises from a caudal extension of the nucleus ambiguus by rootlets below and in series with those of IX and X. It joins X, from which it is functionally indistinguishable (its name means accessory vagus). This book considers the cranial accessory no more *and neither need you.*
- Spinal accessory: this is the one to remember (Fig. 14.9). This is motor to the muscles bounding the posterior triangle of the neck: sternocleidomastoid and trapezius.

Origin and course: there are *two* foramina
- Rootlets from the upper four or five segments of the spinal cord (in series with those of IX, X and cranial

XI) emerge between the ventral and dorsal spinal nerve roots.
- The spinal accessory *ascends through the foramen magnum* to enter the posterior cranial fossa and briefly runs with cranial XI before it (the cranial) joins the vagus.
- XI *descends through the jugular foramen* into the neck and passes deep to sternocleidomastoid, which it supplies.
- XI enters the posterior triangle of the neck about one-third of the way down the posterior border of sternocleidomastoid and passes across to enter trapezius about one-third of the way up its anterior border.

The nerve contains
- Motor fibres: cell bodies are in the lateral part of the ventral grey horn of cervical cord segments 1–5.

Clinical testing
- Ask your patient to move his chin up to one side against resistance (contralateral sternocleidomastoid).
- Ask your patient to shrug his shoulders (trapezius) against resistance.
- Ask your patient to put his hand on his head (trapezius: shoulder abduction beyond 90°).

Hypoglossal nerve: XII   (Fig. 14.13)

The hypoglossal nerve supplies the muscles of the tongue. Movements of the tongue are important in chewing, in the initial stages of swallowing, and in speech.

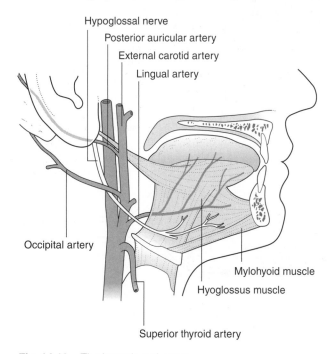

Fig. 14.13   The hypoglossal nerve.

It also conveys fibres from C1 which contribute to the innervation of the strap muscles.

Origin, course and branches

- XII arises from the medulla by rootlets between the pyramid and olive.
- It passes through the hypoglossal (condylar) canal in the occipital bone.
- It receives motor fibres from C1 and descends to the submandibular region.
- It turns forwards, lateral to the external carotid artery and hooks beneath the origin of the occipital artery.

- It gives a branch to the ansa cervicalis, which carries some fibres from C1 to the strap muscles; other C1 fibres remain with XII to supply geniohyoid.
- It enters the tongue from below passing lateral to hyoglossus and supplies the muscles of the tongue.

The nerve contains

- Motor fibres: from the hypoglossal nucleus in the floor of the fourth ventricle in the medulla, to the tongue muscles.

Clinical testing

- Ask your patient to protrude the tongue. If it

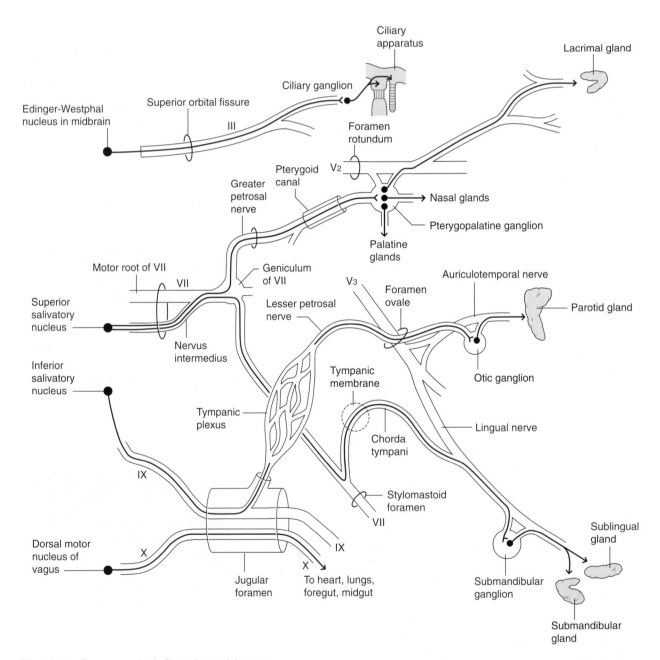

Fig. 14.14 Parasympathetic fibres in cranial nerves.

deviates to one side, then the nerve of that side is damaged – the tongue is pushed to the paralysed side by muscles of the functioning side.

- Ask the patient to push the tongue into the cheek, then palpate the cheek to feel tone and strength of tongue muscles.

Parasympathetics and taste in cranial nerves

Parasympathetic and taste components in cranial nerves, although one is efferent and the other afferent, share some peripheral pathways when crossing from branches of one cranial nerve to another (e.g. chorda tympani, petrosal nerves). These pathways provide material for nit-picking examinations, and are of embryological interest, but from a functional point of view they are insignificant. They may have to be interrupted, for example in ear surgery, and although food and drink may lose some savour, and the patient may subsequently suffer from a dry mouth, life continues much as before. This may be a nuisance but could never be described as life-threatening.

Parasympathetic components   (Fig. 14.14)

- Edinger–Westphal nucleus – III – ciliary ganglion (synapse) – branches of Va – iris, ciliary body.
- Superior salivatory nucleus – VII – greater petrosal nerve – pterygopalatine ganglion (synapse) – branches of Vb – lacrimal, nasal, palatine glands.
- Superior salivatory nucleus – VII – chorda tympani – submandibular ganglion (synapse) – branches of Vc – submandibular, sublingual glands.
- Inferior salivatory nucleus – IX – lesser petrosal nerve – otic ganglion (synapse) – branches of Vc – parotid gland.
- Dorsal motor nucleus of the vagus – X – gut tube derivatives and heart (synapses in or near destination).

Taste fibres   (Fig. 14.15)

- Taste sensation from palate – branches of Vb – greater petrosal nerve – VII (cell bodies in geniculate ganglion) – solitary tract of brain stem.
- Taste sensation from anterior tongue and mouth – branches of Vc – chorda tympani – VII (cell bodies in geniculate ganglion) – solitary tract of brain stem.
- Taste sensation from posterior tongue – IX (cell bodies in sensory ganglia of IX) – solitary tract of brain stem.
- Taste sensation from pharynx – X (cell bodies in sensory ganglia of X) – solitary tract of brain stem.

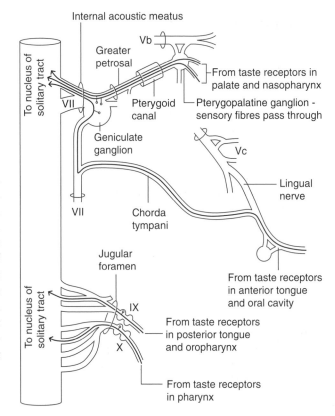

Fig. 14.15   Taste pathways in cranial nerves.

Clinical testing

- Pupillary light reflex: this tests parasympathetic fibres from the Edinger–Westphal nucleus (see 14.11, pp. 268, 269).
- Salivary glands. Ask your patient to suck something bitter (e.g. a lemon) to provoke salivary secretion. This is more usually done to try to locate the position of a calculus in the duct of a salivary gland, usually the submandibular.
- Taste. Testing taste is possible but hardly worth the trouble.

14.5 Neck

Overview

Fascial sheets surround various structures in the neck and are important in the spread of disease. Bones and cartilages in the anterior neck form the visceral skeleton of the larynx. Arteries and veins travel anterior to, or through the vertebral column. The neck is divided into posterior and anterior triangles.

You should:

- know the fascial layers: investing layer, carotid sheath, pretracheal

- know the features and surface markings of the visceral skeleton

- know the main arteries and their branches

- know the surface markings of the internal and external jugular veins

- know the disposition of the deep cervical chain of lymph nodes

- know the contents of the posterior triangle of the neck, and the surface markings of XI within it

- know the position and blood supply of the thyroid gland.

Fascial layers (Fig. 14.16)

- The investing layer of cervical fascia encloses the deep structures like a sleeve. It is attached posteriorly to the nuchal ligament and splits around trapezius and sternocleidomastoid. Cutaneous nerves are superficial to it.

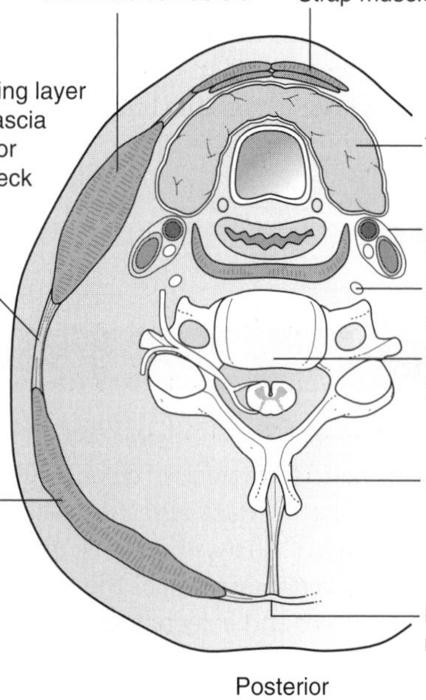

Anterior

Sternocleidomastoid   Strap muscles

Deep investing layer of cervical fascia over posterior triangle of neck

Thyroid gland

Carotid sheath

Sympathetic chain

Vertebral body

Bifid spine

Trapezius

Ligamentum nuchae

Posterior

Fig. 14.16   Cross-section through the neck.

- The carotid sheath is a vertical fascial tube deep to the investing layer of fascia. It contains the common and internal carotid arteries, the internal jugular vein, the vagus nerve and the deep cervical chain of lymph nodes.

- The prevertebral 'space' is the area between the prevertebral muscles and the pharynx/oesophagus containing loose connective tissue and lymph nodes. It allows disease to spread from one side of the neck to the other. The cervical sympathetic chain is found here, immediately posterior to the carotid sheath.

- The pretracheal fascia in front of and to the sides of the trachea encloses the thyroid gland and with the investing layer of cervical fascia anteriorly forms sheaths around the strap (infrahyoid) muscles of the neck.

- Platysma muscle is directly subcutaneous. When it contracts it raises ridges in the skin of the neck and is useless except for those who shave. It is supplied by VII and is a now-redundant muscle of 'facial' expression.

Visceral skeleton of the neck

- Hyoid bone. This is palpable immediately underneath, almost inside, the mandible at the top of the neck. The greater horns (cornua) extend backwards from the sides of the body (be careful when palpating these – too much pressure will fracture the bone).

- Thyroid cartilage. Right and left laminae join in the midline to form the thyroid prominence or Adam's apple. Superior horns extend up towards the hyoid bone, and inferior horns articulate with the cricoid cartilage below.

- Cricoid cartilage. This is a cartilaginous ring at the top of the trachea. It has a lamina posteriorly and facets for synovial joints with the inferior horns of the thyroid cartilage at the sides.

- Membranes attach these cartilages to each other so that they move as one.
  - thyrohyoid membrane, palpable between hyoid bone and thyroid cartilage
  - cricothyroid membrane, palpable between thyroid and cricoid cartilages. Laryngotomy is performed here.

Clinical box

Vertebral levels of the visceral skeleton of the neck
Despite movement during swallowing, these vertebral levels are worth remembering:

- hyoid bone: about C2

- thyroid cartilage, upper margin of lamina (surface marking of bifurcation of common carotid artery): about C3

- vocal cords: about C4
- thyroid cartilage, lower margin of lamina: about C5
- cricoid cartilage (surface marking of beginning of trachea and oesophagus): C6.

Arteries of the neck (Figs 14.17, 14.18)

Common carotid artery. This ascends in the carotid sheath, behind and medial to the internal jugular vein and vagus nerve, to the level of the upper border of the thyroid cartilage (vertebra level about C3) where it bifurcates.

Internal carotid artery This has no branches in the neck, but enters the skull through the carotid canal. It is called internal because it passes into the cranium, not because of its position in the neck.

External carotid artery (Fig. 14.18). This gives branches as follows:

- Superior thyroid: to thyroid gland, larynx, pharynx. This may arise from the bifurcation or even from the common carotid artery.
- Ascending pharyngeal (not important).
- Lingual: to the tongue.

- Facial: to the face. The lingual and facial may arise by a common trunk.
- Occipital: to the back of the head. The occipital comes off the posterior border at about the same level as the lingual and facial arise anteriorly, and at its origin is intimately related to XII.
- Posterior auricular: to the region around the ear.

The two terminal branches, arising behind the neck of the mandible, are:

- superficial temporal: to the side of the head and scalp, usually visible and palpable
- maxillary: to the mandible, maxilla, cheek, nasal cavity, skull bones and cranial meninges.

Clinical box

Carotid pulse
Press posteriorly lateral to the upper border of the thyroid cartilage. You are compressing the common carotid artery against the anterior aspect of the transverse process of vertebra C3. Do not push too hard, and do not palpate both sides together.

Superficial temporal pulse
Place your fingers about 2 cm above the middle of a line joining the top of the pinna to the side of the orbit.

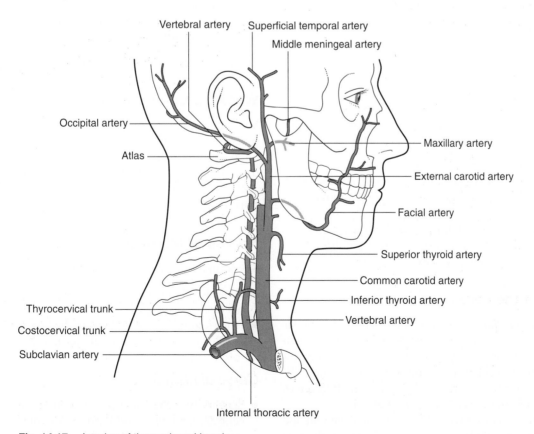

Fig. 14.17 Arteries of the neck and head.

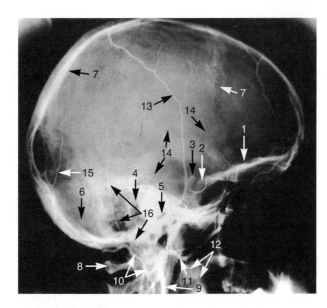

Fig. 14.18 External carotid arteriogram, lateral view: 1, orbital plate of frontal bone; 2, pituitary fossa; 3, dorsum sellae; 4, mastoid air cells; 5, external acoustic meatus; 6, occipital bone; 7, parietal bone (if you look closely you can see the two layers of the diploë); 8, posterior arch of the atlas; 9, external carotid artery; 10, occipital artery; 11, maxillary artery; 12, palatal branches of the maxillary artery; 13, superficial temporal artery; 14, meningeal arteries; 15, branches of occipital artery; 16, posterior auricular artery; 17, coronal suture (faintly visible).

Vertebral artery. This is a branch of the first part of the subclavian artery. It ascends through the foramina transversaria of vertebra C6 (usually) to C1, then turns medially, grooving the upper surface of the atlas behind the atlanto-occipital joint facet, pierces the meninges and enters the subarachnoid space. It passes through the foramen magnum, ascends on the anterior aspect of the brain stem and unites with its opposite number to form the basilar artery.

- Branches in the neck supply deep neck structures and give twigs through intervertebral foramina to the spinal cord.
- Branches in the cranium supply the spinal cord, brain stem, vital centres, vestibular apparatus and the posterior cerebral cortex.

Veins of the neck

Internal jugular vein. This emerges from the jugular foramen of the skull and descends in the carotid sheath with the common carotid artery and X. It terminates behind the sternoclavicular joint where it joins the sub-clavian to form the brachiocephalic vein. It receives tributaries from the face and thyroid gland.

External jugular vein. This is formed behind the angle of the mandible from superficial veins of the face

and passes obliquely towards the midpoint of the clavicle. It receives tributaries from superficial neck tissues and terminates by joining the subclavian vein either directly or indirectly.

Anterior jugular veins. These are situated near the medial (anterior) border of sternocleidomastoid and form a venous arch that drains to the brachiocephalic veins.

Clinical box

Surface markings of neck veins
- Internal jugular: ear lobe (roughly) – sternoclavicular joint. It is deep to sternocleidomastoid, so is neither visible nor palpable.
- External jugular: angle of mandible to midpoint of clavicle. This is superficial and is visible throughout its length.

Jugular venous pulsation
A routine part of the examination of the cardiovascular system is an assessment of jugular venous pulsation. The height of the column of blood in the jugular veins reflects pressure changes in the right side of the heart. The internal jugular veins are more accurate in this respect than the external as there are no valves between the right atrium and internal jugulars, but unfortunately pulsations in them are hidden by sternocleidomastoid. In a healthy person the top of the column of blood should be at the sternal angle although the pulsations may be just visible above the clavicle. In heart failure the column of blood will be taller, so the pulsations will be visible higher than normally. In superior vena cava obstruction the pulsations will be lost and the vein will be engorged. Exaggerated pulsations will be visible in tricuspid disease.

Words: jugular, carotid

Veins are jugular (Latin: throat, yoke); arteries are carotid (Greek: drowsiness). Compression of the arteries for long enough would certainly cause something like drowsiness: this method of inducing anaesthesia was prevalent before drugs were introduced for this purpose.

Nerves of the neck

See dermatome map (Fig. 6.6, p. 36).

- Posterior skin is supplied by dorsal rami of cervical nerves.
- Anterior and lateral skin is supplied by ventral rami of C2–4 through the cervical plexus.

Cervical plexus C2–4

- Sensory branches emerge from behind the central region of the posterior border of sternocleidomastoid. They are:

- lesser occipital (C2, 3)
- great auricular (C2, 3)
- transverse (or anterior) cutaneous of the neck (C2, 3)
- supraclavicular nerves (C3, 4), passing down and laterally over the clavicle to meet the dermatome of T2 over the second rib (C5–T1 dermatomes are in the upper limb)
- branches to the phrenic nerve C3–5 for thoracic viscera and central diaphragmatic sensation.
- Muscular branches:
  - to the phrenic nerve C3–5 for the diaphragmatic muscle
  - to the strap (infrahyoid) muscles attached to the hyoid bone and thyroid cartilage. Fibres from C1 travel briefly with XII, and then join fibres from C2 and C3 to form the ansa cervicalis, which supplies the strap muscles. It may have to be cut in surgery: we can live without both it and the muscles it supplies
  - from C4 to levator scapulae, rhomboids etc., of no clinical importance.

Posterior triangle of the neck (Fig. 14.19)

Boundaries

- Posterior border of sternocleidomastoid.
- Anterior border of trapezius.
- Middle portion of clavicle.

The apex of the triangle is at the mastoid process. The external jugular vein and supraclavicular nerves run over the triangle, and deep to them the roof of the triangle is formed by the investing layer of cervical fascia between sternocleidomastoid and trapezius.

Contents

- Upper trunk of the brachial plexus inferomedially.
- Apex of the lung extending above the middle third of the clavicle for about 2 cm.
- Lymph nodes around the edges of the triangle.
- Accessory nerve (XI). Its approximate surface markings are: one-third of the way down sternocleidomastoid to two-thirds of the way down trapezius.

Clinical box

At risk in the posterior triangle
- The accessory nerve (XI) is easily damaged and is at risk in malignant involvement of lymph nodes, careless biopsy of enlarged lymph nodes, and stab wounds. It would result in weakness of trapezius with impaired shoulder abduction, leading to difficulty in hair grooming etc.
- Stab wounds may damage the brachial plexus (upper trunk injury leading to Erb's palsy) and the apex of the lung (leading to a pneumothorax).

Anterior triangle of the neck

Boundaries

- The anterior border of sternocleidomastoid.
- The midline.
- The lower border of the mandible.

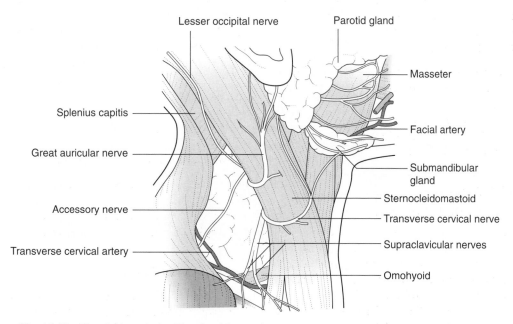

Fig. 14.19 The right posterior triangle of the neck.

Contents

- Superficial: anterior jugular veins, cutaneous branches of cervical plexus.
- Strap muscles: thyrohyoid, sternohyoid, sternothyroid, omohyoid. Nerve supply: cervical plexus C1–3 through ansa cervicalis. Their names give their attachments, omo- (Greek: shoulder) -hyoid coming from the upper border of the scapula just medial to the scapular notch. Sternohyoid overlies both sternothyroid and thyrohyoid; sternothyroid is immediately anterior to the thyroid gland.
- Larynx and trachea (described in 14.8, p. 252).
- Thyroid gland.

Thyroid gland (Fig. 14.20)

The thyroid gland has two lateral lobes and a central isthmus. The isthmus overlies tracheal rings 2–4 and the lateral lobes extend up to about the middle of the thyroid cartilage. Note that the bulk of the thyroid gland is significantly lower than the thyroid cartilage.

Relations, enlargement of the thyroid gland

The thyroid gland is enclosed within the pretracheal fascia, and immediately above the gland, thyrohyoid muscle is attached to the thyroid cartilage. This means that when the gland enlarges (goitre) its expansion above is limited by this attachment. At the sides, expansion is limited by the fusion of the pretracheal fascia with the carotid sheath, so that apart from some generalised swelling, gross enlargements of the gland expand inferiorly where there is nothing to stop the gland growing down into the mediastinum (mediastinal goitre). Such mediastinal masses may compress the jugular and brachiocephalic veins leading to venous engorgement of the neck and face.

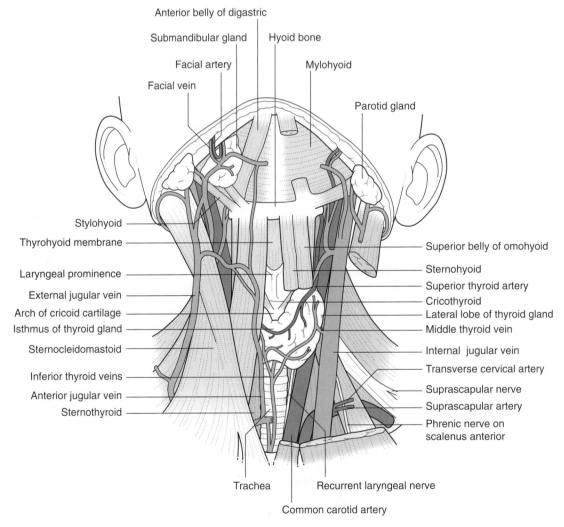

Fig. 14.20 Thyroid gland and relations.

Arteries

- Inferior thyroid: from the thyrocervical trunk of the first part of the subclavian artery. It loops behind the carotid sheath before turning upwards once more to branch as it enter the lower pole of the lateral lobe.
- Superior thyroid: from the external carotid artery.

The territories of both arteries communicate with each other and across the midline with their opposite numbers. There is often a posterior anastomotic artery between branches of the superior and inferior thyroid arteries.

- Thyroidea ima artery: from the brachiocephalic artery or aortic arch; infrequent (less than 10%).

Relationship of arteries to the laryngeal nerves

- The superior thyroid artery is closely related near its origin to the superior laryngeal nerve (branch of X). Section of the nerve would anaesthetise the laryngeal mucosa and abolish the cough reflex, so increasing the risk of food or a foreign body entering the trachea.
- The inferior thyroid artery is closely related to the recurrent laryngeal nerve (branch of X) as it enters the gland. Section of this would result in paralysis of the muscles that move the vocal cords on that side. Any patient for thyroid surgery should have the vocal cords inspected beforehand so that, in the event of any suspicion of the surgeon having damaged the nerve during surgery, there is a record of their preoperative state.

Veins

- Inferior thyroid veins: numerous vessels drain into the brachiocephalic veins.
- Middle and superior thyroid veins, usually one each on each side, pass anterior to the common carotid artery and drain into the internal jugular vein.

Clinical box

Development, thyroglossal cysts, ectopic thyroid tissue

The thyroid gland develops as an exocrine downgrowth from the foramen caecum of the tongue, its duct, the thyroglossal, closing with increasing vascularisation of the gland. The attachment of the duct to the gland may be marked by a pyramidal lobe on the upper aspect of the isthmus. Ectopic thyroid tissue can be found at the foramen caecum (lingual thyroid) or along the course of the duct. Thyroglossal cysts may develop in the track of the duct and cause sufficient trouble for them to require excision. In such cases it is usually necessary to remove the central part of the hyoid bone as well, since the thyroglossal duct may be attached to its posterior surface before continuing its downwards journey.

How do you distinguish between a thyroglossal cyst and, say, a sebaceous cyst that just happens to be in the midline? The thyroglossal cyst will be pulled up when the patient swallows or protrudes the tongue.

Parathyroid glands

There are usually two small parathyroid glands on each side, but their position is not constant. The superior parathyroids are on, or in, the posterior surface of the lateral lobes of the thyroid gland, often somewhere near the anastomotic artery joining the inferior and superior thyroid arteries. The inferior parathyroids are close to the lower pole of the thyroid gland and supplied by branches of the inferior thyroid artery.

14.6 Face, parotid, VII, scalp

Overview

Muscles of facial expression are supplied by VII. This nerve is intimately related to the parotid gland on the side of the face. Sensory nerves of the face and anterior scalp are branches of V; those of the posterior scalp are from spinal nerve C2. Vessels and nerves of the scalp are superficial to the epicranial aponeurosis, and bleeding after scalp injuries is usually profuse.

Learning Objectives

You should:

- know the approximate position of the parotid gland
- understand how and why diseases of the parotid gland can affect VII
- know the principal muscle groups supplied by VII
- know the main cutaneous nerves supplying the face and scalp
- understand why scalp injuries bleed profusely, and why they may result in subaponeurotic haematomas and black eyes.

Muscles of facial expression

The muscles of facial expression are attached to the deeper layers of the skin. They mimic emotion and so are called the mimetic muscles, and they are used in speech and for eye protection. They are all supplied by the facial nerve (VII).

There are many individual muscles, some with charming names, but it is not necessary to know most of them. Think of them collectively as the muscles of facial expression, and know the names of:

- orbicularis oculi
- orbicularis oris
- buccinator.

(You have already met platysma: it is unimportant.)

Some muscles supplied by VII remain deep, attached to the temporal bone, and are involved in movements of the pharynx: posterior belly of digastric (mastoid process – hyoid – mandible); stylohyoid (styloid process – hyoid).

Cutaneous innervation of the face

(Fig. 14.21)

Note the following:
- Eyes and above: Va.
- Between palpebral fissure and mouth, and malar (over the cheekbone) skin: Vb.
- Chin and 'beard area' except skin over the angle of the mandible: Vc (from top down: auriculotemporal, buccal, and mental branches).
- Neck, skin over angle of mandible and area between 'beard area' and ear: cervical plexus C2, 3.

Clinical box

Miscellanea
- The auriculotemporal nerve accompanies the superficial temporal artery on the temple. In cases of temporal arteritis, the nerve is anaesthetised so that the overlying skin can be incised to obtain a biopsy of the artery.
- Trauma to the infraorbital margin may cause sensory loss in infraorbital skin as a result of damage to the infraorbital nerve (branch of Vb)

Parotid gland and VII   (Fig. 14.22)

The parotid salivary gland lies at the side of the face behind the mandible, which it may overlap. It lies superficially and parotid swellings (e.g. mumps, tumours) produce an obvious retromandibular bulge. It is partially enclosed by the investing layer of cervical fascia, the superficial layer fusing with the fascia over masseter, and the deep layer having a free anterior edge (known misleadingly and inaccurately as the stylomandibular ligament).

The parotid duct emerges from the anterior border of the gland and passes forwards on masseter. It then turns medially, penetrates buccinator and opens into the mouth opposite the second upper molar tooth. The duct is found by palpating the anterior border of a tensed masseter. Detached islands of secretory tissue may be found scattered along the duct.

Other structures that pass through the substance of the gland are the retromandibular vein, the auriculotemporal nerve and the termination of the external carotid artery (sometimes).

Parasympathetic supply. Secretomotor impulses to the gland come from the inferior salivatory nucleus and travel by way of IX, the lesser petrosal nerve and the otic ganglion (see p. 235 and Fig. 14.14).

Facial nerve. The single most important thing about the parotid gland is its relationship to the branches of the facial nerve. The single most important thing about the extracranial facial nerve is its relationship to the parotid gland.

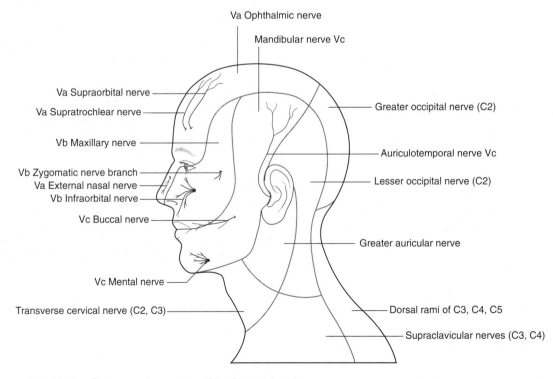

Fig. 14.21 Cutaneous innervation of the face and scalp.

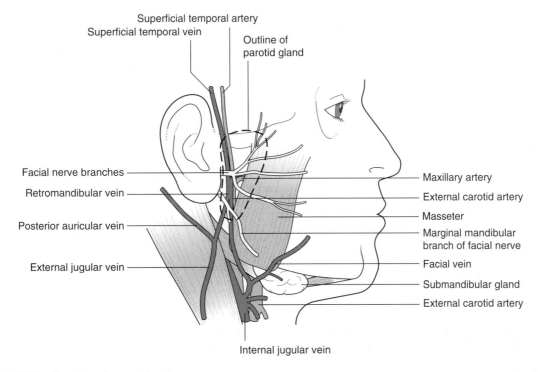

Fig. 14.22 Parotid region and facial nerve.

The facial nerve emerges from the skull at the stylomastoid foramen in the temporal bone, behind the ear. It immediately turns forwards and superficially to enter the parotid gland in which it forms a complex and variable plexus. It is superficial in the gland. This means that the nerve is liable to damage (trauma, parotid tumour) leading to a facial palsy.

Branches of VII emerge from the anterior margin of the gland usually in five groups, the pattern being known as the pes anserinus (Latin: foot of the goose):

- temporal: to frontal belly of occipitofrontalis
- zygomatic: to orbicularis oculi and upper face
- buccal: to buccinator, orbicularis oris and mid-face
- marginal mandibular: to orbicularis oris and the corner of the mouth
- cervical: to platysma.

Watch out particularly for the marginal mandibular nerve that passes on or just below the lower margin of the mandible. It is superficial even to the palpable facial pulse, and is thus liable to injury from, for example, trauma or careless incisions. Damage would result in weakness of the muscles of the corner of the mouth resulting in drooling of saliva.

Clinical box

Facial palsy, Bell's palsy
A lower motor neuron lesion of VII is called a facial palsy. It may be a lesion of the cell bodies in the facial motor nucleus, or of the nerve itself, and the muscle fibre(s) supplied by the affected neuron(s) will be paralysed. Facial wrinkles disappear, and there will be facial asymmetry so it is usually easy to spot. Bell's palsy is a facial palsy of unknown cause.

Facial nerve in the newborn baby
The mastoid process is almost non-existent in a newborn baby and the stylomastoid foramen is superficial. The facial nerve may be damaged here as a result of manipulation of the baby's head during birth. This is serious: VII supplies buccinator, which the baby needs for feeding.

Frey's syndrome
After parotidectomy, cut ends of postganglionic parasympathetic fibres begin to grow. If these sprouting fibres find their way into Schwann cells sheaths occupied before surgery by sympathetic fibres, stimuli normally producing salivation will instead induce sweating over the site of the parotid.

Scalp

The layers of tissue forming the scalp are:

- skin
- connective tissue containing vessels and nerves
- aponeurosis of occipitofrontalis muscle (epicranial aponeurosis or galea aponeurotica)
- loose areolar tissue.

Add the 'p' for periosteum of the cranial bones and the initial letters spell 'scalp'. The areolar tissue gives a natural cleavage plane between the aponeurosis and the bone.

Occipitofrontalis muscle and its aponeurosis

This forms a helmet over the vault of the skull. Occipital muscle fibres are attached to the superior nuchal line, and anteriorly, frontalis is attached to the skin of the forehead: these fibres crease the skin. Laterally, the aponeurosis is attached to the superior temporal line, and some people have muscles fibres here so are able to wiggle their pinnas. The muscle fibres are supplied by VII: occipitofrontalis is a mimetic muscle.

Vessels and cutaneous nerves of the scalp

These are in the connective tissue layer, superficial to the aponeurosis.

- Arterial blood. There is a profuse supply to the scalp from:
  - the supraorbital artery from the orbit (a branch of the ophthalmic and internal carotid)
  - branches of the external carotid artery at the sides and back, in order from the front: superficial temporal, posterior auricular, occipital.

    The rich anastomosis means that scalp wounds bleed profusely, and from the point of view of the casualty officer trying to stem the flow, this is not helped by the tension exerted on the margins of the wound by occipitofrontalis pulling in both directions at once.
- Venous blood drains externally to internal and external jugular veins (see above) and by connections through the orbit, diploic cavities and elsewhere to intracranial venous sinuses.
- Cutaneous nerves of the scalp (see Fig. 14.21):
  - anterior to the vertex: Va (supraorbital and supratrochlear branches)
  - posterior to the vertex: greater occipital nerve, dorsal ramus of C2
  - at the sides there are small areas supplied by: zygomatic (Vb), auriculotemporal (Vc) and lesser occipital (C2, 3 from cervical plexus) nerves.

14.7 Anatomy of mastication

Overview

Movements of mastication occur at the temporo-mandibular joint. Muscles of mastication are supplied by Vc. The infratemporal fossa, deep to the mandible contains the maxillary artery and some of these muscles. Sensory nerves to the oral cavity are branches of Vb and Vc. Muscles on the tongue are supplied by XII and it receives sensory fibres through Vc and IX. The submandibular and sublingual glands are in the floor of the mouth. The tonsils are at the posterior limit of the oral cavity, at the oropharyngeal isthmus.

Learning Objectives

You should:

- know how the mandible moves, and the nerve supply of the muscles that move it
- understand that other muscles are required for chewing
- know the sensory innervation of the oral cavity and teeth
- know the innervation and lymph drainage of the tongue
- know the position of the submandibular and sublingual salivary glands
- know the position and significance of the tonsils.

Temporomandibular joint and mandibular movements

The temporomandibular joint is divided into two separate synovial cavities by a fibrocartilaginous disc. The sensory supply to the joint comes from the auriculotemporal nerve (Vc), which is why pain from the joint, like that from the teeth and tongue, can be referred to the skin of the external acoustic meatus and tympanic membrane (they are all supplied in whole or in part by branches of Vc).

The mandibles are tethered by the attachment of the sphenomandibular ligament extending from the spine of the sphenoid to the lingula of the mandible, and the two mandibles move by pivoting on an axis passing through the lingula, adjacent to the mandibular foramen on each side.

As the mouth opens, the head of the mandible moves forwards, and this is how lateral pterygoid acts as a depressor of the mandible: it exerts forward traction on the head, neck and joint capsule. You will be able to deduce what happens when the mandible closes. Protraction is the action that results in the entire mandible being pulled anteriorly; retraction is the opposite. Masticatory movements involve mandibular depression, elevation, protraction, retraction and side-to-side grinding.

Muscles   (Fig. 14.23)

- Temporalis. Attachments: a wide area of temporal bone and fascia – coronoid process and anterior border of ramus of mandible, passing deep to the zygomatic arch.
- Masseter. Attachments: zygomatic arch – lateral aspect of angle of mandible.
- Lateral pterygoid. Attachments: lateral side of lateral pterygoid plate of sphenoid – head and neck of mandible, joint capsule, articular disc. It is a 'front-to-back' muscle.
- Medial pterygoid. Attachments: medial side of lateral pterygoid plate of sphenoid – medial aspect of angle of mandible. It is a 'top-to-bottom' muscle.
- Mylohyoid. Attachments: mylohyoid line on medial aspect of mandible – median raphe between hyoid bone and midpoint of posterior surface of mandible.
- Digastric, anterior belly. Attachments: hyoid – digastric fossa of mandible; below mylohyoid.

These muscles are all supplied by Vc.

Movements

- Elevation. The mandible is suspended from the skull by a muscular sling formed internally by medial pterygoid and laterally by masseter. From directly above, temporalis is a powerful elevator of the mandible.
- Depression. This is brought about in two ways:
  - by anterior traction on the head of the mandible by lateral pterygoid
  - by inferior traction on the mandible by the anterior belly of digastric and mylohyoid.

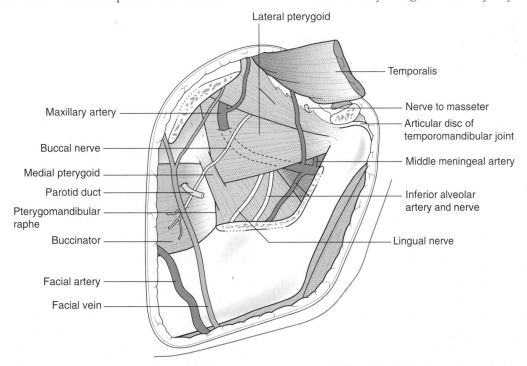

Fig. 14.23   Infratemporal fossa. Part of the mandible has been cut away.

- Grinding. Lateral and rotatory movements are produced by muscles of the two sides working cooperatively. For example, moving the mandible to the left involves the left masseter and the right medial pterygoid.
- Protraction: lateral pterygoid, anterior fibres of temporalis.
- Retraction (not powerful): posterior fibres of temporalis.

Infratemporal fossa   (Fig. 14.23)

The area beneath and in front of the temporal bone, bounded also by the ramus of the mandible, the maxilla and the pterygoid plates of the sphenoid, is the infratemporal fossa. It contains the pterygoid muscles and venous plexus, and branches of Vc and the maxillary artery.

Mandibular nerve

The mandibular nerve enters the roof of the fossa through the foramen ovale. The inferior alveolar and lingual nerves descend between the two pterygoid muscles, and the buccal nerve aims laterally for the skin of the cheek, passing between the two heads of lateral pterygoid. From its origin at the foramen ovale, the auriculotemporal nerve passes laterally directly underneath the skull. In the fossa, the chorda tympani emerges from the temporal bone and joins the posterior aspect of the lingual nerve.

Maxillary artery, pterygoid venous plexus

- The maxillary artery is one of the terminal branches of the external carotid artery and arises posterior to the neck of the mandible. It runs medially and forwards, and disappears medially through the slit between the lateral pterygoid plate of the sphenoid and the maxilla, the pterygomaxillary fissure (see below). It has several branches, the two most important being:
  - the middle meningeal, which ascends to the foramen spinosum (usually passing between the roots of the auriculotemporal nerve)
  - the inferior alveolar, which joins the nerve of the same name and enters the mandibular foramen.
- The pterygoid venous plexus in and around lateral pterygoid communicates with facial veins superficially and through skull foramina with intracranial venous sinuses.

Fissure, fossa, foramen …

If you study the bony skull from the side and look through the pterygomaxillary fissure, you will be able to see directly into the nasal cavity. From lateral to medial you see:

- pterygomaxillary fissure, between the lateral pterygoid plate and maxilla
- pterygopalatine fossa: a small recess deep to the fissure into which the foramen rotundum opens from behind
- sphenopalatine foramen, through which you see the nasal cavity.

Pterygopalatine fossa

The relations of the pterygopalatine fossa are as follows: the maxillary sinus is anterior, the inferior orbital fissure is anterosuperior, the nasal cavity is medial, the foramen rotundum (Vb enters here) and the pterygoid canal are posterior, the infratemporal fossa is lateral (the maxillary artery enters here) and the palatine canals are inferior. In the fossa the maxillary nerve and artery divide into their terminal branches. These pass to:

- the nose
- the maxillary sinus and skin of the cheek
- upper teeth
- palate
- nasopharynx.

Pterygopalatine ganglion

The pterygopalatine fossa also contains the pterygopalatine ganglion, a parasympathetic ganglion on the pathway from the superior salivatory nucleus to nasal, palatine and lacrimal glands (Fig. 14.14). The ganglion is attached to one or more branches of the maxillary nerve and because of this you might be misled into thinking that it is an integral part of the maxillary nerve. It is not: any sensory fibres belonging to the maxillary nerve that approach the ganglion, for example those from the palate, pass through the ganglion without taking any part in its morphology. It is purely a parasympathetic ganglion that has attached itself to branches of the maxillary nerve for the convenience of distributing its postganglionic fibres. It receives preganglionic fibres from the nerve of the pterygoid canal (from the superior salivatory nucleus and VII).

Mouth   (Fig. 14.24)

- The vestibule is the area external to the teeth and gums. The midline fold between the inner aspect of the upper lip and gum is the frenulum.
- The oral cavity is the area internal to the teeth, alveolar processes and gums. The midline fold between the inner aspect of the lower gum and the tongue is the frenulum of the tongue.

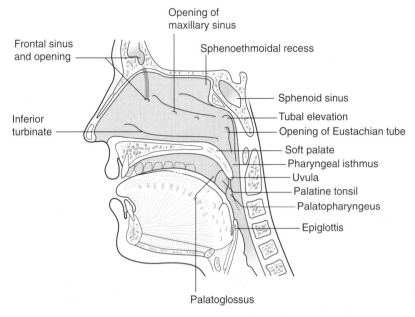

Frontal sinus
and opening

Opening of
maxillary sinus

Sphenoethmoidal recess

Sphenoid sinus

Tubal elevation

Inferior
turbinate

Opening of Eustachian tube

Soft palate

Pharyngeal isthmus

Uvula

Palatine tonsil

Palatopharyngeus

Epiglottis

Palatoglossus

Fig. 14.24   Mouth and nasal cavity, sagittal section.

- The muscles of the wall of the mouth are:
  - orbicularis oris, which forms the oral sphincter
  - buccinator, which forms the muscle of the cheek.
    These are muscles of facial expression and are supplied by VII.
    Buccinator is attached posteriorly to the pterygomandibular raphe, which is attached to the hamulus of the sphenoid and the mandible just behind the third lower molar tooth.
- The parotid duct opens opposite the second upper molar tooth. The submandibular duct opens on either side of the frenulum of the tongue and the sublingual ducts open nearby.
- The sensory innervation of buccal skin and mucosa is from branches of Vc, particularly the buccal.

- The arterial supply is from branches of the external carotid, particularly the facial, and venous drainage is to the facial vein and tributaries of the external jugular.

Tongue and floor of the mouth   (Fig. 14.25)

The tongue has two parts: the oral, or anterior two-thirds; and the pharyngeal, or posterior one-third. The boundary is the sulcus terminalis, visible on the dorsum (superior surface) of the tongue as a V-shaped sulcus with its apex pointing backwards. The foramen caecum, at the apex of the sulcus, marks the site of origin of the thyroglossal duct forming the thyroid gland.

The anterior portion of the tongue is covered by papillae of various shapes. The posterior part has lymphoid follicles, often visible, which are parts of Waldeyer's ring of lymphoid tissue guarding the oropharyngeal isthmus, and large circumvallate papillae arranged in line with and in front of the sulcus terminalis. Taste buds are present in all areas.

Muscles of the tongue

- Intrinsic muscles alter the shape of the tongue.
- Extrinsic muscles move the tongue bodily:
  - hyoglossus, attached to the length of the greater horn of the hyoid bone
  - genioglossus, attached to the mandible; and
  - styloglossus, attached to the styloid process.
    If the extrinsic muscles are paralysed, the tongue falls back and may block the airway.

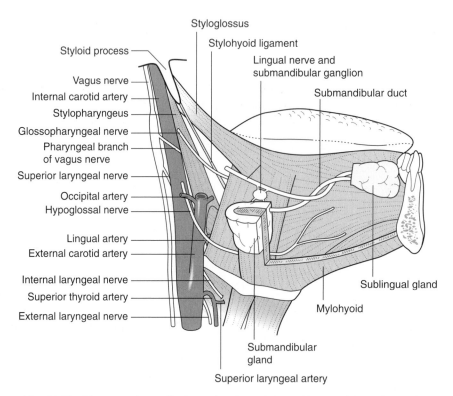

Styloglossus

Stylohyoid ligament

Styloid process

Lingual nerve and submandibular ganglion

Vagus nerve

Internal carotid artery

Submandibular duct

Stylopharyngeus

Glossopharyngeal nerve

Pharyngeal branch of vagus nerve

Superior laryngeal nerve

Occipital artery

Hypoglossal nerve

Lingual artery

External carotid artery

Internal laryngeal nerve

Superior thyroid artery

External laryngeal nerve

Sublingual gland

Mylohyoid

Submandibular gland

Superior laryngeal artery

Fig. 14.25   Tongue, submandibular region, lateral view with mandible and part of mylohyoid cut away.

- The muscles of the tongue rest upon the floor of the mouth formed by geniohyoid (genial tubercle of mandible – hyoid) and mylohyoid.

Nerves of the tongue

- Motor to all tongue muscles: hypoglossal nerve (XII). It descends in the neck to the level of the hyoid bone, then passes lateral to the internal carotid artery hooking under the origin of the occipital artery. It approaches the tongue from below and passes lateral to hyoglossus.
- Motor to anterior belly of digastric and mylohyoid: Vc.
- Sensory innervation of the anterior two-thirds of the tongue:
  - 'ordinary' sensation (tactile, pain, temperature, etc.): lingual nerve (branch of Vc), with cell bodies in the trigeminal ganglion
  - taste sensation: lingual nerve, chorda tympani, VII, with cell bodies in the geniculate ganglion (of VII).
- Sensory innervation of the posterior one-third of the tongue: IX for all types of sensation, with cell bodies in the sensory ganglion of IX. The quality of sensation from this area is different from that in the anterior portion: anything more than a brief touch elicits the gag reflex (see p. 232).

- For sensory innervation, the boundary between the anterior two-thirds and posterior one-third is an imaginary line in front of the circumvallate papillae, which are supplied by IX.
- The lingual nerve (branch of Vc), having descended between the pterygoid muscles, where it is joined by the chorda tympani, lies adjacent to the third lower molar tooth.
  - In the floor of the mouth the submandibular ganglion is attached to the nerve, which then enters the tongue lateral to hyoglossus.
  - The lingual nerve passes forwards from lateral to medial under the submandibular duct.

Arteries

Arterial blood comes from the lingual artery, which enters the tongue from behind, lateral to hyoglossus.

Lymph drainage of the tongue

- From the tip: to submental nodes, in the midline below the middle of the mandible.
- From the body: to submandibular nodes, with the midline portion of the tongue draining to both sides.
- From the posterior third: to the deep cervical chain.

The message is: if you have a patient with a tongue tumour, check the nodes on both sides of the neck.

Submandibular and sublingual glands

(Fig. 14.25)

The submandibular salivary gland lies beneath and medial to the angle of the mandible. The posterior border of mylohyoid indents the anterior surface of the gland, partially dividing it into superficial (below) and deep (above) portions. The submandibular duct passes forwards, lateral to hyoglossus, to open into the mouth on either side of the frenulum of the tongue. The duct is prone to blockage by submandibular stones, largely because the duct is long and the secretions sticky, the gland being rich in mucous secretory acini. In its course in the floor of the mouth the duct is intimately related to the lingual nerve (see above).

Sublingual salivary glands are scattered along the submandibular duct, into which some of them open, others opening directly into the oral cavity.

Secretomotor impulses to both glands originate in the superior salivary nucleus and pass by way of VII, the chorda tympani, lingual nerve and the submandibular ganglion (see Fig. 14.14).

Clinical box

Facial pulse
The facial pulse is palpable as the artery crosses the mandible. The facial artery has a tortuous course (to allow for mandibular movements) and passes through the submandibular gland.

Inferior alveolar nerve
The inferior alveolar nerve in the mandibular canal may be damaged by a mandibular fracture leading to sensory loss distally. This can be assessed by testing sensation over the chin (mental nerve, a continuation of the inferior alveolar).

Oral anaesthesia
Injection of local anaesthetics into the oral mucosa on the medial side of the mandible, aiming for the inferior alveolar nerve, can also involve the nearby lingual nerve causing numbness of the tongue and oral mucosa. In wisdom tooth extractions, the buccal nerve may also be involved giving numbness of the cheek.

Lingual nerve damage
Damage to the lingual nerve in the floor of the mouth would cause loss of sensation of all types from the anterior two-thirds of the tongue. It may result from careless extractions of the third lower molar (wisdom) tooth, fractures of the angle of the mandible, or manipulation or surgery of the submandibular duct.

Referred pain to the ear
Any area supplied by the mandibular nerve may give referred pain to the ear. Beware of patients with cotton wool in the external acoustic meatus – look in the mouth for the disease (e.g. oral or lingual cancer).

Palate and tonsillar bed

- The hard palate is formed by parts of the maxilla and palatine bone.
- The soft palate is muscular and formed by tensor palati, levator palati, palatoglossus and palatopharyngeus, the last two forming the palatoglossal and palatopharyngeal arches, visible in the mouth.
  - Tensor and levator palati: base of lateral pterygoid plate – soft palate (details not necessary).
- The palatal arches (faucial arches, or fauces):
  - The palatoglossal arch (with the uvula), the more anterior of the two, passes from the palate to the tongue and marks the posterior limit of the oral cavity.
  - The palatopharyngeal arch, the more posterior of the two, passes from the palate to the side of the pharynx, and marks the anterior boundary of the oropharynx.
  - The region between the two arches is the oropharyngeal isthmus.
- The tonsillar bed is at the side of the tongue between the two arches. Its principal artery is the tonsillar artery (a branch of the facial), which enters from below. Infection of the palatal mucosa above the tonsillar bed between the arches may lead to an abscess in these peritonsillar tissues and cause bulging of the arches. This is a quinsy. An incision is required to drain the pus.
- The motor innervation of these muscles is X except for tensor palati, which is Vc.
- The sensory innervation is from palatine branches of Vb and, in the tonsillar bed, branches of IX.
- The lymph drainage passes to the tonsillar (jugulodigastric) node at the top of the deep cervical chain.

Clinical box

Nerves of ingestion and chewing: functional considerations
Opening the mouth depends upon the mandibular and facial nerves: the mandibular nerve supplies the muscles that open the jaw, and the facial supplies the muscles that part the lips. Food processing in the mouth is, like chewing itself, served by the same nerves together with the hypoglossal: in simple language, facial keeps the lips closed, the mandibular innervates the muscles that chew and grind the food, and both the facial and hypoglossal nerves maintain the food in the occlusal plane by innervating buccinator and the tongue. Furthermore, in a baby before weaning, the facial and hypoglossal nerves supply the principal muscles of sustenance producing the necessary sucking forces: buccinator and the tongue. This is why damage to the facial nerve in a baby is serious.

Sensory components of ingestion and chewing are also served by the trigeminal and facial nerves. Both the mandibular and maxillary nerves sense the position and consistency of the food and regulate the force of contraction of the muscles, and taste perception in the mouth is served by various branches of the trigeminal and the facial nerves.

As we chew, it is necessary that the strength of contraction in muscles like masseter and temporalis is monitored. Were these muscles to exert undue force, and they are very powerful muscles, teeth and gums would be damaged. Proprioceptive impulses from the upper jaw are carried in branches of Vb and from the lower jaw in branches of Vc. The fibres which carry them are unique in that their cell bodies are not in a peripheral (in this case the trigeminal) ganglion: they have been 'sucked' into the brain stem to form the nucleus itself: the mesencephalic trigeminal sensory nucleus. Onward connections from this nucleus are not well established, but some pass to the trigeminal motor (mandibular) nucleus for direct control of the motor impulses to the muscles.

14.8 Anatomy of swallowing and phonation

Overview

The pharynx is divided into, from above down, nasopharynx, oropharynx and hypopharynx (laryngopharynx). Its walls are formed by constrictor muscles. The larynx opens from the anterior pharyngeal wall and contains the vocal cords. All movements of the pharynx and larynx, for swallowing and phonation, are supplied by the nucleus ambiguus of the brain stem, principally through cranial nerve X. The anatomy of the laryngeal skeleton is important for intubation and access to the airway in an emergency.

Learning Objectives

You should:

- understand the basic construction of the pharynx and larynx
- understand the anatomy of vocal cord movements
- know the motor and sensory innervation of the pharynx and larynx, and the areas to which pain may be referred
- know the lymph drainage of the pharynx and larynx
- know the surface anatomy of the larynx, particularly with regard to laryngotomy and tracheostomy.

Pharynx

Parts of the pharynx (Fig. 14.26)

- Nasopharynx: above the level of the palate (see 14.9, p. 256).
- Oropharynx: between the levels of the palate and the tip of the epiglottis. This is anterior to vertebrae C1, 2. Its anterior boundary is the palatopharyngeal arch.
  - The mucosal fold in the midline between the posterior surface of the tongue and the base of the epiglottis is the median glosso-epiglottic fold. The small recess on each side is the vallecula.
- Hypopharynx, or laryngopharynx: between the tip of the epiglottis and the cricopharyngeal sphincter (vertebral level C6) at the top of the oesophagus.
  - The larynx opens from the anterior wall of the hypopharynx.
  - The piriform fossas are the lateral portions of the hypopharynx, on either side of the laryngeal opening. They are the pathways taken by swallowed material on its way from mouth to oesophagus, thus avoiding the laryngeal opening.

Walls of the pharynx

The constrictor muscles form the walls of the pharynx and are attached posteriorly to the median pharyngeal raphe. This hangs down from the pharyngeal tubercle underneath the basi-occiput just anterior to the foramen magnum, and blends inferiorly with the posterior wall of the hypopharynx and oesophagus.

The constrictors are arranged as three overlapping units: superior, middle and inferior. Between muscle and pharyngeal epithelium is the pharyngobasilar fascia, which is attached to the base of the skull and the medial pterygoid plates. Fibres of the constrictors pass down and laterally to attach to various skeletal elements in front. From above down:

- Superior constrictor: this is attached to the lower half of the medial pterygoid plate, the pterygomandibular raphe and the adjacent lingula. It continues forwards as buccinator. It is not attached to the upper part of the medial pterygoid plate: the Eustachian tube opens here.
- Middle constrictor: this is attached to the side of the body and lesser horn of the hyoid bone.
- Inferior constrictor: this is attached to the lateral surface of the thyroid and cricoid cartilages.
- Cricopharyngeus is part of the inferior constrictor that forms a sphincter at the level of the cricoid cartilage (vertebral level C6), controlling entry to the oesophagus.

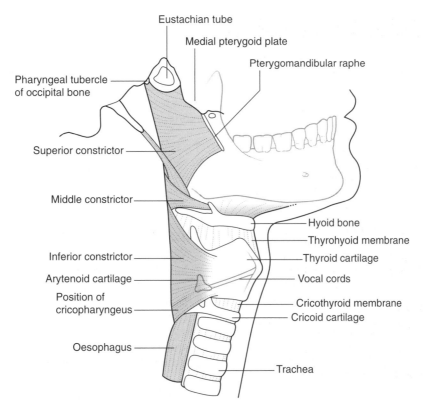

Fig. 14.26 Muscles of the pharynx, lateral view.

- Other muscles, details are not important:
  - Palatopharyngeus has no skeletal attachments. Part of it passes up to the nasopharynx to surround the orifice of the Eustachian tube (see p. 256).
  - The movements of the pharynx are assisted by other muscles from above, such as stylohyoid (VII), stylopharyngeus (IX), and styloglossus (XII).
- Killian's dehiscence. This is a potential weak spot in the posterior wall of the pharynx where the obliquely orientated fibres of the inferior constrictor and the transverse cricopharyngeus fibres leave a triangular defect. A pharyngeal diverticulum may arise here.

Nerves

The pharyngeal plexus in the pharyngeal wall receives fibres as follows:

- Motor: fibres from the nucleus ambiguus in X supply all pharyngeal muscles, unless otherwise stated.
- Sensory:
  - nasopharynx: fibres from Vb and IX
  - oropharynx: fibres from IX and X; scattered taste buds in the epiglottic region are supplied by X
  - hypopharynx and below: fibres from X.

Blood and lymph vessels

Arteries. Blood supply is from local branches of the external carotid artery: ascending pharyngeal, superior thyroid, lingual, facial.

Veins. Venous blood drains to tributaries of the internal and external jugular veins.

Lymph. Lymph drainage is to the deep cervical chain and retropharyngeal nodes.

Swallowing

Once the bolus of food has been propelled to the posterior third of the oral cavity by buccinator (VII) and the tongue (XII):

- The soft palate rises to close off the nasopharynx (palatal muscles, X).
- The Eustachian tube orifice opens (X).
- The laryngeal entrance is reduced in size to minimise the likelihood of material entering it. This involves narrowing of the laryngeal entrance (laryngeal muscles, X), elevation of the larynx (stylo- muscles, VII, IX, X; posterior digastric, VII, mylohyoid Vc, etc.) and the epiglottis momentarily flips down during the act of deglutition.
- The cricopharyngeal sphincter opens (X).

I think I have something stuck in my throat
Foreign bodies, such as fish or chicken bones, sometimes become impaled in the vallecula. These are easy to get at. More often, they are arrested in the piriform fossa or at the cricopharyngeal sphincter, with the patient requiring anaesthesia for laryngoscopy. A lateral radiograph of the neck may display such a foreign body, but remember that calcification of the laryngeal cartilages may confuse you. Often, when a patient thinks there is something stuck, it is simply that a sharp object has scratched the mucosa on the way down and the patient is misled by the dull visceral pain of a scratch.

Earache and pharyngeal tumours
The vagus supplies a large area of pharyngeal mucosa and also skin of the posterior wall of the external acoustic meatus and posterior tympanic membrane. Pharyngeal tumours may present as earache (referred pain).

Piriform fossa tumours
These can become fairly large before they start to cause obstruction and dysphagia. Although they may give rise to referred earache, they do not always cause pain, and by the time the patient notices anything the disease may be well advanced. Enlarged lymph nodes may the first sign.

Vagal reflexes
Irritation of the skin on the posterior wall of the external acoustic meatus (supplied by the vagus) can cause coughing, vomiting, or syncope (as a result of reflex bradycardia).

Larynx

Parts of the larynx   (Figs 14.27, 14.28)

Revise the anatomy of the hyoid bone, thyroid and cricoid cartilages (14.5, p. 236).

Parts of the larynx, described from superior to inferior, are:

● Resting on the (posterior) lamina of the cricoid cartilage are the right and left pyramidal-shaped arytenoid cartilages. The mucosal ridges that connect these to the base of the epiglottis are the aryepiglottic folds and they form the upper margin of the laryngeal opening (or aditus).
● The laryngeal vestibule is below the aryepiglottic folds and is limited inferiorly by two mucosal bulges, the vestibular folds or false vocal cords.
● The vocal cords (true vocal cords, or vocal folds) are below the vestibular folds, at about vertebral level C4, just below the level of the thyroid prominence.
● The two vocal cords as a unit constitute the glottis, and the aperture between them is the glottic aperture.
● The subglottic area of the larynx is below the vocal cords and extends down to the cricoid cartilage at vertebral level C6, at which point the trachea begins.

Vocal cords and movements: a simplified account

From the anterior (vocal) process of each arytenoid, a fibrous bands extends forwards, attached in front to the posterior surface of the lamina of the thyroid cartilage. This is covered by laryngeal epithelium and forms the vocal cord. The two cords oscillate against one another,

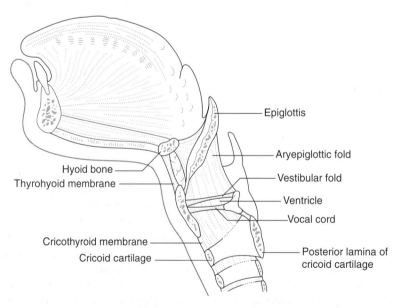

Fig. 14.27   Cross-section through the larynx.

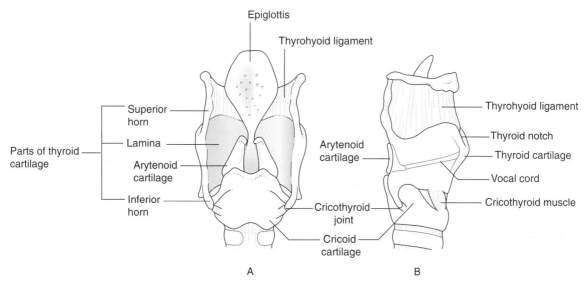

Fig. 14.28 Laryngeal skeleton: (**A**) from behind; (**B**) from the side.

setting up a vibrating column of air above – phonation – which is transmuted into speech by movements of other head and neck structures.

The sides of the glottic aperture are formed by the vocal cords (anterior two-thirds) and the medial border of the arytenoid cartilage from which they extend (posterior one-third). The cords can be abducted in two ways:

- The arytenoid cartilages can simply be pulled apart, creating a triangular-shaped glottic aperture.
- The arytenoid cartilages can swivel on the lamina of the cricoid at the synovial cricoarytenoid joints. If the lateral processes of the arytenoids are pulled backwards, their anterior processes and vocal cord attachments swing laterally to produce a diamond-shaped aperture.

The movements of adduction are the opposite of these.

The tension of the vocal cords affects the pitch of the voice. If the cords are stretched, the pitch rises. This occurs when the thyroid cartilage is tilted forwards on the cricoid.

Muscles that move the vocal cords

- Abduction: posterior cricoarytenoid.
- Adduction: lateral cricoarytenoid, thyroarytenoids.
- Tensing: cricothyroid (Fig. 14.28), and muscle fibres attached to the cords themselves.

Nerves

- Motor: X. All muscles are supplied by the recurrent laryngeal nerve, except for cricothyroid, which is supplied by the external branch of the superior laryngeal nerve.

- Sensory: X. Laryngeal mucosa above the cords is supplied by the internal branch of the superior laryngeal nerve, and below by the recurrent laryngeal nerve.

Blood and lymph vessels

Arteries. The larynx is supplied by laryngeal branches of the superior and inferior thyroid arteries.

Veins. Blood drains to tributaries of the thyroid and internal and external jugular veins.

Lymph drainage and tumour spread. Lymph drains to the deep cervical chain and retropharyngeal nodes. However, the vocal cords themselves, where the stratified squamous epithelium is tightly bound on to the underlying fibrous tissue, have no submucosa. They therefore have no lymphatics. A tumour of the vocal cords themselves will not spread into the lymphatic system until it has invaded locally beyond the vocal cords.

Speaking

Noise production – phonation. The vocal cords create the narrow slit through which air is directed to make a sound, much as in an oboe, recorder or organ pipe. Muscles which move the cords are supplied by the recurrent laryngeal nerve (X). Pitch is modulated principally by tensing (cricothyroid) and relaxing the vocal cords through the superior and recurrent laryngeal nerves (X). It is unnecessary to learn individual laryngeal muscles or their attachments: it is enough to know of their innervation.

Making the noise intelligible – articulation. The pharyngeal muscles (X), the tongue (XII), the muscles of facial expression (VII), mandibular movements (Vc) and the palate (X, V) all modify the crude noise produced by the larynx to create speech.

Movements of the pharynx and larynx: swallowing and phonation

The cell bodies of the peripheral motor neurons supplying the muscles of the pharynx and larynx are in the nucleus ambiguus in the medulla. You will be able to imagine what the effect would be of a lesion of the nucleus ambiguus: profound swallowing and speech disorders – bulbar and pseudobulbar palsies (see Ch. 15, p. 298).

Clinical box

Laryngeal tumours
Tumours which are restricted to the cords are likely to be picked up early because a voice change is an early presenting feature and the combination of an early presentation with no local lymphatics means that survival rates are good. In contrast, tumours of the subglottis are not good. This area has lymphatics (to local deep cervical nodes) and a tumour here will not only spread, but also will present late. It will have to grow large before it is visible beyond the vocal cords on laryngoscopy, and it may not cause voice changes.

Laryngotomy (tracheotomy), tracheostomy
- Emergency: laryngotomy. The problem is usually that the glottic aperture is blocked (foreign body, swollen cords, etc.), so there is no point inserting a hollow needle above the cords. Insert the needle in the midline of the cricothyroid membrane, below the thyroid prominence. (This is sometimes called tracheotomy – wrongly, since the needle is inserted into the larynx not the trachea).
- More permanent: tracheostomy. Divide the isthmus of the thyroid gland (much lower than a laryngotomy) and remove part of the anterior tracheal wall (in the region of tracheal rings 2–4). Note that stoma means orifice, -tomy means cut (as in anatomy).

Referred pain and laryngeal tumours
The vagus supplies a large area of laryngeal mucosa, whether by the internal or the recurrent laryngeal nerves. As with pharyngeal tumours, and for the same reason, laryngeal tumours often present as earache.

Mediastinal tumours
Because of the thoracic course of both recurrent laryngeal nerves, mediastinal tumours may present as voice changes. This is more common on the left than the right because the nerve is lower on the left.

Thyroid arteries
The arteries of the thyroid gland are closely related to the laryngeal branches of X, as described on page 241. Damage to the recurrent laryngeal nerves at this point nearly always affects fibres innervating the vocal cord abductors before those affecting adductors. This is serious, since if abduction is lost, the cords will be adducted and breathing will be difficult.

14.9 Nose, nasal sinuses and the sense of smell: cranial nerve I

Overview

The nasal cavity is divided by three turbinate bones (conchae) into inferior, middle and superior meatuses, and, at the top, the sphenoethmoidal recess. Nasal sinuses open into the lateral wall of the nasal cavity, ethmoid sinuses separating the nasal cavity from the orbit. The nasal cavity receives arterial blood mainly from the maxillary artery and is innervated mainly by the maxillary nerve. Olfactory mucosa is confined to the sphenoethmoidal recess. This is separated from the anterior cranial fossa by the cribriform plate of the ethmoid bone, sometimes fractured in head injuries.

Learning Objectives

You should:

- know the superior and lateral relations of the nasal cavity

- know the anatomy and innervation of the nasal sinuses

- understand why head injuries may lead to anosmia and CSF rhinorrhoea.

External nose

The skeleton of the external nose is mainly cartilaginous. The overlying skin is supplied laterally by branches of Vb and in the midline by the external nasal nerves (continuations of the anterior ethmoidal branches of Va), which become superficial at the junction of cartilage and nasal bone, easily palpable. Fractures of the nasal bridge may damage this nerve resulting in sensory loss in skin down to the nasal tip.

Nasal cavity   (Figs 14.24, 14.29, 14.30)

The nasal cavity extends between the anterior nasal aperture (naris) and the posterior nasal aperture (choana), which opens into the nasopharynx. The cavity and the paranasal sinuses or air cells that communicate with it are all components of the upper respiratory tract and are lined by respiratory epithelium.

The nasal septum separates the two cavities. The anterior portion is cartilaginous, the central portion is formed by the perpendicular plate of the ethmoid, and

Superior, middle and inferior turbinates (or conchae) project into the nasal cavity from the lateral wall. The superior and middle turbinates are parts of the ethmoid, but the inferior turbinate is a separate bone. The epithelium of the turbinates is highly vascular, almost erectile, for the purpose of humidifying inspired air, and is frequently the site of inflammatory reactions to allergens. The turbinates divide the nasal cavity into four parts as follows:

- inferior meatus, below the inferior turbinate
- middle meatus, between inferior and middle turbinates
- superior meatus, between middle and superior turbinates
- sphenoethmoidal recess, between the superior turbinate and the cribriform plate of the ethmoid.

Openings on the lateral wall of the nose

- Into the inferior meatus: nasolacrimal duct, anteriorly, draining tears from the orbit.
- Into the middle meatus: frontal and maxillary sinuses, respectively at the anterior and posterior ends of a crescentic groove, the hiatus semilunaris. Behind this is the sphenopalatine foramen, which admits branches of the maxillary artery and nerve from the pterygopalatine fossa. This is covered by mucosa in the live specimen.
- Into the middle and superior meatuses: numerous ethmoid air cells.
- Into the sphenoethmoidal recess: sphenoid air sinus. This cavity in the body of the sphenoid bone is immediately in front of and below the pituitary fossa and a transnasal or trans-sphenoidal approach to the pituitary may be used.

Arteries and nerves

- Upper third of nasal cavity and ethmoid sinuses: ethmoidal branches of the ophthalmic artery and Va.
- Lower two-thirds of nasal cavity and maxillary sinus: branches of the maxillary artery and Vb. These come mainly through the sphenopalatine foramen.
- Anteriorly, branches of the facial artery enter.
- For the septum, the pattern is as for the lateral wall. Structures entering through the sphenopalatine foramen gain access to the septum by passing across on the roof of the nasal cavity.

Venous drainage

This is to local venous networks including facial veins and the pterygoid venous plexus. About a centimetre

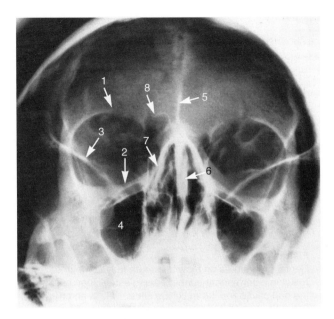

Fig. 14.29 Radiograph of head, frontal view: 1, supraorbital margin (frontal bone); 2, infraorbital margin (maxilla); 3, greater wing of sphenoid; 4, maxillary sinus; 5, cribriform plate of ethmoid; 6, nasal septum, bony part (ethmoid, vomer); 7, position of ethmoid sinuses; 8, part of outline of frontal sinus (other walls of sinus are obscured).

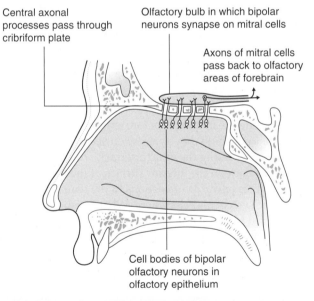

Fig. 14.30 Olfactory pathways.

the posterior portion, separating the two choanae, is formed by the vomer. A deformed or deviated nasal septum may interfere with nasal breathing and the cartilaginous portion can be removed in whole or in part by an operation called a submucous resection (SMR). The floor of the cavity is formed by the palatal shelf of the maxilla and the palatine bone, and the roof by the cribriform plate of the ethmoid.

inside the naris on the septum, close enough for a finger to reach, is Little's area, the site of a rich venous anastomosis between tributaries of facial veins and veins draining deeply. It is often the site of bleeding and is frequently cauterised (often unnecessarily).

Lymph drainage

This is mainly to retropharyngeal nodes and the deep cervical chain, with the anterior region draining to superficial facial lymph vessels and the submandibular nodes.

Maxillary sinus (antrum)

This, the largest of the nasal sinuses, is in the maxilla between the upper teeth and the orbit. The infraorbital nerve (Vb) runs in its roof and supplies it. Its floor is intimately related to the roots of the maxillary teeth, particularly the second molar. In young children, this area is occupied by the as yet unerupted permanent dentition and the maxillary sinus is rudimentary.

Nasopharynx

The nasal cavities open into the nasopharynx through the two choanae. Its features are:

- the opening of the Eustachian tube
- the fossa of Rosenmüller, of no significance in itself except as the site of the adenoids (nasopharyngeal tonsils). These are components of Waldeyer's lymphoid ring, which may be particularly large in children and block the Eustachian tube orifice.

The sensory innervation of the nasopharynx is from branches of Vb that pass back from the pterygopalatine fossa, and from branches of IX. It is included here as a reminder that it is part of the upper respiratory tract, as are the Eustachian tube and tympanic cavity, described in 14.10 (p. 259).

Clinical box

Maxillary sinus washout
The orifice between the maxillary sinus and the middle meatus is high on the medial wall of the sinus and it is said that the sinus is therefore badly drained. (This may be so when we stand, but not when we are lying or reading with our head dependent, and neither is it badly sited in quadrupeds). It is sometimes thought appropriate to wash out the sinus. This is done by forcing a cannula through the bony lateral wall of the inferior meatus, and injecting fluid at pressure, which then, with the head in a dependent position, flows out through the natural orifice together with whatever was in the sinus beforehand.

Clinical box (*cont'd*)

Ethmoid sinus pain
Pain from the ethmoid sinuses may be referred to the forehead (branches of Va).

Sinus cancers and proptosis
Epithelial cancers of the lining of the ethmoid and maxillary sinuses may invade the orbit causing proptosis (protruding eyes). Diplopia (double vision) results as the eyes become increasingly displaced.

Maxillary sinus pain
Infections of the maxillary sinus may cause referred pain to other structures supplied by Vb, e.g. upper teeth, infraorbital skin.

Fistula
Dental procedures on maxillary teeth may sometimes result in a permanent opening being established between the oral cavity and the maxillary sinus. This is an oro-antral fistula and it is a nuisance since pieces of food lodge in the sinus, become infected and give off offensive odours.

Olfaction, cranial nerve I (Fig. 14.30)

Olfactory epithelium is confined to the spheno-ethmoidal recess, underneath the cribriform plate of the ethmoid.

- Olfactory receptors are the peripheral processes of bipolar sensory neurons, the cell bodies being deeper in the epithelium.
- Central axonal processes of the bipolar cells pass through the cribriform plate of the ethmoid and penetrate the meninges before entering the olfactory bulb. In the bulb they synapse on secondary sensory neurons forming the olfactory tract, which tract passes back on the inferior surface of the frontal lobe and gives onward connections to the temporal lobe, limbic system and elsewhere. What is usually referred to as the first cranial nerve, the olfactory tract, is not properly a *nerve* at all since it is part of the central nervous system. There are, in fact, many olfactory nerves on each side, not just one.

Clinical box

Anosmia, CSF rhinorrhoea
Head injuries which fracture the cribriform plate may tear olfactory axons resulting in post-traumatic anosmia. Such injuries may also lead to cerebrospinal fluid dripping from the nasal cavity (CSF rhinorrhoea) as a result of also tearing the dura mater and arachnoid.

Thanks for the memory
Olfaction and taste are two aspects of the same thing and both neural systems share common links. These

---

include those to the limbic system of the brain, which is why smells and tastes can evoke memories, emotions and sexual responses, and also why there is some basis to aromatherapy and the ritual use of aromatics such as incense.

Clinical testing of I
It is hardly worth the trouble; you might just as well rely on the subjective opinion of the patient, which is, after all, what matters most.

14.10 Ear, hearing and vestibular function: cranial nerve VIII

Overview

The ear is in three parts: external, middle and internal. The external and middle ears, separated by the tympanic membrane, conduct sound waves to the inner ear by means of the ossicular chain. The middle ear is part of the upper respiratory tract. The inner ear contains the auditory and vestibular organs in a common hydraulic system, so inner ear disease often leads to both auditory and vestibular symptoms.

Learning Objectives

You should:

- understand the organisation of the three parts of the ear, the tympanic membrane and the ossicles
- know the innervation of the external ear and middle ear
- understand that the middle ear is part of the upper respiratory tract and liable to respiratory tract disease
- know the basic organisation of the inner ear
- understand why disease of the external ear and middle ear causes conductive deafness
- understand why disease of the inner ear causes sensorineural deafness
- understand that inner ear disease may case both auditory and vestibular symptoms.

Parts of the ear

The complex evolutionary history of what we call the

ear has resulted in a three-part structure: external ear, middle ear, and inner ear.

- The external ear consists of the pinna (or auricle), which focuses sound waves from the environment into the external acoustic meatus and on to the tympanic membrane. This membrane (commonly known as the ear drum) has air on each side, air on the medial side being in the middle ear cavity, which is a lateral extension of the nasopharynx.
- The middle ear or tympanic cavity contains the ossicles, three small bones that transmit vibrations from the tympanic membrane to the inner ear in the petrous temporal bone.
- The inner ear is an enclosed hydraulic system within the petrous temporal bone. The vibrations in the fluid of the inner ear act upon hair cells that send electrical impulses to the brain in the cochlear portion of the eighth cranial nerve.
- The inner ear has another, more important, function. It contains vestibular organs for registering movement of the head with respect to gravity. These movements, too, are picked up by hair cells with nerve impulses being conveyed to the brain in the vestibular portion of the eighth cranial nerve. In this regard, you may be able to understand why the petrous bone is rock-like (for protection), and why it is important that it is firmly fixed to the sphenoid and occipital bones, indeed fused in adult life, so that the right and left vestibular organs do not vary in position relative to each other.

The frequency of general medical consultations about the ear justifies consideration of the clinical anatomy of the ear in some detail.

External ear

Pinna or auricle

The elastic cartilages of the pinna are arranged in a number of curved ridges which include the helix (outer rim) and the tragus (the small flap 'guarding' the external acoustic meatus anteriorly). The lobule (ear lobe) is fatty and apparently functionless except in some people as a hook to hang things on.

- Sensory nerves: cervical plexus C2, 3 except for the concavity (the concha) opposite the tragus, which is supplied by the auricular branch of X.
- Arteries, veins, lymph: as for the external acoustic meatus (see below).

External acoustic meatus   (Fig. 14.31)

Laterally (about two-thirds), the external meatus is a cartilaginous tube; medially it is a bony canal in the

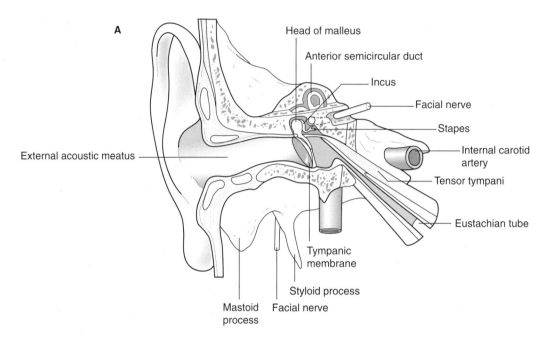

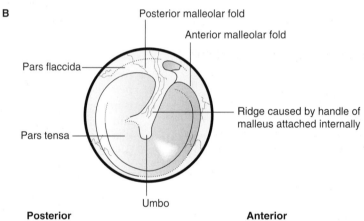

Fig. 14.31 External and middle ear, tympanic membrane: (**A**) schematic view; (**B**) lateral aspect of tympanic membrane (as viewed through an otoscope).

temporal bone. It curves forwards and downwards as it approaches the tympanic membrane, so in the adult it can be straightened by pulling the pinna up and back: this gives a better view when you use an otoscope. In a young child, pull the pinna down and back (this is because the external meatus is shorter, there is virtually no bony portion, and the orientation of the cartilaginous part is different). The cross-sectional diameter of the meatus, and the diameter of the tympanic membrane, are much the same in the child as in the adult.

The meatus is lined by skin secreting cerumen, modified sebum with protective properties for the delicate meatal skin. Epithelial cells migrate externally as they are replaced by new ones and the combination of discarded cells and cerumen is wax. This is a naturally regulated process and *never* requires assistance from cotton buds. Unless you are examining someone's

ear, never put anything in the external acoustic meatus that is any smaller than an elbow.

- Sensory innervation:
  - anterior three-quarters (roughly): branches of the cervical plexus laterally, and auriculotemporal nerve (Vc) medially
  - posterior quarter: auricular branch of X.
- Arteries: posterior auricular and other branches of the external carotid artery.
- Veins: to tributaries of the external jugular vein.
- Lymph: to parotid and mastoid nodes and the deep cervical chain.

Tympanic membrane   (Fig. 14.31)

This is a three-layered structure.

- The outer layer is modified skin, continuous with that of the external acoustic meatus and sharing the pattern of cell renewal and disposal. Should this pattern fail, or be disrupted by cotton buds, disease results.
- The middle layer is connective tissue through which the chorda tympani passes.
- The inner layer is respiratory epithelium of the middle ear cavity.

The membrane is arranged as a shallow cone with the apex, umbo, pointing medially. It faces slightly downwards and laterally, the anterior wall of the external meatus being longer than the posterior. This apparently trivial detail is responsible for the cone of light that you see when using an otoscope.

Sensory nerves:
- Anterior three-quarters: branches of the auriculotemporal nerve (Vc).
- Posterior quarter: auricular branch of X.

Arteries, veins, lymph. Blood supply and blood and lymph drainage are as for the middle ear (see below).

Clinical box

Features of the tympanic membrane visible externally
- The membrane is roughly circular. The handle of the malleus (see later) is attached to the internal surface of the membrane and this is visible externally as a ridge pointing backwards from about 2 o'clock to the umbo. When examined with an otoscope the cone of reflected light is visible pointing downwards and forwards from the umbo.
- The membrane is divided approximately one-quarter of the way down into a smaller upper sector, the pars flaccida, and a larger lower sector, the pars tensa, the dividing line being the anterior and posterior malleolar folds. Disease in the pars flaccida should be treated seriously because of what lies behind it.

Middle ear cavity, mastoid antrum, ossicles, oval window

Imagine that you are miniaturised in the nasopharynx. The orifice of the Eustachian (pharyngotympanic, auditory) tube is level with the posterior end of the inferior turbinate. The cartilaginous walls of the tube project into the nasopharynx somewhat, and the tubal orifice is surrounded by fibres of an extension of palatopharyngeus muscle (called salpingopharyngeus) which is responsible for opening the orifice during swallowing.

- You proceed along the Eustachian tube laterally, upwards and backwards, through the temporal bone. The tube opens into the middle ear or tympanic cavity, very narrow (1–2 mm) from side to side, but quite tall. On its lateral wall you see the tympanic membrane with the malleus attached to its medial surface and the chorda tympani running from front to back (or back to front) near the top of the membrane, lying between the membrane and the respiratory epithelium. Above, you see the ossicular chain.
- Continue backwards through an orifice into a smaller chamber with a large number of air cells opening from it. This is the mastoid antrum, the entrance into it is the aditus of the mastoid antrum, and the many small cells are the mastoid air cells in the mastoid process of the temporal bone. Now return to the main chamber.
- The upper part of the tympanic cavity contains the ossicles. It is quite extensive and its roof is formed by a thin plate of bone, the tegmen tympani, separating it from the middle cranial fossa and the temporal lobe of the brain. The handle of the malleus, attached to the tympanic membrane, is continuous above with the body of the malleus, and this articulates (a synovial joint) with the body of the incus. The long process of the incus descends medially to articulate with the stapes at the incudostapedial joint (also synovial). The stapes is stirrup-shaped: the neck, which articulates with the incus, gives two crura (there used to be an artery between them) with a medially facing footplate attached to their ends. The footplate fits into the oval window (fenestra ovalis, fenestra vestibuli) in the medial wall of the middle ear, which, were it not closed by the footplate of the stapes, would allow us to proceed through it into yet another cavity in the temporal bone, the inner ear. Vibrations of the tympanic membrane and ossicular chain cause the footplate of the stapes to move back and forth in the oval window, the edges being sealed by connective tissue.
- The inner ear is a closed, fluid-filled system and so when the footplate of the stapes moves medially there must be a compensatory mechanism in the inner ear to take account of the fact that fluids are not compressible. A secondary membrane bulges laterally into the middle ear cavity when the footplate of the stapes moves medially, and vice versa. This is the round window (fenestra rotundum, fenestra cochleae) situated below the oval window.
- Two muscles are attached to the ossicles:
  - Tensor tympani runs from the bone near the Eustachian tube to the handle of the malleus. It is supplied by Vc and if you try chewing whilst listening to someone, you will see, or rather hear, what it does.

- Stapedius is attached to the neck of the stapes. It arises from the medial wall of the middle ear cavity and dampens the movements of the stapes. It protects the delicate inner ear hair cells from being mechanically overstimulated. Before considering its nerve supply, the single most important relationship of the middle ear cavity needs to be mentioned: the facial nerve.
- The facial nerve passes from the posterior cranial fossa into the internal acoustic meatus, at the lateral end of which it turns backwards into the facial canal. This is separated from the middle ear cavity by only the thinnest (at most 1 mm) of bony partitions, absent in some people. The facial canal then turns laterally and down towards the stylomastoid foramen, forming the lower border of the aditus into the mastoid antrum. It gives a branch to supply stapedius, and just before emerging at the stylomastoid foramen it gives off the chorda tympani.
- Other relationships of the middle ear cavity:
  - The tegmen tympani, which may be very thin (1 mm or less), separates the middle ear cavity from the middle cranial fossa and the temporal lobe of the brain.
  - The internal carotid artery and internal jugular vein are very close to the floor.

Nerves and vessels of middle ear and Eustachian tube

- Sensory nerves to the mucosa: mainly branches of IX.
- Arteries: direct branches of the internal carotid (through the roof of the carotid canal), pharyngeal vessels.
- Veins: to the internal jugular vein.
- Lymph: to the deep cervical chain.

Clinical box

Vagal reflexes
Irritation of the skin on the posterior wall of the external acoustic meatus (supplied by the vagus) can cause coughing (X: bronchial tree sensation), vomiting (X: alimentary canal sensation), or syncope (reflex bradycardia).

Referred pain to the ear
The nerve supply of the external ear from the cervical plexus, the auriculotemporal and vagus nerves means that earache may be caused by referred pain from:
- cervical nerve entrapment resulting from disease of the cervical spine
- disease of the mouth and tongue (Vc)

Clinical box (*cont'd*)

- disease of the pharynx, oesophagus, larynx and trachea (X).

Conductive deafness
Deafness resulting from diseases of the external and/or middle ear is called conductive deafness because the conduction of mechanical impulses to the footplate of the stapes is defective. It may be caused by:
- A blocked external acoustic meatus (e.g. inspissated wax, foreign body, inflammation).
- A perforated tympanic membrane reducing the effective area for the reception of sound waves.
- Dislocation of the ossicular chain (e.g. after a head injury).
- Synovial joint disease (e.g. rheumatoid arthritis) of the ossicular chain.
- Reduced ossicular movement as a result of the middle ear cavity being full of mucus, overproduced by its lining respiratory epithelium. This is glue ear. It may be caused by the pharyngeal orifice of the Eustachian tube being blocked by enlarged adenoids.
- Fixation of the footplate of the stapes in the oval window as a result of calcification at the margins.
  All these causes of deafness are treatable.

Facial nerve
Because of the proximity of the middle ear cavity to the facial canal, a middle ear infection may cause a lesion of VII.

Hyperacusis
If stapedius is inactive (e.g. as a result of lesion of VII), movements of the stapes are not dampened, and sounds are distorted and echoing. This is hyperacusis.

Brain abscess
Because of the proximity of the middle ear cavity to the middle cranial fossa and temporal lobes, a middle ear infection may give rise to a temporal lobe abscess.

Inner ear (Fig. 14.32)

The inner ear has two parts: the osseous labyrinth and the membranous labyrinth.

Bony labyrinth

The bony (osseous) labyrinth is a single cavity in the petrous temporal bone containing perilymph, which would drip out through the oval and round windows were the windows not occluded. The cavity has three parts:

- The vestibule is the central ovoid part.
- The two and a half turns of the cochlea extend anteriorly, coiled around the central modiolus.
- The anterior (or superior), lateral and posterior semicircular canals extend from the vestibule

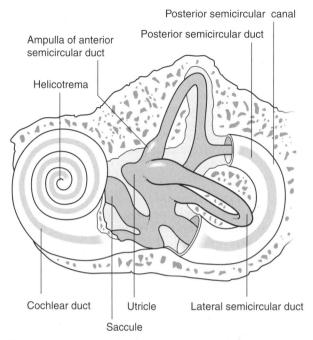

Posterior semicircular canal

Posterior semicircular duct

Ampulla of anterior
semicircular duct

Helicotrema

Cochlear duct Utricle Lateral semicircular duct

Saccule

Fig. 14.32 Inner ear showing membranous labyrinth inside bony labyrinth.

posteriorly. They are disposed at right angles to each other for the purposes of registering movements in all planes.

Membranous labyrinth

The membranous labyrinth is a fluid-filled tube within the bony labyrinth. It contains endolymph and does not communicate with perilymph.

Hearing

Within the bony cochlea is the membranous cochlear duct, echoing the shape of the bony cochlea around it. The cochlear duct is wedge-shaped in cross-section and is attached to the walls of the bony cochlea so that the perilymph-containing area does not surround the cochlear duct, but is above and below it in, respectively, the scala vestibuli and the scala tympani. The membranous cochlear duct between is the scala media. The scala vestibuli and scala tympani communicate at their origin from the vestibule and at the apex of the cochlea, the helicotrema. The partition between the scala media (cochlear duct) and the scala tympani is the basilar membrane and the sensory hair cells form the organ of Corti resting on this membrane.

- The side wall of the scala media is composed of epithelial cells and melanocytes making up the stria vascularis, which produces endolymph.
- Vibrations of the footplate of the stapes set up vibrations in perilymph which in turn impinge upon

endolymph, the basilar membrane and the organ of Corti.

Vestibular function

The membranous labyrinth within the bony vestibule is more complex in its anatomy than that of the cavity around it.

- It has two chambers, saccule and utricle, joined by connecting ducts from which the endolymphatic duct extends through the temporal bone. This terminates in the endolymphatic sac lying between the dura and the bone in the posterior cranial fossa. This is the pressure-release chamber for endolymph.
- Semicircular ducts (membranous) open from the utricle and are disposed in more or less the same way as the semicircular canals in which they are situated (anterior or superior, lateral and posterior).
- At several sites in the walls of the utricle and saccule, and in a dilatation (ampulla) at the base of each semicircular duct, hair cells extend into a gelatinous cap which 'floats' in the endolymph and moves in response to postural changes, thus distorting the hairs of the hair cells.
- The precise functions of the vestibular components of the membranous labyrinth are not clear.

Arteries and veins of middle ear and Eustachian tube

- Arteries: labyrinthine artery (from vertebrobasilar system through internal acoustic meatus), direct branches of the internal carotid (through the temporal bone).
- Veins: to internal jugular vein.

VIII: auditory pathways and reflexes

- From the organ of Corti, nerve impulses pass in bipolar neurons with cell bodies in the cochlear (spiral) ganglion in the modiolus (central pillar) of the cochlea. The central processes of these axons form the cochlear portion of VIII, which joins the vestibular portion at the lateral extremity of the internal acoustic meatus to form the eighth cranial nerve.
- VIII passes medially alongside VII in the meatus, across the posterior cranial fossa and is attached to the brain stem at the cerebellopontine angle, the most lateral of the nerves attached at that site.
- Axons pass to the cochlear nuclei of the lateral medulla.
- Secondary sensory neurons pass bilaterally to the midbrain (for auditory reflexes), medial geniculate bodies, and thence to the auditory cortex in the upper part of the temporal lobe (see Ch. 15).

- Some secondary sensory neurons pass elsewhere, e.g. to the medial longitudinal fasciculus (see below).

  Auditory reflexes. When a loud noise is heard:

- Extrinsic ocular muscles turn the eyes towards the source of the sound. Connections responsible for this include those to the nuclei of III, IV and VI in the medial longitudinal fasciculus.
- There may be a sudden inspiration and/or exclamation (startle reflex). This illustrates connections to the spinal cord and nucleus ambiguus from the midbrain.
- There may be tensing of the tympanic membrane by tensor tympani and stabilisation of the stapes, which directly impinges on the cochlea, by stapedius. This illustrates connections to the trigeminal motor nucleus (for tensor tympani) and the facial motor nucleus (for stapedius).
- You may be awoken because of connections to the brain stem reticular formation.

VIII: vestibular pathways

- From the hair cells of the utricle, saccule and semicircular ducts, nerve impulses pass in bipolar neurons with cell bodies in the vestibular ganglion adjacent to the vestibule in the petrous temporal bone. The central processes of these axons form the vestibular portion of VIII, which joins the cochlear portion at the lateral extremity of the internal acoustic meatus to form the eighth cranial nerve.
- VIII passes medially alongside VII in the meatus, across the posterior cranial fossa and is attached to the brain stem at the cerebellopontine angle, the most lateral of the nerves attached at that site. Most axons pass directly to the cerebellum.

Clinical box

One closed system
The cochlear duct is continuous with the saccule, utricle and semicircular ducts: they form an enclosed endolymph-containing system derived from the otocyst. Cochlear disorders, therefore, may affect the vestibular system, and vice versa.

Sensorineural deafness
Sensorineural deafness results from disease of the cochlea, the vestibulocochlear nerve or the auditory pathway. It includes the deafness of old age (presbyacusis). It is clinically distinguishable from conductive deafness and is largely untreatable except by hearing aids, although cochlear implants may work if the fault is in the cochlea.

Clinical box (*cont'd*)

Nystagmus
The vestibular system (including the cerebellum) is connected to the nuclei of cranial nerves III, IV and VI and the spinal cord neurons by the medial longitudinal fasciculus, a brain stem tract. Disorders of the vestibular system may therefore result in jerky eye movements: nystagmus. A patient who has nystagmus when looking straight ahead most definitely needs to be investigated. Nystagmus at the extremes of lateral vision is not necessarily abnormal.

Travel sickness
Travel sickness illustrates the connections from the vestibular pathways and cerebellum to the vomiting centre in the medulla.

Ménière's disease
Prosper Ménière described a condition consisting of attacks of deafness, vertigo and tinnitus (noises in the head). It arises from an endolymph disorder and its symptoms reflect the endolymphatic continuity between cochlea, saccule, utricle and semicircular ducts.

Endolymph and Dalmatian dogs
Endolymph production from the stria vascularis requires melanocytes. Pigment disorders (such as albinism) and deafness are associated: did you know that Dalmatian dogs, with their extensive albino patches, are hard of hearing?

Cerebellopontine angle tumours
These cause signs and symptoms of damage to VII and VIII and possibly cerebellar signs. An acoustic neuroma is a tumour of Schwann cells on VIII. If it extends into the internal acoustic meatus it will compress VII and VIII causing a nerve deafness and an ipsilateral facial palsy.

Clinical testing of VIII
- Simple tuning fork tests and audiometry distinguish between external and middle ear deafness (conductive) and inner ear and nerve deafness (sensorineural).
- Vestibular function can be tested by:
  - electrical neurophysiological testing
  - a long-established and still performed test, the caloric test, which involves irrigating the external acoustic meatus with warm and cold water. Convection currents affect the lateral semicircular duct (the nearest to the tympanic membrane), which provokes nystagmus. The duration of this can be measured and compared with results from a normal subject.
- But the best and easiest way to test the function of the vestibulocochlear nerve is to send the patient to the ENT clinic with, of course, a polite request.

14.11 Orbit, eye movements, vision, visual reflexes; cranial nerves II, III, IV, VI

Overview

The bony orbit contains the eyeball and muscles that move it. The muscles are innervated by cranial nerves III, IV and VI. Within the eyeball, the anterior chamber contains aqueous humour produced by the ciliary body and absorbed at the canal of Schlemm. Visual impulses are generated in the retina and transported to the brain by the optic nerve (II). This is a brain outgrowth and is surrounded by meninges and CSF throughout its course from the back of the eyeball to the brain. One of the most commonly performed clinical tests is the pupillary light reflex.

Learning Objectives

You should:

- know the basic relations of the orbit, particularly superior and medial

- understand in simple terms the action of muscles that move the eyeball, and their innervation

- know the structure of the eyeball

- understand the circulation of aqueous humour

- know the course taken by visual impulses, and details of the pupillary light reflex

- understand that the optic nerve is surrounded by meninges and CSF

- know the simple testing methods for II, III, IV and VI, and for the pupillary light reflex.

Orbit (Fig. 14.3)

The bony orbit contains the visual apparatus together with the nerves, vessels and lacrimal apparatus that maintain it, the muscles that move it, and the orbital fat pad that cushions it.

The orbital walls are formed by the frontal bone, the zygoma, the maxilla and the ethmoid. Of the other bones that contribute to the walls, the sphenoid contributes to the posterior walls, and it surrounds all the important structures that enter or leave. The involvement of the orbit in facial and anterior cranial fossa fractures is obvious, and its involvement in tumours of the ethmoid and maxillary sinuses has been mentioned above.

- Superior orbital margin. The supraorbital nerve (from Va) and artery (from the maxillary) may be damaged by injuries to this region. Nerve damage would result in sensory changes in the skin of the anterior scalp.

- Medial wall of the orbit. The ethmoidal nerves (from Va) and artery (from the ophthalmic) pass from orbit to ethmoid sinuses and nose. Nerve damage would result in sensory changes in the upper nasal mucosa and skin of the dorsum of the nose. This part of the orbital wall is very thin (it is called the lamina papyracea, sheet of paper) and easily damaged.

- Inferior orbital margin. The infraorbital nerve (from Vb) and artery (from the maxillary) may be damaged by injuries to this region. Nerve damage would result in sensory changes in the skin of the maxillary region and upper lip.

Foramina

- Superior orbital fissure (in the sphenoid). This transmits, from lateral to medial:
  - lacrimal nerve (branch of Va)
  - frontal nerve (branch of Va)
  - IV
  - III, superior division
  - nasociliary nerve (branch of Va)
  - III, inferior division
  - VI.

  It also transmits several veins draining to the cavernous and other dural venous sinuses.

- Inferior orbital fissure (between maxilla and sphenoid). This transmits the infraorbital and zygomatic nerves (branches of Vb) and veins draining to the pterygoid venous plexus.

- Optic foramen (in the sphenoid): transmits II, and the ophthalmic artery (branch of internal carotid).

Extrinsic ocular muscles

The muscles that move the eyeball are all supplied by cranial nerves III, IV and VI. Most of them arise from a fibrous ring at the back of the orbit so placed that it includes within it the optic foramen and the medial portion of the superior orbital fissure (including III, the nasociliary nerve and VI).

- The muscles (with innervation) that are attached to the fibrous ring are:
  - superior rectus (III)
  - lateral rectus (VI)
  - inferior rectus (III)
  - medial rectus (III).

Muscles are named according to their position and they are attached to the sclera of the eyeball, a few millimetres behind the corneoscleral junction (nearer the front of the eyeball than the back). The action of each muscle is largely predictable, but the lines of pull of superior and inferior rectus muscles are not directly anteroposterior, so the muscles have secondary actions. Superior rectus, for example, is certainly an elevator, but also adducts and medially rotates (intorts).

- Superior and inferior oblique muscles approach the eyeball from the anteromedial corner of the orbit. Inferior oblique (III) is attached to the maxilla anteromedially. Superior oblique (IV) is attached at the *back* of the orbit near the optic foramen outside the common tendinous ring. Its belly runs forwards in the upper medial part of the orbit, and its tendon passes around a fibrous 'pulley' at the front, then turning back and laterally to approach the eyeball from above, more or less mirroring that of inferior oblique below.
  - Inferior oblique turns the eye up and out.
  - Superior oblique turns the eye down and out.
- Levator palpebrae superioris is above superior rectus, between it and the frontal bone. Its fibres are attached to the subcutaneous tissues of the upper eyelid, the superior tarsal plate; and to the skin of the forehead and upper eyelid by fibres passing amongst the circular fibres of orbicularis oculi. It elevates the upper eyelid and acts with superior rectus – when you look up your eyelid rises – and is supplied by the same nerve (III, superior division). It also receives sympathetic innervation, so when the sympathetic pathways are interrupted the upper eyelid droops (ptosis, see Horner's syndrome, p. 273).

Eyelids (palpebrae) and lacrimal apparatus

- The eyelids contain fibrous tarsal plates that provide firmness to the lids and protect the eye when the palpebral fissure is closed. The tarsal plates contain tarsal glands opening by ducts at the palpebral margin of the eyelids. These ducts may become blocked leading to cyst formation.
  - Levator palpebrae superioris is attached to the superior tarsal plate and pulls it up. The superficial tissues of the eyelids also contain the circular fibres of orbicularis oculi muscle, a muscle of facial expression supplied by VII.
  - The space between the eyelids and the eyeball, which extends back for about 10 mm behind the edge of the cornea, is the conjunctival sac into which tears drain. It is lined by conjunctiva, a secretory mucosa with a function similar to that of synovium.

- The lacrimal gland is a small exocrine gland at the upper outer part of the orbit. It is arranged around the edge of the anterior portion of levator palpebrae superioris. Its secretomotor innervation originates in the superior salivatory nucleus and passes by way of VII, the pterygopalatine ganglion and branches of Vb and Va (Fig. 14.14). Numerous ducts open into the conjunctival sac, tears lubricating and protecting the eyeball, then passing medially over the surface of the eyeball to the lacrimal canaliculi, then draining through the nasolacrimal duct into the inferior meatus of the nasal cavity. Infection of the lacrimal canaliculi and/or ducts may block them, leading to tears dripping down the cheeks.

Sensory nerves and vessels of the orbit

- Sensory nerve supply: branches of Va.
- Arteries: almost exclusively from the ophthalmic artery. Some branches supply the nasal cavity (ethmoidals) and scalp (supraorbital and supratrochlear).
- Veins: to the cavernous (venous) and other dural sinuses, the pterygoid venous plexus and facial veins.

Moving the eye: cranial nerves III, IV, VI

III: Oculomotor nerve

- From the midbrain, III passes forwards in the cranial cavity to the lateral wall of the cavernous sinus. It enters the orbit through the superior orbital fissure and supplies levator palpebrae superioris (also supplied by sympathetic fibres), superior rectus, medial rectus, inferior rectus and inferior oblique.
- It conveys parasympathetic impulses for pupilloconstriction and focusing of the lens.

The nerve contains

- Motor fibres: from the oculomotor nucleus in the periaqueductal grey matter of the midbrain.
- Parasympathetic impulses: from the Edinger-Westphal nucleus (adjacent to the above) in the midbrain to the ciliary ganglion (synapse), proceeding to the eyeball in branches of Va.

IV: Trochlear nerve

- From the dorsal aspect of the midbrain, IV passes round the side of the midbrain then forwards to the lateral wall of the cavernous sinus. It passes through the superior orbital fissure and supplies superior oblique.

The nerve contains
- Motor fibres: from the trochlear nucleus in the periaqueductal grey matter of the lower midbrain. Axons pass dorsally, decussating before emerging.

VI: Abducens nerve

- From the pontomedullary junction, VI passes up to the apex of the petrous temporal bone and through (rather than in the lateral wall of) the cavernous sinus on the internal carotid artery. It passes through the superior orbital fissure and supplies lateral rectus.

The nerve contains
- Motor fibres: from the abducens nucleus in the upper medulla, close to the facial motor nucleus.

Clinical box

Oculomotor
III may be stretched in raised intracranial pressure. Nerve damage would cause ptosis (weak levator palpebrae superioris), lateral squint (unopposed superior oblique and lateral rectus), pupillary dilatation (unopposed sympathetic activity), and loss of accommodation and light reflexes. Close to the midbrain, III is related to the posterior cerebral artery, aneurysms of which may compress the nerve.

Trochlear
IV is the thinnest and most fragile nerve and is vulnerable to trauma. Section of the nerve would result in the affected eye being turned medially.

Nuclei of VI and VII
The nucleus of VI and the axons of VII are closely related in the medulla. A brain stem lesion may cause facial weakness in association with a paralysis of the ipsilateral lateral rectus muscle of the eye.

Abducens
VI has the longest intracranial course of any cranial nerve and therefore it is often the first cranial nerve to be affected by intracranial disease. So, if you could only test one cranial nerve as part of a neurological investigation, VI would be it. Damage would result in a medial or convergent squint (the eye abductor being paralysed).

VI passes over the apex of the petrous temporal bone and may be affected by infections of the bone (petrositis) causing weakness of lateral rectus with medial deviation of the ipsilateral eye. This is Gradenigo's syndrome: rare but interesting.

Cavernous sinus thrombosis
This may result from an infection of any part of the head that drains through veins communicating with it (e.g. face, ear, etc.). It would affect III, IV, Va, and VI, but VI is usually affected first because it passes *through* the sinus.

Clinical box (*cont'd*)

Clinical testing of III, IV, VI
- Eye movements. With his head stationary, ask your patient to keep both eyes on an object moving not too quickly (e.g. finger or pen) as it describes a large square with both diagonals. Should any abnormality be observed, or the patient report double vision, each eye may be tested more carefully. Or, if you want it done properly, send your patient to an optician or ophthalmologist.
- Testing III and VI. Ask your patient to look to one side: this tests medial rectus of one side (III) and lateral rectus of the other (VI).
- Testing IV. Although the superior oblique turns the eye down and out, these movements can be performed by other muscles in combination, so simply asking your patient to do this will not adequately test IV. Superior oblique is the only muscle that depresses the eye that has first been adducted, so this is a better test of IV.
- Look for a squint. A lesion of the main trunk of the oculomotor, trochlear or abducens nerves will be obvious.
- Nystagmus. Do not forget the connections of the nuclei of III, IV and VI with the medial longitudinal fasciculus (see 14.10, above).

Eyeball   (Fig. 14.33)

The eyeball is maintained in position by:

- the lateral check ligament – from the sclera near the lateral rectus attachment to the lateral orbital margin
- the medial check ligament – from the sclera near the medial rectus attachment to the medial orbital margin
- the suspensory ligament – between the two check ligaments like a sling
- the rectus muscles
- the orbital fat pad.

Coats of the eyeball

- Outer coat: sclera and cornea. This fibrous layer is protective and provides attachment for the rectus and oblique muscles. The change of orientation at the corneoscleral junction is the limbus.
- Middle coat: choroid, ciliary body, iris, collectively known as the uvea. It contains rich networks of blood vessels.
- Inner coat: retina, described later.

Parts of the eyeball

- In front of the lens:
  - anterior chamber: between cornea and iris
  - posterior chamber: between iris and lens.

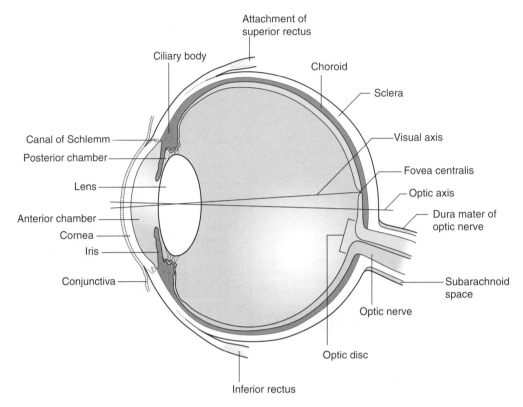

Ciliary body

Attachment of
superior rectus

Choroid

Sclera

Canal of Schlemm

Posterior chamber

Lens

Anterior chamber

Cornea

Iris

Conjunctiva

Visual axis

Fovea centralis

Optic axis

Dura mater of
optic nerve

Subarachnoid
space

Optic nerve

Optic disc

Inferior rectus

Fig. 14.33 Eyeball.

Aqueous humour is secreted into the posterior chamber by the ciliary body and flows through the pupil to the anterior chamber. Here it passes through small defects at the iridocorneal angle (between iris and cornea) to the sinus venosus sclerae, or canal of Schlemm, which is a circumferential venous channel that drains to anterior ciliary veins. Any alteration on the iridocorneal angle, such as may be caused by inflammation of the iris (iritis), might interfere with the passage of aqueous humour into the canal of Schlemm. This causes a rise in intra-ocular pressure, and is one of the causes of glaucoma.

- Iris:
  - radial smooth muscle fibres (dilator pupillae) are supplied by the sympathetic nervous system
  - annular smooth muscle fibres (sphincter pupillae) are supplied by parasympathetic impulses from the Edinger–Westphal nucleus and III.
- Ciliary body: smooth muscle fibres (for accommodation) are supplied by parasympathetic impulses from the Edinger–Westphal nucleus and III.
- Lens: attached to the ciliary processes of the ciliary body by the suspensory ligament of the lens.
- Behind the lens: occupied by vitreous humour.

Vessels and sensory nerves of the eyeball

- Arteries: from branches of the ophthalmic artery:

  - posterior and anterior ciliary vessels
  - the central artery of the retina passes up the centre of the optic nerve to the retina (see below).
- Veins: drain to the venous network of the orbit.
- Sensory innervation (pain, tactile, etc.): nasociliary nerve (Va). The cornea is extremely sensitive. Local anaesthetic drops are used to abolish sensation for ocular procedures (e.g. minor surgery, measurement of intra-ocular pressure). The corneal reflex (p. 228) tests Va and VII.
- Pupillary dilatation results from sympathetic activity, or a loss of parasympathetic activity (fear, surprise, distant vision, lesion of III, darkness, drugs, death).
- Pupillary constriction results from parasympathetic activity, or a loss of sympathetic activity (Horner's syndrome, bright lights, near vision).
- Unequal pupils may signify a unilateral lesion in the autonomic pathways.

Retina, optic nerve (II), optic tract
(Fig. 14.34)

The retina and optic nerve are formed by the optic vesicle, an outgrowth of the embryonic brain containing an extension of the ventricular system. The optic vesicle is subsequently invaginated to form the two-layered retina with a potential space, formerly the cavity, between the layers. The cavity in the optic nerve

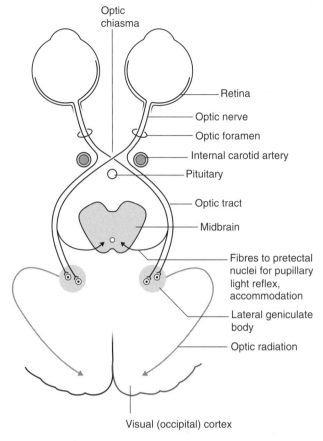

Optic chiasma

Retina

Optic nerve

Optic foramen

Internal carotid artery

Pituitary

Optic tract

Midbrain

Fibres to pretectal nuclei for pupillary light reflex, accommodation

Lateral geniculate body

Optic radiation

Visual (occipital) cortex

Fig. 14.34 Visual pathways.

is obliterated but its position is occupied by the central artery and vein of the optic nerve, the artery being a branch of the ophthalmic artery that enters the nerve in the orbit.

Optic disc, macula

- The optic nerve is attached to the inferomedial part of the eyeball, and the head of the optic nerve is marked on the retina by the optic disc, a pale area surrounded by the much pinker retina. In the centre of the optic disc is the blind spot (no light-sensitive cells) and this is the point at which the central artery and vein give into (usually) four branches disposed as an X on the retinal surface. All this is obvious on retinoscopy, particularly the sharp margin between the pale optic disc and its pink surroundings.
- About 4 mm lateral to the optic disc is the fovea centralis, the most light-sensitive part of the retina, which with its surrounding area constitutes the

macula. The eye is usually positioned so that light rays from the object in the centre of the view fall upon the macula.

Retinal layers

- The outer layer of the retina, adjacent to the choroid, is the pigment layer. This extends on to the posterior aspect of the ciliary body and iris. It contains melanocytes and is reflective.
- The inner layer is the neural layer. In the postnatal eye it stops short of the ciliary body at the ora serrata.
- Rods and cones are in the deepest parts of the neural layer with processes in contact with the pigment layer. Light rays must penetrate the full thickness of the retina before reaching these light-sensitive components: because of this the retina is described as inverted (unlike that of some other vertebrates).
- Rods and cones excite bipolar cells (the primary sensory neurons), which synapse in the retina on ganglion cells.
- Axons of ganglion cells pass on the surface of the retina to the optic disc of the eyeball and then turn posteriorly, piercing the sclera to enter the optic nerve.

Optic nerve, chiasma, tract

- At the external surface of the eyeball the optic nerve acquires meningeal coverings as befits part of the brain: it is surrounded by meninges, subarachnoid space and CSF.
- The optic nerve passes through the optic canal.
- In the anterior cranial fossa the optic nerve meets its opposite number to form the optic chiasma in the anterior wall of the third ventricle of the brain, anterior to the pituitary gland. At the chiasma, fibres from the nasal portion of each retina cross to the optic tract of the opposite side, fibres from the temporal portion of the retina passing to the optic tract of the same side. Light rays from the temporal (lateral) visual field fall on the nasal retina; light rays from the nasal (medial) visual field fall on the temporal retina.
- Some optic tract axons bifurcate sending branches to the midbrain for visual reflexes.
- The optic tract extends from the chiasma to the lateral geniculate body with onward connections to the visual cortex in the occipital lobe (see Ch. 15).

Clinical box

Exophthalmos

In some conditions the eyeball protrudes slightly. To accommodate this the eyelids have to part slightly more than normal so that, unusually, the whites of the sclera are visible all around the cornea and iris, and not just at the sides. This is exophthalmos. The reason for it in thyroid disease is not known, but it is easy to explain in conditions like ethmoid tumours that invade the orbit and displace the eyeball.

Papilloedema

Since the optic nerve is surrounded by meninges and cerebrospinal fluid in the subarachnoid space, if pressure in the subarachnoid space rises, it will compress the optic nerve. This in turn compresses the central artery and vein, the vein being occluded before the artery because venous blood pressure is lower and venous walls are thinner. Blood will be able to enter the retina through the central artery but not leave through the central vein. This leads to venous engorgement and swelling of the head of the optic nerve which bulges into the vitreous, and a blurring of the edge of the optic disc. This is papilloedema. It is a reliable sign of raised intracranial pressure and is visible on retinoscopy, the only investigation where the clinician can directly inspect the central nervous system.

Retinal detachments

The two layers of the optic vesicle that give rise to the neural and pigment layers of the retina are contiguous rather than firmly attached. The potential space between them can open up in certain conditions, e.g. poor vascular perfusion. This is called retinal detachment, and it causes blindness.

Multiple sclerosis

In the optic nerve, which is a brain outgrowth, myelin is produced by oligodendrocytes. The nerve may thus be affected in demyelinating diseases such as multiple sclerosis. This is not so for other cranial nerves in which myelin is manufactured by Schwann cells.

Visual field defects

- Section of one optic nerve causes blindness in the ipsilateral eye. This is not common.
- Destruction of the crossing fibres in the chiasma, for example by an expanding pituitary tumour, causes blindness in the nasal retina of both eyes which gives a bitemporal hemianopia (field loss).
- Pressure on the lateral aspect of the chiasma (e.g. an internal carotid artery aneurysm) affects fibres from the temporal retina of the ipsilateral eye, giving an ipsilateral nasal hemianopia: this is uncommon. Bilateral internal carotid artery aneurysms would cause a binasal hemianopia: even more uncommon.
- Destruction of the pathway behind the chiasma would interrupt pathways from the temporal retina of the ipsilateral eye and the nasal retina of the contralateral eye. This would cause blindness in the same side of both visual fields: a homonymous hemianopia.

Clinical testing of II

So-called testing of the optic nerves usually means testing visual acuity and the visual fields. Visual acuity is tested with charts using print in standard sizes. Visual field assessments may be done by confrontation tests in which the examiner compares the patient's visual fields with his own by moving the fingers in and out of the field of vision. They assume that the examiner's visual fields are normal.

Visual reflexes

Pupillary light reflex (Fig. 14.35).　A light shone into either eye causes both pupils to constrict. This reflex is a crude test of brain stem function. It involves the optic nerve, optic chiasm, optic tract, midbrain and oculomotor nerve (parasympathetic components), ciliary ganglion and iris muscle. The reflex is described as consensual because commissural connections mean that when light is shone into one eye both pupils respond. The reflex does not involve cortical activity and may be performed on an unconscious subject: only at the deepest levels of unconsciousness is there no response. Fixed dilated pupils are those which do not respond to light: they are a likely indicator of brain death.

Accommodation reflex.　Focusing on a near object and then looking away (or vice versa) results in changes of the size of the pupil (near: constricted; far: dilated) and the lens (near: fatter; far: thinner). In the accommodation reflex there is some degree of perception, unlike the pupillary light reflex, and thus the cerebral cortex is involved. There is also some voluntary control since you can decide to focus on a particular object. The precise pathways are not fully understood, but those given below are probable.

Retina → optic nerve → optic chiasma → optic tract → lateral geniculate bodies → visual cortex → frontal cortex → midbrain Edinger–Westphal nuclei → III → ciliary ganglion → ciliary and iris muscles.

Argyll Robertson pupil (note: no hyphen).　This is a pupil that accommodates but does not react to light. A comparison of the pathways for the accommodation reflex, which functions normally, and the pupillary light reflex, which does not, indicates that the lesion could be in (a) the fibres that pass from the optic tract to the midbrain, or (b) the midbrain.

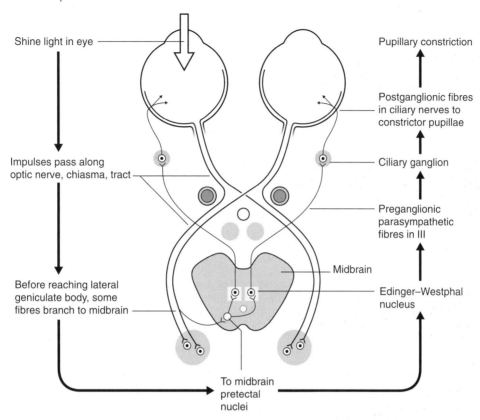

Start at top left and follow arrows

Shine light in eye

Pupillary constriction

Impulses pass along optic nerve, chiasma, tract

Postganglionic fibres in ciliary nerves to constrictor pupillae

Ciliary ganglion

Preganglionic parasympathetic fibres in III

Before reaching lateral geniculate body, some fibres branch to midbrain

Midbrain

Edinger–Westphal nucleus

To midbrain pretectal nuclei

Fig. 14.35 Pupillary light reflex.

14.12 Inside the skull, haemorrhages

Overview

Skull bones and meninges are supplied by meningeal vessels, the largest being the middle meningeal. These pass deep to the pterion and are vulnerable there, bleeding at that site leading to an extradural haematoma. The brain is supplied by the internal carotid and vertebrobasilar systems that together form the arterial circle of Willis. Venous blood drains to sinuses in the margins of dural folds projecting into the cranial cavity. These sinuses eventually join to form the sigmoid sinuses and internal jugular veins. The meninges surrounding the brain are similar to those of the spinal cord except that there is no cranial extra(epi)dural space. Cisterns are dilated areas of the cranial subarachnoid space containing CSF. Other intracranial haemorrhages are subdural, subarachnoid and intracerebral.

Learning Objectives

You should:

- understand the layout of the cranial meninges and venous sinuses

- know the principal arteries supplying skull bones, meninges and brain

- understand venous return from the cranial cavity

- know the anatomy of extradural, subdural, subarachnoid and intracerebral haemorrhages

- know the principal cisterns of the cranial subarachnoid space.

Arteries

Meningeal arteries, extradural haemorrhage

Grooves are visible on the internal aspect of the skull bones. These are for meningeal veins and accompanying arteries that run between the dura and the periosteum of the skull bones. Although called meningeal, in fact these vessels are more important for supplying skull bones and diploic cavities than meninges. Several arteries give meningeal branches, but one in particular is important: the middle meningeal artery. It is a branch of the maxillary artery and enters the middle cranial fossa through the foramen spinosum. The anterior division of the artery passes deep to the pterion where the cranium is thinnest and an injury at this site may tear the artery causing an extradural haemorrhage. This may become quite large before it causes symptoms, and the interval between the injury and the appearance of symptoms is called the lucid interval. This is why patients with head injuries are often admitted to hospital for a brief period.

Internal carotid artery

At the top of the neck, the internal carotid artery enters the carotid canal in the temporal bone. In the canal the artery passes medially before turning upwards once more to enter the cranial cavity at the side of the sphenoid air sinus.

In the middle cranial fossa, the artery runs through the cavernous (venous) sinus, in and above which it describes an S-shaped course with VI on its lateral wall for a short distance. Above the sinus it gives off the ophthalmic artery to the orbit and eye and divides into its terminal branches, the anterior and middle cerebral arteries, as part of the arterial circle of Willis.

Vertebral artery

Having emerged from the transverse foramina of the cervical vertebrae, the vertebral arteries pass medially between vertebra C1 and the occipital bone, penetrate the dura and ascend through the foramen magnum. On the front of the brain stem they unite to form the basilar artery, which supplies the brain stem and inner ear. It terminates in the circle of Willis by dividing into the right and left posterior cerebral arteries.

Meninges, venous sinuses, subdural and subarachnoid haemorrhages
(Fig. 14.36)

The meninges form sacs around the brain, the outer layer being the dura mater, the middle layer the arachnoid mater, and the inner layer, inseparable from the brain itself, the pia mater. Between the arachnoid and the pia is the subarachnoid space, which, like the spinal subarachnoid space with which it is continuous, contains cerebrospinal fluid. The arachnoid is a thin layer, loosely adherent to the inner aspect of the dura.

There is no cranial equivalent of the spinal extra-dural space. Unlike the spinal dura, the cranial dura is firmly adherent to the periosteum of the skull bones except at certain sites where they part company to enclose large endothelial venous channels, the venous sinuses. These are the principal collecting channels for venous blood from the brain. The margins of their attachment are clearly visible on the inside of the skull.

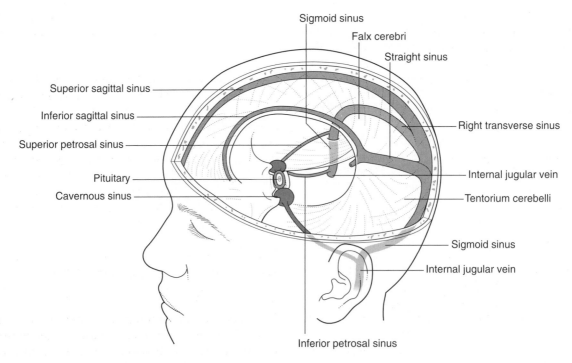

Sigmoid sinus
Falx cerebri
Straight sinus
Superior sagittal sinus
Inferior sagittal sinus
Superior petrosal sinus
Pituitary
Cavernous sinus
Right transverse sinus
Internal jugular vein
Tentorium cerebelli
Sigmoid sinus
Internal jugular vein
Inferior petrosal sinus

Fig. 14.36 Dural reflections and venous sinuses.

Beware. Regrettably, some people call the dura the 'meningeal layer of dura' and the periosteum of the skull bones the 'periosteal layer of dura'. This terminology has nothing to recommend it.

Falx cerebri, tentorium cerebelli

From the larger venous sinuses at several sites, a double layer of dura projects into the cranial cavity. These dural folds form:

- The falx cerebri in the midline, which partially separates the cranial cavity into right and left halves and lies between the two cerebral hemispheres. It is attached to the ethmoid bone in front, the vault of the skull above and behind, and has a free inferior edge.
- The tentorium cerebelli, which is a more or less horizontally arranged sheet extending back from the ridge of the petrous temporal bone and the clinoid processes to the internal occipital protuberance. It forms a complete diaphragm over the posterior cranial fossa except for the tentorial notch, an anterior defect, through which the brain stem and surrounding nerves and vessels pass.

Venous sinuses

- The superior sagittal sinus is in the midline at the attachment of the falx cerebri to the skull vault. Blood in it drains posteriorly and at the internal occipital protuberance it normally turns to the right, becoming the transverse sinus. This passes forwards in the lateral attachment of the tentorium cerebelli to the edge of the petrous temporal bone. Here it curls down as the right sigmoid sinus, passes through the jugular foramen and becomes the right internal jugular vein.
- The inferior sagittal sinus is in the midline in the inferior free margin of the falx cerebri. Blood in it drains posteriorly and is joined at the tentorium/falx junction by blood from the great cerebral vein emerging from the back of the brain stem. These unite to form the straight sinus, which passes back in the attachment of the falx and the tentorium, and at the internal occipital protuberance normally turns to the left, becoming the left transverse sinus. The pattern then mirrors that on the right side, eventually forming the left internal jugular vein. Sometimes the pattern is reversed with the superior sagittal sinus turning left and the straight sinus turning right. At the internal occipital protuberance, the venous channels may communicate: this is the confluence of sinuses. The right-sided venous channels (from the superior

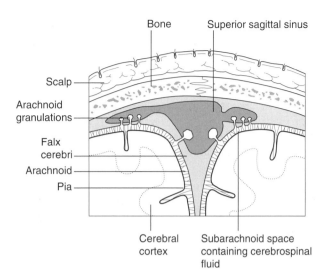

Fig. 14.37 Coronal section through superior sagittal sinus.

sagittal sinus) are usually bigger than the left, with the right internal jugular vein bigger than the left. Indeed, the left internal jugular vein may even be absent altogether.

Arachnoid granulations (Fig. 14.37)
The dural walls of the sinuses, particularly the superior sagittal sinus, possess small defects which allow the underlying arachnoid to billow through into the sinus. These are the arachnoid granulations where only arachnoid and the endothelium of the sinuses separate cerebrospinal fluid from venous blood: they are the sites of reabsorption of cerebrospinal fluid. If the sinuses become thrombosed, reabsorption will be prevented and the pressure of cerebrospinal fluid in the subarachnoid space will rise.

Diaphragma sellae, pituitary fossa (Figs 14.5, 14.38)
This midline fossa directly above the sphenoid (nasal) sinus is guarded by the anterior and posterior clinoid processes to which is attached the diaphragma sellae, a sheet of dura pierced by the pituitary stalk and isolating the pituitary gland below from the subarachnoid space above. There is neither subarachnoid space nor cerebrospinal fluid below the diaphragma, a fact that surgeons are glad of when performing transnasal approaches to the pituitary (see 14.9, p. 255).

Cavernous sinus (Fig. 14.38)
The cavernous sinus is formed in the embryo from the coalescence of several venous channels, giving a system of interconnecting caverns around the internal carotid artery. The right and left cavernous sinuses lie on either side of the pituitary fossa, and communicate with the transverse sinuses and internal jugular veins through petrosal sinuses, and with each other by

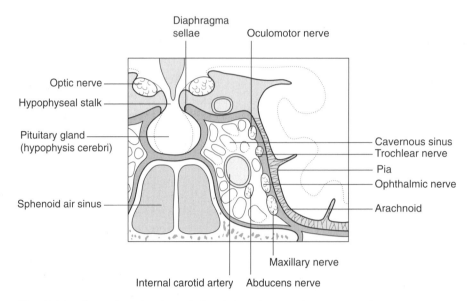

Fig. 14.38 Coronal section through the pituitary fossa and cavernous sinus.

connections across the midline. Cranial nerves III, IV and Va pass in the lateral wall of the sinus on their way to the superior orbital fissure, and VI passes through the sinus on the internal carotid artery. The cavernous sinus is connected through various skull foramina to facial and other external veins, and these may allow a superficial infection to spread to the sinus with the risk of cavernous sinus thrombosis.

Venous blood from the cranial cavity also passes through the foramen magnum to join the internal vertebral venous plexus of the spinal column. This is important if the internal jugular veins become blocked or if they have to be ligated.

Sensory innervation of the dura

Sensory fibres from several nerves innervate the dura. These may be given off as they leave the skull, or they may re-enter the skull through small foramina. The dura is sensitive to pain and stretching. Meningeal branches of the following nerves supply the dura:

- anterior cranial fossa: ethmoidal nerves Va; branches of Vb
- middle cranial fossa: branches of Vb, Vc
- posterior cranial fossa: branches of X and C1, 2.

Clinical box

Intracranial haemorrhages
  Subdural.   The walls of the venous sinuses are pierced by numerous small veins which pass directly from the brain substance into the sinuses. With advancing years, the brain shrinks so these veins become stretched, rendering them more susceptible in

---

Clinical box *(cont'd)*

the old than in the young to tearing as a result of sudden jolts of the head. In such cases, the veins rupture immediately before entering the venous sinuses so blood seeps between the dura and arachnoid (which are normally in contact). This is a subdural haemorrhage.
  Subarachnoid.   Subarachnoid haemorrhages occur when an artery in the subarachnoid space (e.g. an artery of the circle of Willis or one of its branches) ruptures, discharging blood into the cerebrospinal fluid. It is sudden and often fatal, and is the commonest cause of sudden death in young adults.
  Cerebral.   And, for the sake of completeness, (intra)cerebral haemorrhages are bleeds of arteries within the brain substance. These may be either imperceptible in their effects, or have devastating effects depending not just on size but also on what structures are damaged or deprived of a blood supply. These are responsible for what is usually called a stroke.

The anatomy of both extracranial and intracranial haemorrhages is summarised in Table 14.4.

Cranial subarachnoid space, cisterns

- The contours of the dura and arachnoid reflect, except at the sinuses, the cranium. The contours of the pia reflect, indeed are, the surface of the brain. At several sites where the surface of the brain is deeply fissured, the subarachnoid space is wider than at other sites. These areas are the subarachnoid cisterns. They include:
  - the tentorial cistern (also ambient cistern or cisterna ambiens), around the brain stem in the tentorial notch

Table 14.4 Anatomy of extracranial and intracranial haemorrhages: a summary

Position	Usual nature (arterial or venous)	Things to remember
Extracranial		
Subaponeurotic	Either	Scalp wound which also tears the epicranial aponeurosis, unlimited except by occipitofrontalis attachment, periorbital tracking
Subperiosteal	Either	Birth injuries, assumes shape of underlying bone
Intracranial		
Extradural	Arterial	Head injury, pterion, middle meningeal artery
Subdural	Venous	Old people
Subarachnoid	Arterial	Anyone, often (?usually) fatal
Cerebral	Arterial	Arterial, stroke, usually disabling

- the cisterna magna, at the back, just above the foramen magnum, between medulla and cerebellum
- the pontine cistern, ventral to the pons.
- The cranial subarachnoid space extends laterally for a short distance as each cranial nerve passes through its skull foramen. This is for no more than a millimetre or so except for two nerves:
  - the trigeminal, where the extension of subarachnoid space partially encloses the trigeminal sensory ganglion and is known as the trigeminal (Meckel's) cave
  - the vestibulocochlear, where the extension passes for some distance into the internal acoustic meatus.

14.13 Sympathetic impulses to the head

Sympathetic impulses do not emerge from the central nervous system in cranial nerves, but only in thoracolumbar segments of the spinal cord.

- Preganglionic impulses to the head arise in the lateral grey horn of spinal cord segments T1 and/or T2. They pass into the spinal nerve(s) and white rami communicantes to the sympathetic chain at the T1 ganglion, adjacent to the neck of the first rib. Preganglionic axons for cranial structures do not synapse here, but ascend in the chain behind the carotid sheath and synapse (usually) in the superior cervical ganglion immediately below the base of the skull.
- Postganglionic fibres reach their target organs by one or more of the following pathways:
  - With arteries and their branches. Fibres pass to the neighbouring carotid and vertebral arteries forming a plexus in their walls, and are distributed with their branches to intracranial structures, the eye, orbit and skin.
  - Cavernous sinus. As the internal carotid artery passes through the cavernous sinus, postganglionic sympathetic fibres may pass to VI (on the artery) or in fibrous strands to the lateral wall and III, IV and Va, providing another route to the orbit and eye and through branches of Va to the scalp.
  - Deep petrosal nerve. The deep petrosal nerve leaves the plexus around the internal carotid artery in the carotid canal, and joins the greater petrosal nerve to form the nerve of the pterygoid canal. It enters the pterygopalatine fossa and is distributed in branches of Vb to the nose, pharynx, palate and face.

Clinical box

Horner's syndrome
Any interruption of the sympathetic pathway to the eye would result in Horner's syndrome. Levator palpebrae superioris would be weakened leading to ptosis. Sympathetic denervation of the iris would lead to unopposed pupillary constriction, and denervation of sweat glands would result in an absence of sweating (anhidrosis). A tumour at the apex of the lung invading the sympathetic chain on the neck of the first rib would result in such signs. It may also damage the T1 root of the brachial plexus, causing weakness or paralysis of the small muscles of the hand.

Self-assessment: questions

Multiple choice questions

1. Concerning the scalp:
   a. Vessels and nerves lie superficial to the epicranial aponeurosis.
   b. It is supplied with blood only from branches of the external carotid artery.
   c. Branches of the ophthalmic nerve supply as far back as the vertex.
   d. A subaponeurotic haematoma is limited to the shape of the underlying bone.
   e. A subaponeurotic haematoma may result days later in a black eye.

2. Concerning the neck and thyroid gland:
   a. The accessory nerve lies deep in the posterior triangle and is not easily damaged.
   b. The bifurcation of the common carotid artery is level with the cricoid cartilage.
   c. Branchial cysts are present in the midline of the neck.
   d. A thyroglossal cyst moves upwards when the tongue is protruded.
   e. The isthmus of the thyroid gland usually overlies tracheal rings 2 to 4.

3. The hypoglossal (12th cranial) nerve:
   a. If sectioned, causes deviation of the protruded tongue to the side of the lesion.
   b. Carries motor fibres to the tongue muscles.
   c. Arises from the medulla oblongata.
   d. Passes lateral to the hyoglossus muscle.
   e. Is vulnerable in carotid artery surgery.

4. In the oral cavity and pharynx:
   a. The parotid duct opens opposite the second upper molar tooth.
   b. Enlarged adenoids may block the internal acoustic meatus.
   c. The submandibular duct is intimately related to the hypoglossal nerve.
   d. Calculi are more likely in the submandibular duct than in the parotid duct.
   e. Lymph from the posterior third of the tongue may drain to nodes on either side.

5. In the nasal cavity and sinuses:
   a. Little's area is on the lateral wall.
   b. The maxillary sinus opens into the middle meatus.
   c. The middle meatus is lined by olfactory mucosa.
   d. The nasolacrimal duct opens into the inferior meatus.
   e. The sphenoid sinus is immediately below the pituitary fossa.

6. Concerning the visual apparatus:
   a. The ophthalmic artery is a branch of the internal carotid artery.
   b. The optic tract consists of axons of retinal bipolar cells.
   c. A lesion of the sixth cranial (abducens) nerve causes lateral deviation of the eyeball.
   d. Alteration of the iridocorneal angle may hinder reabsorption of aqueous humour.
   e. The posterior chamber of the eye is posterior to the lens.

7. A left pupil that does not respond to shining a light into the right eye might signify:
   a. An opaque right cornea and/or lens.
   b. Damage to the right lateral geniculate body.
   c. A severed left optic nerve.
   d. Damage to the left Edinger–Westphal nucleus.
   e. A severed left oculomotor nerve.

8. Concerning the larynx and associated structures:
   a. The true vocal cords are at the level of the cricoid cartilage.
   b. The true vocal cords are below the false cords (vestibular folds).
   c. The sensory nerve supply of the larynx is entirely from the vagus nerve.
   d. The piriform fossa is part of the hypo(laryngo)pharynx.
   e. During quiet breathing the vocal cords are fully abducted.

9. The following are on or related to the medial wall of the tympanic cavity:
   a. The footplate of the stapes.
   b. The tympanic membrane.
   c. The facial nerve.
   d. The chorda tympani.
   e. The stylomastoid foramen.

10. Section of the left facial nerve at the stylomastoid foramen:
    a. Prevents parotid secretion on the left side.
    b. Abolishes the corneal reflex on the left side.
    c. Causes hyperacusis on the left side.
    d. Paralyses frontalis on the left side.
    e. Prevents lacrimation on the left side.

11. The following contribute sensory fibres to the oral cavity:
    a. Maxillary nerve.
    b. Lingual nerve.
    c. Chorda tympani.
    d. Vagus nerve.
    e. Inferior alveolar nerve.

12. The external carotid artery gives rise to the following arteries:
    a. Occipital.
    b. Posterior auricular.
    c. Ascending pharyngeal.
    d. Inferior thyroid.
    e. Facial.

13. The cerebral subarachnoid space:
    a. Lies between the arachnoid mater and dura mater.
    b. Contains cerebrospinal fluid.
    c. Contains blood vessels.
    d. Surrounds the optic (second cranial) nerve.
    e. Is continuous with the spinal subarachnoid space.

14. The straight sinus:
    a. Is formed by the union of the great cerebral vein and the inferior sagittal sinus.
    b. Contains venous blood.
    c. Enters the confluence of sinuses.
    d. Occupies the line of attachment of falx cerebri to tentorium cerebelli.
    e. Has forward blood flow within it.

15. The following nerves pass through, or in the lateral wall of, the cavernous sinus:
    a. Oculomotor (III) nerve.
    b. Trochlear (IV) nerve.
    c. Abducens (VI) nerve.
    d. Greater petrosal nerve.
    e. Ophthalmic (Va) nerve.

16. The cavernous sinus:
    a. Contains venous blood.
    b. Contains the internal carotid artery.
    c. Communicates with the facial veins.
    d. Lies immediately medial to the trigeminal ganglion.
    e. Is lateral to the sphenoid sinus.

17. The anterior fontanelle:
    a. Lies between parietal and occipital bones.
    b. Is present at birth.
    c. Closes within 6 months of birth.
    d. Overlies the superior sagittal sinus.
    e. Is a cartilaginous joint.

18. An intact corneal reflex depends upon the integrity of:
    a. The facial motor nucleus.
    b. The lateral geniculate body.
    c. The trigeminal ganglion.
    d. The oculomotor nerve.
    e. The ciliary ganglion.

19. The pupillary light reflex depends upon the integrity of:
    a. The trigeminal ganglion.
    b. The optic nerve.
    c. The lateral geniculate body.
    d. The Edinger–Westphal nucleus.
    e. The ciliary ganglion.

Matching item questions

Questions 1–5

Match the numbered item to the lettered response. Each lettered response may be used once, more than once, or not at all.
    a. maxillary nerve (Vb)
    b. mandibular nerve (Vc)
    c. facial nerve (VII)
    d. glossopharyngeal nerve (IX)
    e. vagus nerve (X)
1. smiling
2. mastication
3. blinking
4. parotid salivation
5. toothache from the upper molars

Questions 6–10

Match the numbered item to the lettered response. Each lettered response may be used once, more than once, or not at all.
    a. injury to the pterion
    b. venous bleed
    c. adopts shape of underlying bone
    d. blood from vertebral artery
    e. extracranial haemorrhage
6. subperiosteal haemorrhage
7. extradural haemorrhage
8. subdural haemorrhage
9. subaponeurotic haemorrhage
10. subarachnoid haemorrhage

Questions 11–15

Match the numbered item to the lettered response. Each lettered response may be used once, more than once, or not at all.

    a. branch of axillary
    b. branch of subclavian
    c. branch of external carotid
    d. branch of internal carotid
    e. branch of common carotid

11. superior thyroid artery
12. maxillary artery
13. facial artery
14. middle cerebral artery
15. vertebral artery

Questions requiring short answers

1. Thugs wielding a knife attack a young lady. She is stabbed in the middle and lower parts of the posterior triangle of the neck. Which structures are at risk of damage? Give surface markings, and symptoms that would result from damage to any nerves you name.

2. A patient has a swelling between the left mandible and the ear, which is increasing in size. After a few weeks, the patient notices difficulty in closing the lips for whistling, and before long starts to dribble from the left corner of the mouth. Explain what is going on, giving as much information as you can about any nerve you name.

3. Give the lymph drainage and innervation of the tongue.

4. Briefly describe or draw the anatomy of the submandibular gland and duct. At operation, the surgeon must be careful of certain nerves when (a) making the incision; and (b) handling the duct. Name the nerves, give their function, and explain the results of damage.

5. Describe the blood supply of the scalp and explain why scalp lacerations can lead to a black eye.

6. A blow on the head results in clear fluid dripping from the nose. Explain what has been fractured and/or torn, what is the fluid and what may be a permanent symptom as a result of this injury.

7. Where are the vocal cords? Explain the anatomy of laryngotomy.

8. A patient presents with a cough and hoarse voice. A chest radiograph reveals a left-sided tumour in the region of the pulmonary artery and aortic arch. Briefly describe the anatomy of this region and explain the voice change. Add a note on relevant embryology.

9. What is the middle ear? What major nerve could be affected by a severe middle ear infection? How would you recognise this?

10. Give the sensory innervation of the external aspect of the tympanic membrane and explain why earache may occur in the absence of ear disease.

Self-assessment: answers

Multiple choice answers

1. a. **True.**
   b. **False.** It is also supplied by the internal carotid artery via branches of the ophthalmic.
   c. **True.** The greater occipital nerve (C2 dorsal ramus) supplies the scalp behind the vertex.
   d. **False.** It is a subperiosteal haematoma that is limited to the shape of the underlying bone.
   e. **True.** There is no anterior bony attachment of the aponeurosis to stop it.

2. a. **False.** The accessory nerve is superficial and easy to damage.
   b. **False.** The common carotid artery bifurcates at the top of the thyroid cartilage.
   c. **False.** They are lateral. Thyroglossal cysts are midline.
   d. **True.**
   e. **True.**

3. a–e. **All true!**

4. a. **True.**
   b. **False.** Ha! The internal acoustic meatus is *not* the Eustachian tube. Do not confuse the two things.
   c. **False.** The lingual nerve is related to the submandibular duct.
   d. **True.** The submandibular gland produces stickier secretions.
   e. **True.**

5. a. **False.**
   b. **True.**
   c. **False.** Olfactory mucosa is limited to the sphenoethmoidal recess.
   d. **True.**
   e. **True.** This enables transnasal surgical approaches to the pituitary.

6. a. **True.**
   b. **False.** The optic tract consists of axons of ganglion cells.
   c. **False.** This would be paralysed. Why do you think VI is called the abducens nerve?
   d. **True.** This is one of the causes of glaucoma.
   e. **False.** It is posterior to the iris, and anterior to the lens.

7. a. **True.** Ha! People sometimes do not think of this.
   b. **False.** Geniculate bodies are not involved in the light reflex.
   c. **True.** Although this is somewhat obvious and even more unlikely.
   d. **True.**
   e. **True.**

8. a. **False.** The true vocal cords are at the middle of the thyroid cartilage.
   b. **True.**
   c. **True.**
   d. **True.**
   e. **False.** The vocal cords are in mid-abduction during quiet breathing.

9. a. **True.**
   b. **False.** The tympanic membrane is on the lateral wall of the tympanic cavity.
   c. **True.**
   d. **False.** The chorda tympani run in the tympanic membrane on the lateral wall of the tympanic cavity.
   e. **False.** It is on the external surface of the temporal bone.

10. a. **False.** This is a function of IX, not VII.
    b. **True.**
    c. **False.** Stapedius has already been supplied.
    d. **True.**
    e. **False.** These fibres have already left VII.

11. a. **True.** It supplies the palate and upper teeth.
    b. **True.** It supplies the anterior tongue and surrounding area.
    c. **True.** It carries taste fibres to the anterior tongue.
    d. **False.** The vagus supplies the pharynx, not the oral cavity.
    e. **True.**

12. a. **True.**
    b. **True.**
    c. **True.**
    d. **False.** This is from the thyrocervical trunk of the subclavian.
    e. **True.**

13. a. **False.** This is the subdural space.
    b. **True.**
    c. **True.**
    d. **True.**
    e. **True.**

14. a. **True.**
    b. **True.**
    c. **True.**
    d. **True.**
    e. **False.** Blood flows backwards.

15. a. **True.**
    b. **True.**
    c. **True.**
    d. **False.** This is in the temporal bone.
    e. **True.**

16. a. **True.**
    b. **True.**
    c. **True.**
    d. **True.** (Difficult!)
    e. **True.**

17. a. **False.** It is between the frontal and parietal bones.
    b. **True.**
    c. **False.** It usually closes by 18 months.
    d. **True.** This is useful: drugs can be injected into the sinus through the fontanelle.
    e. **False.** It is not a joint at all.

18. a. **True.** The corneal reflex depends on Va, brain stem and VII.
    b. **False.** This is concerned with vision; the corneal reflex has nothing to do with vision.
    c. **True.**
    d. **False.** This is not concerned at all.
    e. **False.** This is not concerned at all.

19. a. **False.**
    b. **True.**
    c. **False.** Impulses leave the optic tract before the lateral geniculate body is reached.
    d. **True.** This nucleus is part of the midbrain connections.
    e. **True.**

Matching item answers

1. c.
2. b.
3. c.
4. d.
5. a.
6. c.
7. a.

8. b.
9. e.
10. d.
11. c.
12. c.
13. c.
14. d.
15. b.

Short answers

1. The following structures are at risk of damage: XI, apex of lung, upper trunk of brachial plexus, branches of thyrocervical trunk, possibly even subclavian vessels. Surface markings of XI are: one-third of way down sternocleidomastoid – one-third of way up trapezius. Damage to this nerve would result in paralysis of trapezius, inability to abduct the shoulder beyond about 90° (although that might be the least of her problems). Pneumothorax and blood loss might be more urgent.

2. VII is the thing that matters. Parotid tumour invades branches of VII causing lower motor neuron lesion of VII and facial paralysis or weakness. You could mention other structures that pass through the parotid if you wish, and give other details of VII (cerebellopontine angle, internal acoustic meatus, temporal bone, middle ear).

3. The important things are:
   - Lymph drainage: from the tip to the submental nodes; from the sides to the submandibular nodes of that side with the central portion to both sides; from the posterior tongue to both sides
   - Innervation: deep cervical chain.

4. You should include the lingual nerve and its relation to the duct. Damage to it would mean loss of all sensation on the anterior tongue, and loss of some salivation in the sublingual glands (would one notice?).

5. There is no bony attachment of the epicranial aponeurosis anteriorly, so there is nothing to stop blood tracking down into the periorbital tissues. It might take a few days.

6. The cribriform plate of ethmoid has been fractured with tearing of the dura and arachnoid mater, so CSF drips out (rhinorrhoea). The olfactory nerve filaments may also be torn, so there may be post-traumatic anosmia (not post-traumatic amnesia as a student once told me, though you might have this as well!).

7. The thing is that the vocal cords are at the level of the middle of the thyroid cartilage. It is usually the vocal cords that are the site of obstruction, so at laryngotomy you need to make a hole below them. It is no use making a hole in the thyrohyoid membrane, above the cords: use the cricothyroid membrane, which is, unfortunately, slightly more difficult to find than the thyrohyoid membrane.

8. There has been damage to the recurrent laryngeal nerve, which arises in the mediastinum. Revise the mediastinum.

9. The middle ear or tympanic cavity is an extension of the upper respiratory tract from the nasopharynx, and includes the Eustachian tube, middle ear proper and mastoid antrum. It contains the ossicles and is bounded laterally by the tympanic membrane. The facial nerve (VII) is closely related to it, and a facial weakness or palsy might be caused by a severe middle ear infection that affects the nerve.

10. Sensory innervation of the external aspect of the tympanic membrane: Vc (about three-quarters), X (about one-quarter). Referred pain can arise from structures supplied by Vc (lower teeth, tongue, mouth); and from structures supplied by X (larynx, pharynx, trachea). Earache in a patient with normal tympanic membranes might result from disease of the mouth, tongue, pharynx, or larynx.

15 Brain

15.1 Brain vesicles, general terms, ventricles, CSF

Overview

The brain develops from the rostral (upper) end of the neural tube as three brain vesicles: hindbrain, midbrain and forebrain. The hindbrain becomes the medulla, pons and cerebellum; the midbrain remains as the midbrain; and the forebrain becomes, in the midline, the thalamus and associated structures, and on each side the cerebral hemispheres. The ventricular system develops from the dilatations of the central canal in the brain vesicles. The brain stem is the medulla, pons and midbrain, and contains nuclei of cranial nerves as well as axons arranged in tracts passing between brain and spinal cord.

Learning Objectives

You should:

- understand the embryological basis of brain nomenclature
- know the main components of the hindbrain, midbrain, diencephalon and cerebral hemispheres
- understand the production, circulation and flow of CSF.

Introduction

Introductory coverage of the brain considers its components from below upwards: hindbrain, midbrain, and forebrain. But for looking at the brain in slightly more detail, beginning at 15.2, it seems better to work down from the cerebral hemispheres to the medulla. Embryological terms are used both descriptively and clinically, so we begin with a brief developmental survey.

Hindbrain, midbrain, forebrain   (Fig. 15.1)

Working up from the embryonic spinal cord, the three brain vesicles are the hindbrain, the midbrain and the forebrain.

Hindbrain. This develops into the medulla, pons, and cerebellum. It contains the vital centres (cardiac, respiratory, etc.) and the nuclei for cranial nerves V–XII (facial sensation, and movements of the upper end of the gut tube for ingestion and phonation). The cerebellum is concerned with balance and position in space, receiving the majority of fibres from the vestibular apparatus, and with the coordination of complex patterns of skilled movement.

Midbrain. This part of the brain changes least during growth and maturation. It contains the nuclei for cranial nerves III and IV and the centres for eye reflexes (e.g. pupillary light reflex) and auditory reflexes.

Forebrain. This gives rise to the diencephalon (thalamic structures), and the right and left telencephalic

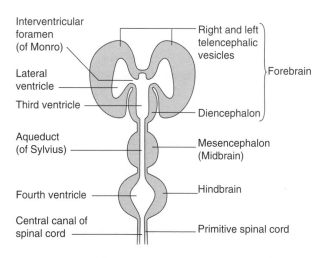

Fig. 15.1 Brain vesicles and ventricles.

derivatives – the cerebral hemispheres. The hemispheres are the only paired elements, all other components of the brain being unpaired. The cerebral hemispheres become very large and grow at first posteriorly, then downwards and forwards so that they are shaped like the horns of a ram, the inferior portions coming to lie on either side of the thalamus and midbrain, which are buried between them. The parts of the hemisphere are named according to the cranial bones to which they are related: the frontal, parietal, occipital and temporal lobes. These are not lobes in the sense of being clearly demarcated anatomical entities, but are simply areas.

- Diencephalic derivatives are concerned with motor and sensory coordination, regulation and control, and include the optic vesicles, which give rise to the optic nerves and retinas.
- Cerebral hemispheres are concerned with so-called 'higher' functions: intellectual, reasoning, long-term memory, conscious perception, and voluntary movement. In the cerebral hemispheres, unlike the spinal cord, grey matter is on the external surface, often called the cerebral cortex, or simply the cortex.

Brain stem. This term is used for the medulla, pons and midbrain together.

Terms derived from Greek:

- Hindbrain = rhombencephalon, rarely used.
- Midbrain = mesencephalon, widely used.
- Forebrain = prosencephalon, rarely used, of which:
  - thalamic structures = diencephalon: widely used, and
  - cerebral hemisphere = telencephalon: sometimes used.

15.2 Neuraxis (axis of the brain): motor and sensory areas

- In the medulla, pons and midbrain the ventral aspect of the neural tube is anterior, and the dorsal aspect is posterior, much as in the spinal cord. Above the midbrain, the axis bends forwards so that in the diencephalon, the ventral aspect is inferior and the dorsal surface superior.
- In the spinal cord, the general rule is that dorsal components tend to be concerned with afferent (sensory) functions, and ventral with efferent (motor) functions. In the medulla it is as if the two dorsal (sensory) components have been dragged laterally so that sensory components are no longer dorsal but lateral, and motor components now not so much anterior as medial. Higher in the brain stem the pattern becomes less and less obvious, and it has all but disappeared in the diencephalon.

Nucleus

A nucleus is a collection in the central nervous system of neuronal cell bodies serving similar functions. A collection of cell bodies in the peripheral nervous system is a ganglion – except that some groups of cell bodies in the brain are known as the basal ganglia, a term sanctified by long-standing use.

Ventricular system, cerebrospinal fluid

Ventricles   (Figs 15.1, 15.2)

Dilatations of the central canal of the neural tube form the cerebral ventricles.

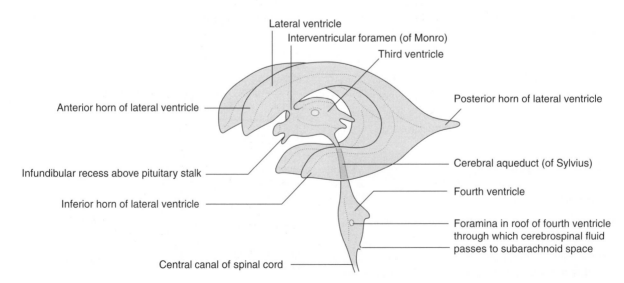

Lateral ventricle
Interventricular foramen (of Monro)
Third ventricle
Anterior horn of lateral ventricle
Posterior horn of lateral ventricle
Infundibular recess above pituitary stalk
Cerebral aqueduct (of Sylvius)
Fourth ventricle
Inferior horn of lateral ventricle
Foramina in roof of fourth ventricle through which cerebrospinal fluid passes to subarachnoid space
Central canal of spinal cord

Fig. 15.2   The ventricular system viewed from the side.

- Hindbrain. The central canal forms the fourth ventricle, continuous below with the central canal of the spinal cord. The ventral surface of the ventricle is the diamond-shaped floor (diamond-shaped brain: rhombencephalon). The thin dorsal surface is the roof and has three openings into the subarachnoid space: one median aperture, the foramen of Magendie, and two lateral apertures, the foramina of Luschka.
- Midbrain. The central canal forms the cerebral aqueduct of Sylvius.
- Diencephalon. The central cavity of the diencephalon forms the third ventricle. This is narrow from side to side (1 or 2 mm) but 10–15 mm in height. Its floor is the hypothalamus and its lateral walls the thalamus of each side, which may touch each other in the midline giving the interthalamic adhesion. You can regard the diencephalon as the structures surrounding the third ventricle or attached to its walls, thus including the optic chiasma, nerve and retina, and the posterior pituitary.
- Telencephalon. The cavities of the cerebral hemispheres are the right and left lateral ventricles. They are adjacent to the midline and are separated from each other by the septum pellucidum, a thin sheet of tissue of no neurological significance. Each lateral ventricle communicates with the third ventricle through an interventricular foramen of Monro, but the two lateral ventricles do not communicate with each other. The lateral ventricle assumes the shape of the hemisphere in which it is situated: there is an anterior (frontal) horn, a posterior (occipital) horn, and an inferior (temporal) horn.

Cerebrospinal fluid

Cerebrospinal fluid is produced by the choroid plexus, a vascular plexus present in all ventricles formed where vessels of the pia mater (external) come into contact with the ependymal lining of the central canal (i.e. there is no intervening neural tissue).

Circulation of cerebrospinal fluid   (Fig. 15.3)
From the lateral ventricles, cerebrospinal fluid flows through the foramina of Monro to the third ventricle. It continues through the cerebral aqueduct to the fourth ventricle where some may enter the central canal of the spinal cord, but most passes to the subarachnoid space through foramina in the roof. It flows around the brain and spinal cord and is absorbed back into the venous system at the arachnoid granulations (see 14.12, p. 271, Fig. 14.37).

Hydrocephalus may be caused by overproduction of cerebrospinal fluid, or reduced absorption (e.g. thrombosis of the superior sagittal sinus). It may be generalised or local, for example blockage of the cerebral aqueduct would cause hydrocephalus in the lateral and third ventricles, but not in the fourth or in the subarachnoid space.

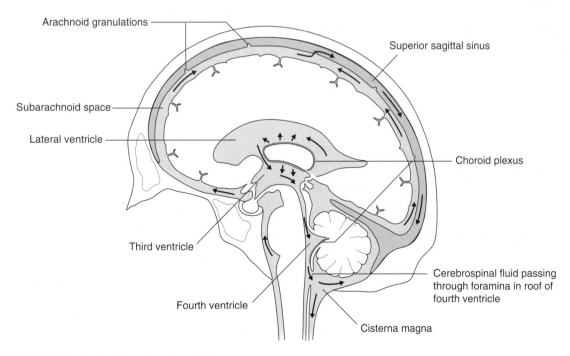

Fig. 15.3   Circulation of cerebrospinal fluid.

Tracts in the central nervous system, internal capsule

The brain stem contains tracts: bundles of myelinated axons (i.e. white matter) all serving similar functions. They can be divided into:

- motor or descending tracts which convey impulses away from the cerebral hemispheres; and
- sensory or ascending tracts which convey impulses towards the hemispheres.

Each of these may be further subdivided into named tracts connecting specific areas, the name of the tract generally being derived from the origin and the destination. Thus, the corticospinal tract conducts impulses from the cortex to the spinal cord – a motor tract; the spinothalamic tract conducts impulses from the spinal cord to the thalamus – a sensory tract.

Internal capsule

In the region where telencephalic and diencephalic regions meet, all the tracts in and out of the cerebral hemispheres are within a fairly small area on each side forming a sheet of white matter. This is the internal capsule, and it is covered in more detail later.

15.3 Forebrain

Overview

The cerebral cortex on each side is shaped like a ram's horn. Its parts are named according to the bones they are related to. The principal functional areas are motor, sensory, auditory, and visual. The limbic system is the area responsible for emotions, short-term memory and instinctual behaviour. The central part of the brain, on either side of the third ventricle, is the diencephalon consisting mainly of the thalamus and hypothalamus. All tracts conveying impulses between cerebral cortex and brain stem pass in the internal capsule, which lies lateral to the thalamus, between it and the cerebral cortex. Lesions here are usually catastrophic because so many axons are packed into such a small area. The basal ganglia are a group of nuclei adjacent to the diencephalon, and in the midbrain.

Learning Objectives

You should:

- know the principal parts of the cortex
- know the site of the motor, sensory, auditory and visual areas
- know the components of the limbic system and their functions, in as far as they are known
- know the components of the basal ganglia and their functions, in as far as they are known
- know the anatomy of the internal capsule, and understand the term 'stroke'.

Cortex   (Figs 15.4–15.8)

The cerebral cortex is shown in Figures 15.4 and 15.5. The numerous small fissures are sulci (singular: sulcus) and the raised areas between them are gyri (singular: gyrus).

- The large fissure between the parietal and temporal lobes is the lateral fissure and its edges are the opercula (singular: operculum). If you separate the opercula you will see a buried area of cortex deep in the lateral fissure: this is the insula.
- The median sagittal fissure separates the right and left hemispheres. It contains the falx cerebri.
- Commissures. Numerous bundles of fibres (white matter) connect the two sides: these are the commissures, and the largest, deep in the sagittal fissure, is the corpus callosum. The anterior portion of the corpus callosum is the genu, the central part the body, and the posterior part the splenium. There are other commissures: the anterior commissure is part of the anterior wall of the third ventricle, and the posterior and habenular commissures are in the posterior wall of the third ventricle.

Functional areas of cortex   (Figs 15.4, 15.5)

Motor, sensory

On the lateral aspect of the cortex is the central sulcus (it is neither central nor easily identifiable), the approximate surface marking of its inferior limit being the pterion. The cortex anterior to the central sulcus, the precentral gyrus, is the main motor area concerned with the initiation of voluntary movement. The cortex posterior to it, the postcentral gyrus, is the main sensory area.

- For both the motor and sensory cortex the inferior (lateral) portion is concerned with the head. The rest

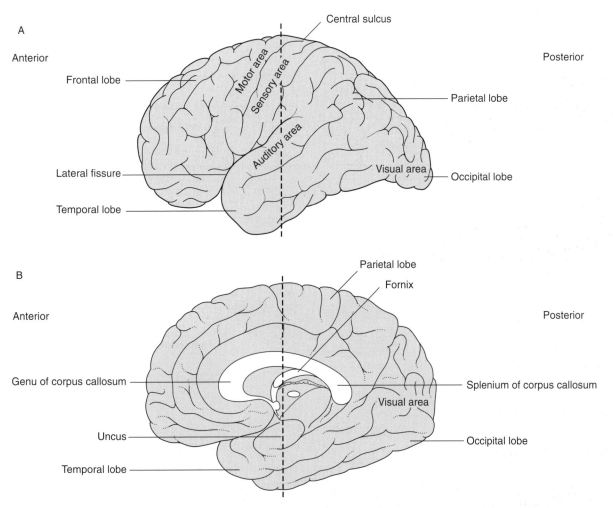

A

Anterior

Central sulcus

Frontal lobe

Motor area

Sensory area

Auditory area

Posterior

Parietal lobe

Visual area

Occipital lobe

Lateral fissure

Temporal lobe

B

Anterior

Parietal lobe

Fornix

Posterior

Genu of corpus callosum

Splenium of corpus callosum

Visual area

Uncus

Occipital lobe

Temporal lobe

Fig. 15.4 The cerebral hemispheres: **(A)** lateral aspect; **(B)** medial aspect. The dotted line indicates the plane of the section in Figure 15.5.

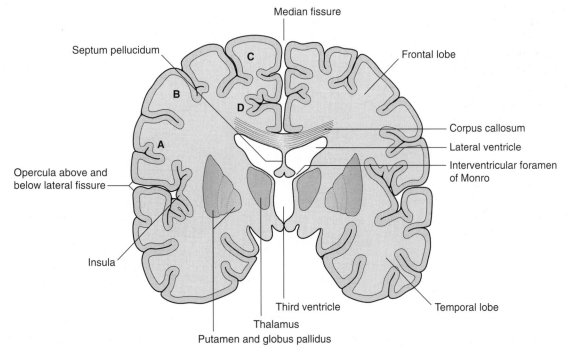

Median fissure

Septum pellucidum

C

Frontal lobe

B

D

Corpus callosum

Lateral ventricle

Interventricular foramen of Monro

A

Opercula above and below lateral fissure

Insula

Putamen and globus pallidus

Thalamus

Third ventricle

Temporal lobe

Fig. 15.5 Coronal section through cerebral hemispheres in the plane of the dotted line in Figure 15.4B.

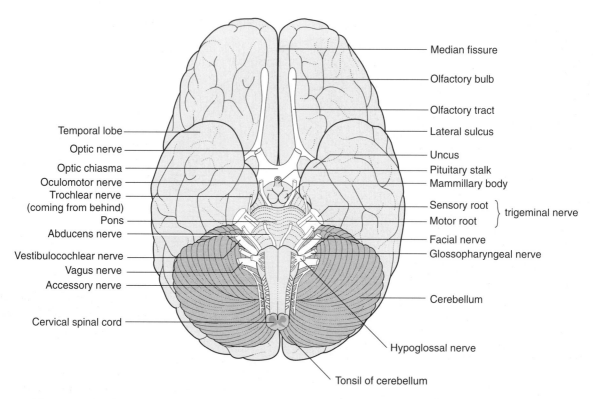

Median fissure

Olfactory bulb

Olfactory tract

Lateral sulcus

Temporal lobe

Optic nerve

Optic chiasma

Oculomotor nerve

Trochlear nerve
(coming from behind)

Pons

Abducens nerve

Vestibulocochlear nerve

Vagus nerve

Accessory nerve

Cervical spinal cord

Uncus

Pituitary stalk

Mammillary body

Sensory root
Motor root } trigeminal nerve

Facial nerve

Glossopharyngeal nerve

Cerebellum

Hypoglossal nerve

Tonsil of cerebellum

Fig. 15.6 Brain, inferior aspect.

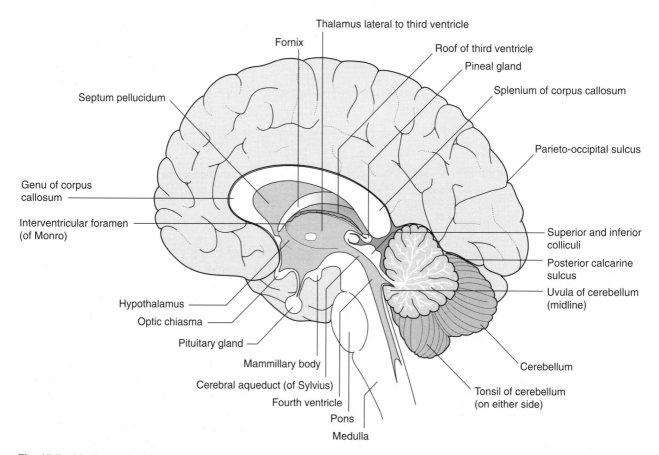

Thalamus lateral to third ventricle

Fornix

Roof of third ventricle

Pineal gland

Splenium of corpus callosum

Septum pellucidum

Parieto-occipital sulcus

Genu of corpus
callosum

Interventricular foramen
(of Monro)

Superior and inferior
colliculi

Posterior calcarine
sulcus

Uvula of cerebellum
(midline)

Hypothalamus

Optic chiasma

Pituitary gland

Mammillary body

Cerebral aqueduct (of Sylvius)

Fourth ventricle

Pons

Medulla

Cerebellum

Tonsil of cerebellum
(on either side)

Fig. 15.7 Median sagittal section through the brain.

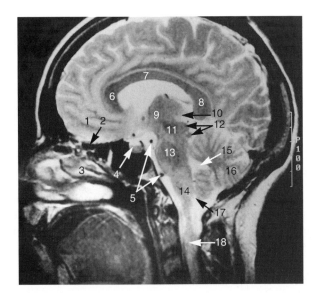

Fig. 15.8 Median sagittal scan through the head: 1, frontal lobe; 2, region of cribriform plate of ethmoid; 3, nose; 4, pituitary fossa; 5, arteries which happen to have been sectioned at right angles to the plane of the section; 6, genu of corpus callosum; 7, body of corpus callosum; 8, splenium of corpus callosum; 9, diencephalon; 10, region of pineal; 11, midbrain; 12, superior and inferior colliculi (so the section is not quite in the midline); 13, pons; 14, medulla; 15, fourth ventricle; 16, cerebellum; 17, region of (median) foramen of Magendie (between fourth ventricle and cisterna magna); 18, spinal cord.

of the body is represented sequentially passing superiorly and medially over the cortex so that the cortical areas for the lower limbs are on the medial aspect of each cerebral hemisphere with the foot area being adjacent to the corpus callosum.

- It is a fact, although one without convincing explanation, that the right cortex serves the left side of the body and vice versa.
- Broca's area is adjacent to the head area of the dominant motor cortex (usually the left in a right-handed person). It is in the frontal lobe, immediately above the lateral fissure, and is concerned with the motor mechanisms of speech. Damage to it (for example occlusion of a branch of the middle cerebral artery) leads to motor speech aphasia (aphasia: wordless): it is not that the patient does not know the word, it is that he can not muster the motor forces to enunciate it.

Visual, auditory, olfactory

- The visual cortex is in the occipital lobe (posterior)
- The auditory cortex is on the superior surface of the temporal lobe.
- The olfactory cortex is on the under surface of the temporal lobe, principally the uncus.

Limbic system (Fig. 15.9)

The Latin word limbus means margin or border. The limbic system develops from the border of the telencephalon adjacent to the diencephalon. Like many other telencephalic derivatives, this assumes the ram's-horn shape. Components of the limbic system include the fornix, the hippocampus (medial to the inferior horn of the lateral ventricle), the amygdala, the uncus and the cingulate gyrus (medially, just above the corpus callosum). The limbic system has connections with olfactory and taste fibres, and with certain diencephalic structures, e.g. the mammillary bodies and anterior thalamic nuclei. Limbic functions include elements of emotion, recent memory, olfaction, taste, sexual urges, and basic instinctive drives: smells and tastes can evoke memories, emotions, mood changes and sexual responses.

Clinical box

Destruction or degeneration of the mammillary bodies
This occurs in alcoholics and as a result of vitamin B1 (thiamine) deficiency. Short-term memory is lost, so patients tend to cover up this defect by inventing fiction: confabulation (Korsakov's syndrome). It has even been known to occur in operations for pituitary tumours that have gone wrong.

Congenital absence of the amygdala
Patients without an amygdala, and such people are rarely found, neither feel rage, nor recognise it in others – a blissful state, one would think. They may also exhibit hypersexuality. It is difficult to think of the amygdala as anything other than the organ of guilt and repression.

Dementias, Alzheimer's disease
Progressive dementias may arise from disorders of the hippocampus and its connections, associated with a loss of cholinergic neurons in Meynert's nucleus in the anterior limbic system.

Diencephalon (Figs 15.5, 15.7, 15.8)

- The thalamus forms the lateral wall of the third ventricle. It is concerned with many functions, one of which is as a relay (synapse) on the main somatosensory pathways. It has several nuclei: the ventral is concerned with somatic sensation, and the anterior with the limbic system.
- The hypothalamus forms the floor of the third ventricle. Its most obvious features when inspecting the brain from below are the pituitary stalk and the mammillary bodies (mammilla = little mamma or breast). The hypothalamus contains the centres regulating appetite and much autonomic activity (e.g. temperature regulation) as well as controlling the activity of the pituitary gland.

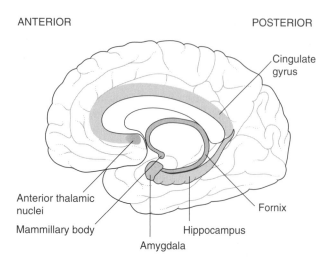

ANTERIOR   POSTERIOR

Cingulate gyrus

Anterior thalamic nuclei

Mammillary body

Fornix

Hippocampus

Amygdala

Fig. 15.9 Components of the limbic system. Note that the mammillary bodies and anterior part of the fornix are adjacent to the midline, but as components of the limbic system pass posteriorly they diverge to enter the temporal lobes in which are the hippocampus and amygdala.

- – The posterior pituitary is a component part of the hypothalamus with direct neural connections from the supraoptic and paraventricular nuclei of the hypothalamus. Hormones released by the posterior pituitary (oxytocin, vasopressin) are manufactured in the cell bodies of neurons in these nuclei, and travel down axons to the posterior pituitary where they are released into the bloodstream.
  - – The anterior pituitary is a separate gland that migrates from the roof of the primitive pharynx. The hypothalamus controls it by releasing hormones into the hypophyseal portal system of veins, through which they are transported to the anterior pituitary to act upon its component cells.
- • The roof of the third ventricle contains no neural tissue except for commissural fibres which arise anteriorly and grow backwards, over the roof of the third ventricle, to form the corpus callosum.
- • The epithalamus is the posterior region of the third ventricle: it contains the pineal gland.
- • The metathalamus, the most lateral part of the diencephalon, consists of the geniculate bodies (lateral: part of the visual pathway; medial: part of the auditory pathway).

Clinical box

Pituitary tumours
Immediately anterior to the pituitary stalk is the optic chiasma, which may be damaged by enlarging pituitary tumours causing a bitemporal hemianopia (see 14.11, p. 268).

Clinical box (*cont'd*)

Pineal
The pineal gland often calcifies with advancing age. The advantage of this is that it provides a landmark for the assessment of whether or not there is any displacement of the brain: the pineal gland is a midline structure.

Internal capsule, basal ganglia

(Figs 15.5, 15.10–15.13)

Lateral to the thalamus is the site of the main ascending and descending tracts of white matter, the internal capsule, and several collections of grey matter collectively known as the basal ganglia.

Internal capsule

The internal capsule is boomerang-shaped on horizontal section with anterior and posterior limbs joined at the genu (pointing medially). The anterior limb contains fibres to and from the frontal lobe, of uncertain function. The genu contains fibres to and from the head and neck cortical areas. The posterior limb contains fibres to and from the cortical areas concerned with the trunk and limbs.

The relations of the internal capsule are:

- • medial to the posterior limb: the thalamus
- • medial to the anterior limb: the caudate nucleus, another of the structures stretched into the shape of a ram's horn by the growth of the brain

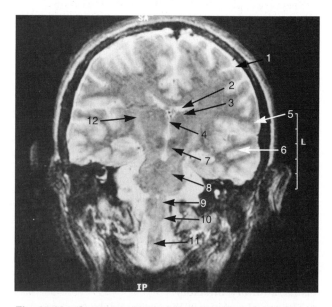

Fig. 15.10 Coronal scan through the head, pinna to pinna: 1, parietal lobe; 2, lateral ventricle; 3, thalamus, lateral to; 4, third ventricle; 5, lateral fissure; 6, temporal lobe; 7, cerebral peduncle of midbrain; 8, pons; 9, medulla; 10, region of decussation of the pyramids; 11, spinal cord; 12, internal capsule.

- lateral to both limbs: the lentiform nucleus, itself composed of a medial globus pallidus and a lateral putamen.

There are numerous fibres crossing the internal capsule linking the thalamus, caudate and lentiform nuclei, and when a fresh or fixed brain is cut, these are evident as

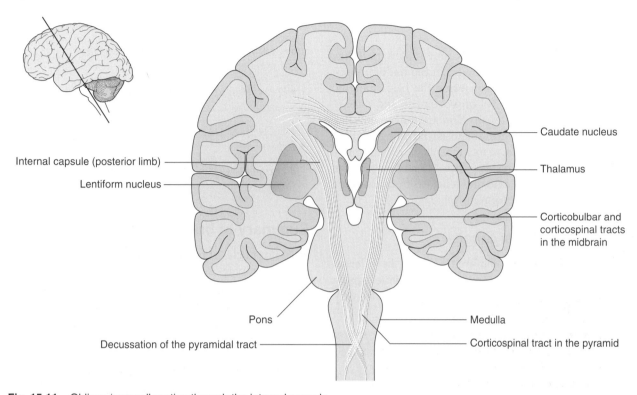

Internal capsule (posterior limb)

Lentiform nucleus

Caudate nucleus

Thalamus

Corticobulbar and corticospinal tracts in the midbrain

Pons

Decussation of the pyramidal tract

Medulla

Corticospinal tract in the pyramid

Fig. 15.11   Oblique 'coronal' section through the internal capsule.

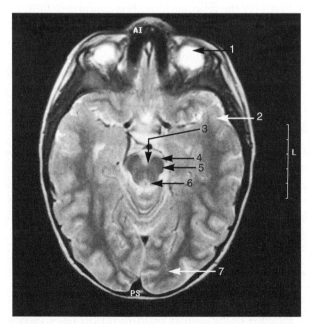

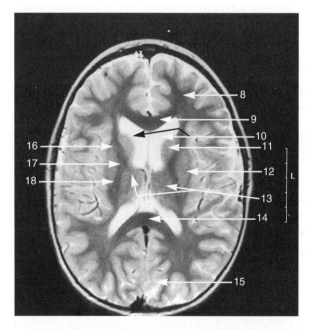

Fig. 15.12   Transverse scan through the head at the level of the eyeballs: 1, eyeball; 2, temporal lobe in middle cranial fossa; 3, interpeduncular fossa of midbrain; 4, cerebral peduncles of midbrain containing descending corticobulbar and corticospinal fibres; 5, substantia nigra of midbrain (appears lighter on scan); 6, periaqueductal grey matter of midbrain (lighter) and aqueduct; 7, occipital lobe.

Fig. 15.13   Transverse CT scan about 2 cm above the level of the eyeballs: 8, frontal lobe; 9, genu of corpus callosum; 10, lateral ventricles with septum pellucidum between; 11, caudate nucleus; 12, lentiform nucleus; 13, thalamus, lateral to midline third ventricle (not clear); 14, splenium of corpus callosum; 15, occipital lobe; 16, anterior limb of internal capsule; 17, genu of internal capsule; 18, posterior limb of internal capsule.

striations. For this reason, this area was originally called the corpus striatum, and this term, although of doubtful validity, is still used.

Basal ganglia

The caudate nucleus, putamen and globus pallidus, together with the substantia nigra in the midbrain (see below) and other nuclei, constitute the basal ganglia. Their function is the control of movement, and disease of them leads to unwanted involuntary movements, for example tremors, writhing (athetosis), fidgeting (chorea) and uncontrolled explosive movements (hemiballismus). Parkinson's disease results from disorders of the substantia nigra, and chorea and athetosis from disorders of the caudate and lentiform nuclei.

Lateral to the basal ganglia

Lateral to the basal ganglia are, in order, the external capsule, the claustrum (grey matter), the extreme capsule and the insular cortex. None of these areas is very important clinically.

Clinical box

Stroke
When disease (such as haemorrhage or arterial occlusion) affects the internal capsule, the result is a profound and often catastrophic loss of function because so many fibres, both motor and sensory, are concentrated into such a small area. This is, in common parlance, a stroke and is discussed in more detail later.

15.4 Brain stem

Overview

The brain stem consists of grey matter made up of cell bodies grouped as nuclei, and white matter: the myelinated axons of fibre tracts. Nuclei of the cranial nerves are prominent in the brain stem. Those of III and IV are in the midbrain, those of V–XII in the pons and medulla. Some of the tracts are short local connections which run in all directions between nuclei, and others are long motor and sensory tracts conveying information between cerebral hemispheres and spinal cord. The midbrain houses nuclei concerned with visual and auditory reflexes. The cerebellum is posterior to the pons and receives most of the information from the vestibular system. Cerebellar lesions are ipsilateral, unlike those of the rest of the brain which are usually contralateral.

Learning Objectives

- know the disposition and principal functions of the midbrain, pons, cerebellum, and medulla
- know the position and significance of the substantia nigra
- know the part of the brain stem to which each cranial nerve is attached
- know the significance and symptoms of disease at the cerebellopontine angle
- know the significance and symptoms of cerebellar disease.

Summary of brain stem nuclei

- Motor nuclei of cranial nerves III–XII.
- Parasympathetic (visceral motor) nuclei: Edinger–Westphal, superior salivatory, inferior salivatory, dorsal motor nucleus of the vagus (Fig. 14.14, p. 234).
- Sensory nuclei: trigeminal sensory nuclei for cutaneous and oral sensation, nucleus of the solitary tract for visceral sensation (e.g. taste).
- Other named nuclei for visual and auditory reflexes, as outlined in the text below.
- Nuclei of the reticular formation concerned with vital centres and arousal. These are hard to pinpoint accurately and for clinical purposes it is unnecessary to do so. One definition of the reticular formation is that it is what is left when you have removed everything else with a specific name.

Midbrain   (Fig. 15.14)

The midbrain passes through the tentorial notch of the tentorium cerebelli. It has a very distinctive shape in cross-section and is easy to draw. This is worth the effort since the midbrain is an important area from the point of view of pupillary and accommodation reflexes, descending motor tracts and other clinical conditions. Its parts are as follows.

- Tectum. This is the area dorsal to the aqueduct. There are four dorsal prominences, two superior colliculi and two inferior colliculi (also known together as the corpora quadrigemina). The superior colliculi are associated with visual reflexes and the inferior colliculi with auditory reflexes. Cranial nerve IV is attached between them.
- Periaqueductal (around the aqueduct) grey matter. This contains the nuclei of cranial nerves III and IV and the medial longitudinal fasciculus, which

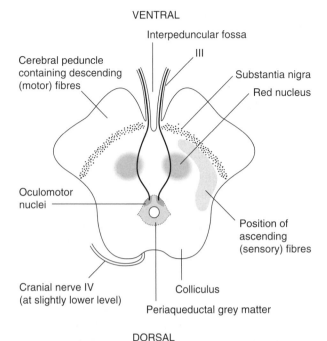

VENTRAL

Interpeduncular fossa

III

Cerebral peduncle containing descending (motor) fibres

Substantia nigra

Red nucleus

Oculomotor nuclei

Position of ascending (sensory) fibres

Cranial nerve IV (at slightly lower level)

Colliculus

Periaqueductal grey matter

DORSAL

Fig. 15.14 Transverse section through the midbrain.

integrates the nuclei of III, IV and VI with vestibular information, amongst other things. In this area, fibres involved in the pupillary light reflex pass from the optic tracts to the Edinger-Westphal nucleus of III.

- The tegmentum is the area ventral to the aqueduct. One of its components is the red nucleus, to all intents and purposes an outpost of the cerebellum (see below).
- Substantia nigra (Latin: black substance). This is a dark area in the ventral tegmentum. The pigment is melanin, a reminder of the amine biochemistry commonly found in derivatives of neuroectoderm. Depleted levels of dopamine in this area lead to symptoms of Parkinson's disease (e.g. resting tremor): functionally, this is one of the basal ganglia.
- Anterior to the substantia nigra are two large projections facing slightly laterally. These contain the main descending motor fibres called, variously, the cerebral peduncles, basis pedunculi, or cerebral crura, each being the crus cerebri. This text uses the first term.
- The fossa between the peduncles is the interpeduncular fossa in which cranial nerve III is attached.
- The long sensory tracts conveying information from the spinal cord and the lower brain stem to the thalamus are just behind the substantia nigra, extending posteriorly on to the lateral aspect of the midbrain. The long motor tracts are in the cerebral peduncles. (Dorsal: sensory; ventral: motor.)

Pons   (Figs 15.6, 15.7)

The pons is that part of the brain stem to which the cerebellum and cranial nerve V are attached. It contains scattered nuclei concerned with cerebellar connections, and nuclei of cranial nerves V, VI and VII, although the course of fibres from VI and VII means that these nerves are attached lower down the brain stem at the pontomedullary junction. For reasons which are not clear, fibres of VII pass at first dorsally before looping round the nucleus of VI and turning anteriorly.

The locus coeruleus (Latin: blue place) is a pigmented area (amines again) in the dorsal pons. It is concerned with the limbic system and autonomic functions and is of interest to neuroscientists as a focus for drug action.

The long motor and sensory tracts are scattered in numerous bundles as they pass through the pontine substance.

Cerebellum   (Figs 15.6, 15.7)

The cerebellum is an outgrowth of the dorsal pons, separated from it by the fourth ventricle. On each side, the white matter connecting the pons and cerebellum forms the superior, middle and inferior cerebellar peduncles. Despite all the work of neuroscientists, the cerebellum remains somewhat mysterious: it is concerned with the coordination of motor activity, the regulation of muscle tone and the maintenance of equilibrium.

Cerebellar cortex. The cerebellar cortex has superficial grey matter, inside which is white matter and, most deeply of all, the four paired cerebellar nuclei. Cerebellar equivalents of the cerebral gyri are folia (thinner and straighter than gyri). The midline portion is the vermis, the most inferior part of which is the uvula and the most superior part (on the roof of the fourth ventricle) the lingula. Laterally, the most inferior parts of the cerebellar hemispheres are the tonsils, so, as at the back of the mouth, the uvula is between the tonsils.

Vestibulocerebellum. The cerebellum, more obviously than other parts of the nervous system, displays its evolution. The earliest part to arise was that concerned with vestibular impulses, the vestibulocerebellum, and it is largely separate from the rest of the cerebellum, although this is not evident to the naked eye. It is the flocculonodular node, the floccules being on either side joined in the midline at the nodule. The deep cerebellar nucleus of the vestibulocerebellum is the fastigial nucleus, which has connections with:

- cranial nerve VIII: most fibres from the vestibular apparatus pass to the cerebellum through the inferior cerebellar peduncle
- the medial longitudinal fasciculus for the coordination of vestibular impulses and eye movements (nuclei of III, IV, VI).

Other parts of the cerebellum. Subsequently (in evolutionary terms), parts of the cerebellum acquired connections with the spinal cord (for movements of the limbs and trunk) and most recently with the cerebral cortex. The deep cerebellar nuclei for spinal connections are the globose and emboliform, and for cerebral connections the dentate nucleus.

- Impulses from the spinal cord arrive in spinocerebellar tracts.
- Impulses to and from the cerebral cortex pass from the dentate nucleus through the superior cerebellar peduncle to the red nucleus (midbrain) and on to the cerebral cortex (dentato-rubro-thalamic tract). Connections from the red nucleus pass to and from the spinal cord (thus rubrospinal, spinorubral) for further integrative activity.

Clinical box

Cerebellar disease
Disease of the cerebellum causes *ipsilateral* symptoms, not contralateral, manifested principally as a lack of coordination called ataxia. This gives rise to an intention tremor; that is to say there is no tremor present at rest, but as soon as any movement is attempted, lack of coordination becomes apparent. This contrasts with the tremor of basal ganglia disease, which is present at rest, but which disappears when purposeful movement is attempted. The resultant speech patterns are called scanning speech (it is as if the person is scanning his vocabulary for the right word, so laboured is the progress); the lack of coordination of eye movement is nystagmus. Cerebellar lesions are perfectly mimicked by drunkenness, which is nothing more or less than cerebellar poisoning by alcohol, and it is not unknown for a person with cerebellar disease to be arrested on suspicion of being intoxicated.

Tonsillar herniation
The tonsils rest upon the dura over the edge of the foramen magnum and in cases of raised intracranial pressure they may be pushed down either through or into the foramen magnum where they compress the posterior aspect of the brain stem and the vital (e.g. respiratory) centres it contains, causing death. This is herniation of the cerebellar tonsils, or coning. It occurs if a lumbar puncture is performed on a patient with raised intracranial pressure. The sudden release of pressure (as a result of the lumbar puncture) in the lumbar region means that the brain is pushed down as described above. This is why you should always test for signs of raised intracranial pressure (e.g. look for papilloedema of the optic disc) before performing a lumbar puncture.

Pontomedullary junction   (Fig. 15.15)

The pontomedullary junction is marked anteriorly by a transverse sulcus where VI is attached medially, and VII and VIII laterally in the cerebellopontine angle.

Medulla   (Fig. 15.15)

Anterior aspect.   Four swellings are visible, two on either side of the midline.

- The medial swelling on each side is the pyramid containing the descending motor corticospinal tracts to the opposite side of the body. The rootlets of XII are attached laterally to these swellings.
- Lateral to the pyramid is the olive containing the inferior olivary nucleus, a convoluted band of grey matter which, like the red nucleus in the midbrain, is an outpost of the cerebellum. Lateral to the olive are the rootlets of, from above down, IX, X and XI.

Posterior aspect.   Two tubercles are visible on each side, the gracile medially and the cuneate laterally. These are concerned with sensation from the spinal cord (see below).

Nuclei.   The hypoglossal nucleus is close to the midline and the floor of the fourth ventricle. The motor nuclei of the vagus nerve are lateral to this (dorsal motor and nucleus ambiguus), and the 'spinal' part of the trigeminal sensory nucleus more lateral still.

Medulla/spinal cord junction.   This is *not* at the foramen magnum, but a few millimetres below. It means that C1 and C2 nerves pass slightly upwards from their spinal cord origin to emerge from the vertebral column.

Some features of the fourth ventricle

- In the floor, the facial colliculus is a small swelling lateral to the central region of the ventral median sulcus. It is caused by the internal genu of the fibres of VII looping around the nucleus of VI. Lower down is the hypoglossal trigone, immediately over the nucleus of XII.
- In the roof, the foramina of Luschka (right and left) and Magendie (median) allow cerebrospinal fluid to pass from the ventricular system to the subarachnoid space.

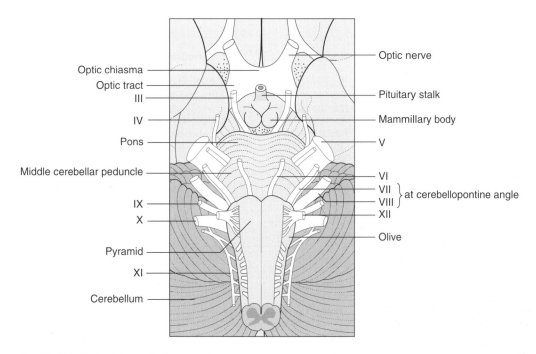

Fig. 15.15   Brain stem, anterior aspect.

15.5 Cranial nerve nuclei

Overview

Cranial nerve nuclei can be grouped by functional type: somatic motor, branchiomotor, visceral motor (parasympathetic), somatic sensory, visceral sensory and special sensory. These groups are disposed vertically in the brain stem, somatic motor being the most medial, with sensory nuclei more laterally sited. Not all nuclei contribute to all cranial nerves, some nerves containing only somatic motor fibres, and some only sensory fibres. Mixed nerves are those that supply the upper end of the gut tube – in embryological terms, these are the nerves of the branchial arches.

Learning Objectives

You should:

- know which nuclei are in which parts of the brain stem

- be able to work out which cranial nerves would be affected by various brain stem lesions: midbrain, pontine, cerebellopontine angle, lateral medullary and medial medullary.

Brain stem nuclei

Lesions of the brain stem give rise to symptoms according to which cranial nerves arise near the lesion. Motor impulses in cranial nerves arise from brain stem motor nuclei, and sensory impulses in cranial nerves pass to brain stem nuclei. Tables 15.1, 15.2 and 15.3 set out these nuclei in detail. As a simplification, it is enough for you to realise that:

- midbrain lesions cause disturbances of eye movements
- pontine lesions cause disturbances of mandibular movement
- medullary lesions cause disturbances of phonation and swallowing.

Table 15.1 Cranial nerve motor nuclei

Nucleus	Position	Nerve	Function
Oculomotor	Upper midbrain	Oculomotor III	Eyeball movements
Trochlear	Lower midbrain	Trochlear IV	Eyeball movements
Trigeminal	Pons	Mandibular Vc	Mastication
Abducens	Pons	Abducens VI	Eyeball movements
Facial	Pons	Facial VII	Facial expression etc., stapedius
Nucleus ambiguus	Medulla	Glossopharyngeal IX Vagus X	Swallowing, phonation
Accessory	See text	Accessory XI	Sternocleidomastoid, trapezius
Hypoglossal	Medulla	Hypoglossal XII	Tongue

Table 15.2 Cranial nerve parasympathetic nuclei

Nucleus	Position	Nerve(s)	Function
Edinger–Westphal	Midbrain	Oculomotor III	Pupilloconstriction, accommodation
Superior salivatory	Pons	Facial VII, Vb	Secretomotor: nasal, palatine, lacrimal glands
Superior salivatory	Pons	Facial VII, Vc	Secretomotor: submandibular, sublingual glands
Inferior salivatory	Upper medulla	Glossopharyngeal IX	Secretomotor: parotid gland
Dorsal motor of vagus	Medulla	Vagus X	Heart, foregut, midgut

Table 15.3 Cranial nerve sensory nuclei

	Source of stimulus	Ganglion	Nucleus and/or connections
Cutaneous and oral sensation			

V	Oral and nasal cavities, teeth, TMJ, skin of anterior scalp, face, most of external ear	Trigeminal	Trigeminal:
			  Spinal (pain, temperature)
			  Principal (tactile)
			  Mesencephalic (proprioception, see text)

X	Some skin of external ear	Sensory ganglia of X	
Visceral sensation			
VII	Taste buds, anterior, tongue, etc.	Geniculate VII	
IX	Mucosa of oropharynx Taste buds, posterior tongue Carotid body	Sensory ganglia of IX	
X	Mucosa of hypopharynx, larynx Taste buds, epiglottic region Aortic body Thoracoabdominal viscera	Sensory ganglia of X	Nucleus of solitary tract
Special sensation			
I	Olfactory epithelium	Olfactory bipolar cells	Olfactory bulb, olfactory cortex, etc.
II	Rods and cones	Retinal bipolar cells	Lateral geniculate body, visual cortex
VIII	Organ of Corti	Cochlear (spiral)	Cochlear nuclei, auditory cortex
VIII	Saccule, utricle, semicircular ducts	Vestibular	Vestibular nuclei, cerebellum

15.6 Vessels of the brain

Overview

The vertebrobasilar system supplies the brain stem and, with the internal carotid system, forms the arterial circle of Willis at the base of the forebrain. This gives rise to the anterior, middle and posterior cerebral arteries. The anterior cerebral artery supplies the medial side of the cerebral hemisphere, including the lower limb area of the motor and sensory cortex. The middle cerebral artery supplies the lateral aspect of the cerebral cortex, including the auditory cortex and the sensory and motor cortex for the rest of the body. The posterior cerebral artery supplies (not exclusively) the visual cortex. The internal capsule is supplied mainly by branches of the middle cerebral artery.

Learning Objectives

You should:

- know the territories of the vertebrobasilar system and the anterior, middle and posterior cerebral arteries

- know the likely effects of blockage of these vessels

- know the vessels that supply the internal capsule and the likely effect of their blockage

- revise the anatomy of the venous sinuses.

Arteries

Vertebrobasilar system, posterior cerebral artery (Fig. 15.16)

The vertebrobasilar system supplies the brain stem and visual cortex.

- After the right and left vertebral arteries have pierced the dura in the region of the foramen magnum they give branches which include:
  - anterior and posterior spinal arteries, which pass down to supply the spinal cord
  - posterior inferior cerebellar artery (PICA), which supplies the lateral medulla and the lower cerebellum.

- The vertebrals unite to form the basilar artery, which ascends on the ventral aspect of the pons giving:
  - pontine branches
  - the labyrinthine artery, which enters the internal acoustic meatus and supplies the inner ear
  - anterior inferior and superior cerebellar arteries.

- The basilar artery terminates by contributing to the arterial circle of Willis, giving:
  - the posterior cerebral arteries, which pass posteriorly lateral to the midbrain supplying it, the geniculate bodies and most of the occipital (visual) cortex of the brain
  - the posterior communicating arteries.

Clinical box

Lateral medullary syndrome (Wallenberg's or PICA syndrome)
This is caused by thrombosis of the posterior inferior cerebellar artery. Since this supplies the upper lateral medulla, some of the symptoms are explicable on the basis of the involvement of the spinal part of the trigeminal sensory nucleus and the nucleus ambiguus: disturbances of facial temperature sensation and paralysis of speech and swallowing. There may also be cerebellar involvement and balance disorders (because of possible involvement of cochlear and vestibular nuclei). The spinothalamic tract conveying pain and temperature sensation from the contralateral trunk and limbs may also be involved.

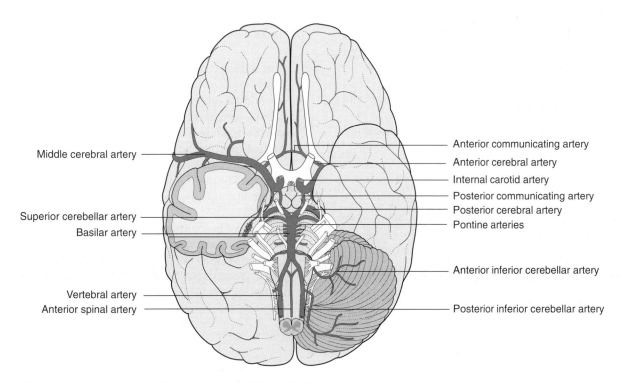

Middle cerebral artery

Superior cerebellar artery
Basilar artery

Vertebral artery
Anterior spinal artery

Anterior communicating artery
Anterior cerebral artery
Internal carotid artery
Posterior communicating artery
Posterior cerebral artery
Pontine arteries

Anterior inferior cerebellar artery

Posterior inferior cerebellar artery

Fig. 15.16 Inferior aspect of brain and arterial circle of Willis.

Internal carotid artery (Fig. 15.16)

The intracranial course of the internal carotid artery was described in Chapter 14 (14.12, p. 270). It terminates by giving the anterior and middle cerebral arteries as part of the arterial circle of Willis.

Arterial circle of Willis (Fig. 15.16)

The circle is formed by: the posterior cerebral arteries, the posterior communicating arteries, the internal carotid artery (briefly), the anterior cerebral artery and the (single) anterior communicating artery. There is much variation and asymmetry. The anastomotic possibilities of the circle are not normally brought into action unless there is some requirement for increased blood flow as a result of disease or blockage elsewhere.

Anterior cerebral artery (Fig. 15.17)

- This passes forwards and medially under the genu of the corpus callosum, then upwards and posteriorly on the superior surface of the corpus callosum between the cerebral hemisphere and the falx cerebri. It runs very close to its opposite number (and would be better called the medial cerebral artery).
- It supplies the optic chiasma, the frontal lobes and the medial aspect of the parietal lobe.
- It supplies the lower limb areas of both motor and sensory cortex.

Middle cerebral artery (Fig. 15.17)

From its origin, the middle cerebral artery passes laterally to the insula and on to the lateral aspect of the cerebral hemisphere through the lateral fissure.

- It supplies most of the parietal lobe, all the temporal lobe and part of the occipital lobe. This includes

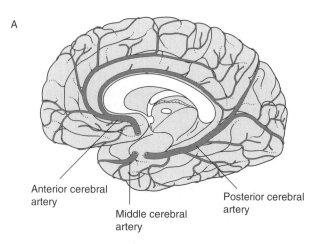

A

Anterior cerebral artery

Middle cerebral artery

Posterior cerebral artery

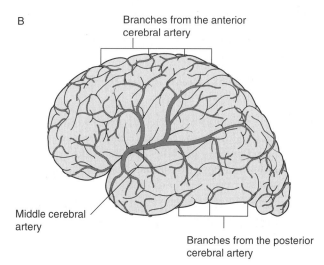

B

Branches from the anterior cerebral artery

Middle cerebral artery

Branches from the posterior cerebral artery

Fig. 15.17 Territories of three main cerebral arteries: **(A)** medial aspect of brain; **(B)** lateral aspect of brain.

most of the sensory, motor and auditory cortical areas.
- The middle cerebral, and the termination of the internal carotid, give off a group of arteries, sometimes known as central arteries, supplying the internal capsule and basal ganglia:
  - lenticulo(thalamo)striate arteries, which supply the basal ganglia and internal capsule, blockage or haemorrhage of which will cause a catastrophic stroke
  - choroidal branches, which supply the choroid plexus and diencephalon.
- As the middle cerebral artery emerges on to the lateral aspect of the hemisphere, it provides a rich arterial supply for Broca's motor speech area and the

head and neck areas of the sensory and motor cortex.

Veins

These were described in Chapter 14 (14.12, p. 271).

15.7 Motor systems and tracts

Overview

Voluntary motor systems pass from the motor cortex to cell bodies of lower motor neurons. Corticobulbar fibres pass to cranial nerve motor nuclei, most decussating towards the end of their journey. Corticospinal fibres pass to spinal cord ventral horn cells. Most decussate in the medulla at the decussation of the pyramids, but some do so just before terminating on the ventral horn cells. Interruption of these pathways gives pyramidal signs and symptoms. Lower motor neuron cell bodies also receive impulses form other brain centres (basal ganglia, reticular formation, etc.) and lesions of these are referred to as extrapyramidal syndromes. Both pyramidal and extrapyramidal lesions are examples of upper motor neuron lesions: such lesions interrupt motor impulses before they reach the cell body of the lower motor neuron.

Learning Objectives

You should:

- understand the layout of the corticobulbar and corticospinal pathways

- know the position of the decussation and the synapse in these pathways

- understand the effects of interrupting these pathways

- understand in simple terms the extrapyramidal system

- know what constitutes an upper motor neuron lesion.

Motor systems

Impulses leave the cortex in corticofugal pathways. Between the motor cortex and skeletal (striated) muscles, the pathways are arranged in two neuronal groups: upper motor neurons and lower motor neurons.

- Upper motor neurons are confined to the central nervous system. Their cell bodies are found in various centres in the brain, but the most important are those in the motor cortex. Axons pass through the brain stem, decussating (crossing the midline) somewhere on the way and terminate by synapsing on to the cell bodies of the lower motor neurons.
- Lower motor neurons have cell bodies in the central nervous system: for spinal nerves these are in the ventral horn of grey matter of the spinal cord, and for cranial nerves, in the motor nucleus of the nerve concerned (III, IV, Vc, VI, VII, nucleus ambiguus, XII). The axons of lower motor neurons pass out in peripheral nerves to the muscle fibres without further synapse.

Corticospinal, corticobulbar, corticonuclear, pyramidal, extrapyramidal pathways: what do these terms mean?

- The corticobulbar or corticonuclear pathway conveys impulses from cortex to cranial nerve motor nuclei. The terms are synonymous even though not all the cranial nerve motor nuclei are in the bulb, an archaic name for the medulla.
- The corticospinal pathway conveys impulses from cortex to ventral horn cells of the spinal cord. Since the corticospinal pathways pass deep to the pyramids of the medulla, they are known as the pyramidal pathways – a widely used clinical term.
- Extrapyramidal pathway. Upper motor neurons include fibres from other brain centres (e.g. basal ganglia, cerebellum, reticular formation) that connect with the lower motor neurons, thus influencing their activity. These do *not* pass through the pyramids – they are *not* components of the corticospinal pathways – and so are grouped together as *extra*pyramidal pathways. It is important to remember these when considering what may go wrong (see later).

Upper motor neurons for cranial nerves: corticonuclear, corticobulbar

For cranial nerves, cell bodies of upper motor neurons are in the head area of the motor cortex. Axons descend through the genu of the internal capsule, decussating just before synapsing with cell bodies of lower motor neurons that make up the motor nucleus of that cranial nerve.

Upper motor neurons for spinal nerves: corticospinal

For spinal nerves, cell bodies of upper motor neurons are in the appropriate area of the motor cortex. Axons descend through the posterior limb of the internal capsule, the cerebral peduncles of the midbrain, the pons and the pyramids of the medulla. Immediately below the pyramids, just above the beginning of the spinal cord, most of them (about 85%) decussate to form the lateral corticospinal tract of the spinal cord. They descend in this tract to the appropriate level in the spinal cord and synapse on the ventral horn cells – the cell bodies of the lower motor neurons. The remainder descend without decussating as the anterior corticospinal tract, but even these decussate at the last minute, just before synapsing on ventral horn cells.

Pyramidal decussation. The decussation is just below the pyramids. There is no synapse here: the axon merely changes sides.

Clinical box

Lower motor neuron lesion – flaccidity, hyporeflexia, wasting, ipsilateral
If all lower motor neurons passing to a muscle are severed, the muscle will be completely paralysed. It will be flaccid (atonic, hypotonic), it will not respond to reflexes (arreflexic, hyporeflexic) since no impulses reach it, and it will fairly quickly atrophy as a result of denervation. The injury and the paralysis are on the same side: they are *ipsilateral* with respect to each other.

Upper motor neuron lesion – spasticity, hyperreflexia, contralateral (usually)
If upper motor neurons to a muscle are severed, the ability to control and initiate movement in the muscle may be lost. However, lower motor neurons are intact, and since some of the fibres to lower motor neurons from elsewhere are inhibitory, other centres which influence lower motor neurons, e.g. basal ganglia, may cause an increase in muscle tone (hypertonic, spastic). Also, reflexes are disinhibited (hyperreflexic, exaggerated). The muscle will not become atrophied except through disuse. Most upper motor neuron lesions are in the internal capsule (strokes) and in this case, since upper motor neurons have not yet decussated, the functional loss will be on the side *opposite* to the site of the lesion: they are *contralateral* with respect to each other.

These characteristics of upper motor neuron lesions (UMNL) and lower motor neuron lesions (LMNL) are clinically very important.

Bulbar palsy: ipsilateral lower motor neuron lesion
This is caused by a lesion of the medulla that involves the nucleus ambiguus and the hypoglossal nucleus. It may arise from blockage of the posterior inferior cerebellar artery (Fig. 15.16). The cell bodies of lower motor neurons are affected, with resultant ipsilateral motor disorders of chewing (to a variable extent), swallowing and speaking. Because the nuclei concerned are in the bulb (medulla), this is a bulbar palsy.

Pseudobulbar palsy: contralateral upper motor neuron lesion
This is caused by interruption of the upper motor neuron

Clinical box (*cont'd*)

pathways, usually in the internal capsule, cerebral peduncles or pons. The contralateral muscles of the tongue and pharynx would be affected. Since this presents as a disorder of the muscles of speech and swallowing, it is at first sight like a bulbar palsy, but being an upper motor neuron lesion, it is caused by a lesion on the opposite side. It is known as a pseudobulbar palsy.

Bilateral upper motor neuron control of cranial nerves III, IV, VI and part of VII
The pattern in the head and neck, as in the rest of the body, is that the motor cortex innervates contralateral motor nuclei. However, muscles which move the eyes, and the eyelids and forehead in association with eye movements, receive bilateral cortical innervation. The nuclei concerned are those of III, IV and VI, and that portion of the facial (VII) motor nucleus that innervates orbicularis oculi and frontalis. This must have evolved in association with, and for the protection of, the sense of sight, by which means we seek sustenance and mates, and avoid danger.

There may be limited bilateral control of the other cranial nerve motor nuclei as is evidenced by partial recovery of function in patients after a stroke.

Upper motor neuron lesions of VII
Because of the bilateral cortical control of the upper facial muscles, in upper motor neuron lesions of VII, the forehead and orbicularis oculi muscles are largely spared. For the lower facial muscles this is not so: the normal pattern prevails with only contralateral control. So: the upper part of the face is spared in upper motor neuron lesions of VII.

Another interesting feature of upper motor neuron lesions of VII is that although the patient may be unable at will to move facial muscles around the mouth, he may smile at something he considers amusing. This is a reminder of the fact that the lower motor neurons are intact and are able to respond to impulses from other than the corticobulbar pathway (in this case presumably from the jocularity centre – if it exists).

Facial palsy (lower motor neuron lesion)
A lower motor neuron lesion of VII, a facial palsy, may result from a lesion of the facial motor nucleus, or the nerve itself, and the muscle fibre(s) supplied by the affected neuron would be paralysed. There is no question of partial preservation of function in this case: if the lower motor neuron is damaged, nothing can reach the muscle. Facial wrinkles disappear if the muscles are paralysed, so it is usually easy to spot. Bell's palsy is a facial palsy of unknown aetiology. See Chapter 14 (14.6, p. 243).

VI and VII
The relationship between the nucleus of VI and the axons of VII means that a brain stem lesion may cause facial weakness in association with a paralysis of the ipsilateral lateral rectus muscle of the eye.

15.8 Sensory systems and tracts

Overview

Sensory impulses are delivered to the central nervous system in neurons with cell bodies in peripheral ganglia. Pathways decussate after the first synapse in the CNS and pass to the contralateral thalamus before being relayed to various parts of the brain. Within the spinal cord, some modalities (e.g. fine touch) are carried by tracts of neurons before decussating, so are ipsilateral with respect to the source of the impulse (dorsal column pathways). Other modalities (e.g. pain, temperature) are carried by fibre tracts of neurons after synapsing, so are contralateral with respect to the source of the impulse (spinothalamic pathways). Sensory information from cranial nerves is handled by brain stem nuclei of V before going on to the thalamus. Visceral sensation, such as taste, or sensation from internal organs, passes to the nucleus of the solitary tract in the brain stem.

Learning Objectives

You should:

- understand the basic plan of sensory systems
- know the dorsal column pathways and the effect of their interruption
- know the spinothalamic pathways and the effect of their interruption
- know the trigeminal sensory systems.

Basic plan of sensory systems

There are three neuronal groups:

- Primary sensory neurons: receptor to central nervous system. These fibres convey impulses in a peripheral nerve from receptors to the central nervous system. The cell bodies are in a peripheral sensory ganglion: a dorsal root ganglion for spinal nerves, or a cranial nerve sensory ganglion for cranial nerves (e.g. trigeminal, geniculate). Once inside the central nervous system, the primary sensory neurons synapse on the cell bodies of secondary sensory neurons.
- Secondary sensory neurons: to the thalamus. The axons of these neurons ascend from the nucleus to the contralateral thalamus (in the diencephalon),

decussating soon after leaving the nucleus. Other fibres from the nucleus pass elsewhere, for example to reticular nuclei and the cerebellum, for the dissemination of information and its integration with other functions and systems.

- Tertiary sensory neurons: thalamus to cortex (thalamocortical) and elsewhere. These pass through the internal capsule.

There are no synapses outside the brain and spinal cord: the first synapse is in the central nervous system between primary and secondary sensory neurons.

From spinal nerves

There are two systems, spinothalamic (or anterolateral) and the dorsal columns. For confirmation of this, consider what happens when you stub your toe. You are aware of something having touched your toe about half a second or so before feeling the pain. The tactile information (dorsal columns) speeds up the spinal cord much more quickly than the pain information (spinothalamic), speed in this case being a result of larger diameter, more heavily myelinated fibres.

Dorsal columns: touch, vibration sense, limb position sense

- From the dorsal rootlets of spinal nerves, fibres pass into the adjacent ipsilateral dorsal column of white matter and ascend to the top of the spinal cord. Fibres from the sacral region lie most medially, the higher the subsequent level of entry, the more laterally placed the fibre. Fibres in the dorsal white column form two bundles, the medial being thin (gracile) and the lateral larger and wedge-shaped (cuneate).
- At the top of the spinal cord these fibres synapse on cell bodies of secondary sensory neurons in the gracile and cuneate nuclei, and axons cross the midline to ascend to the contralateral thalamus through the medulla, pons and midbrain in a tract called the medial lemniscus.
- The spinal cord tract in this system is made up of primary sensory neurons and is *ipsilateral* with respect to the source of the impulse.

Spinothalamic (anterolateral): pain, temperature

- From the dorsal rootlets of spinal nerves, fibres enter the adjacent dorsal horn of grey matter and synapse in this region within a segment or two.
- Axons of secondary sensory neurons cross the midline and ascend in the spinothalamic tracts in the

lateral white column to the ventral nucleus of the thalamus.

- The spinal cord tract in this system is made up of secondary sensory neurons and is *contralateral* with respect to the source of the impulse.

From cranial nerves

Most somatic sensory fibres are carried in V and a small number enter the brain stem in X, but within the central nervous system all somatosensory fibres pass to the trigeminal sensory nuclei.

Trigeminal sensory nuclei

The trigeminal sensory nucleus has three parts, each for different modalities.

- Principal or chief nucleus: tactile sensation. This is in the pons and receives the central processes of primary sensory neurons transmitting tactile sensation. From the nucleus, axons decussate and ascend in the trigeminal lemniscus to the contralateral thalamus. A small proportion of fibres may also pass to the ipsilateral thalamus.
- The spinal nucleus: pain and temperature sensation. This is so called because it extends down through the medulla into the cervical spinal cord and is continuous with the dorsal horn of spinal grey matter (which also receives pain and temperature fibres). From the nucleus, axons decussate and ascend in the trigeminal lemniscus to the contralateral thalamus.
- The mesencephalic nucleus: proprioceptive sensation etc. This is in the upper pons and lower midbrain and receives proprioceptive information from masticatory muscles, and deep pressure sensation from the teeth and gums (see 14.7, pp. 249, 250). The mesencephalic nucleus is unique since it houses primary sensory nerve cell bodies which, for all other sensory fibres, would be in a peripheral ganglion. Details of its connections are not clear, but some pass to the motor nucleus of V, the salivatory nuclei, and the nucleus ambiguus, for chewing and swallowing.

Visceral sensation (e.g. taste, internal organs)

Much less is known about visceral sensation pathways. All that you need to know is that it is all handled by the nucleus of the solitary tract in the lateral medulla, no matter how it gets there (see Fig. 14.15, p. 235). Axons from the nucleus of the solitary tract pass to the salivatory nuclei (for salivation reflexes) and also rostrally by multisynaptic pathways, to the thalamus, and probably the insula and uncus for connections with olfactory centres. As pointed out earlier (p. 235), none of this matters clinically.

15.9 Special sensation

Overview

Olfactory impulses pass to components of the limbic system and the temporal lobe. Visual impulses pass to the occipital cortex for vision and to the midbrain for visual reflexes. Auditory pathways pass to the temporal lobe. Vestibular impulses pass mainly to the cerebellum. There are numerous other connections allowing for integration between systems, both within the brain and from brain to spine cord. A good example of such a pathway is the medial longitudinal fasciculus that coordinates cranial nerve nuclei of III, IV and VI with vestibular and cerebellar function.

Learning Objectives

You should:

- know in outline the olfactory, auditory and vestibular pathways
- know in some detail the pathways for vision and visual reflexes
- understand the anatomy of nystagmus.

Olfactory pathways in the brain

The olfactory epithelium and nasal cavity were considered in Chapter 14 (14.9, p. 254).

The connections of the olfactory bulb are not fully established. Olfactory impulses pass posteriorly from the olfactory tract to the limbic system, particularly the uncus and amygdala of the temporal lobe, thus providing connections with memory circuitry and much else.

Olfaction and taste. The pleasures of eating and drinking lie as much with smell as with taste: it is a common experience that an upper respiratory tract infection which interferes with the sense of smell impairs the enjoyment of food. Olfaction and taste are clearly closely linked and it is thought that from the nucleus of the solitary tract, to which taste fibres pass, axons project to the uncus to connect with olfactory centres.

Temporal lobe tumours. Diseases such as epilepsy in the areas to which the olfactory impulses project (e.g.

the temporal lobe) may cause olfactory hallucinations. The smells are usually unpleasant and are often accompanied by pseudo-purposeful movements associated with tasting such as licking the lips. Temporal lobe tumours may also present as mood or memory disturbances – more evidence of limbic functions.

Visual pathways in the brain

The visual pathways as far back as the lateral geniculate bodies were considered in Chapter 14 (14.11, p. 263).

Lateral geniculate body, optic radiation, visual cortex

In the lateral geniculate body, axons of retinal ganglion cells synapse with cell bodies of neurons forming the optic radiation. This passes backwards, skirting the posterior limb of the internal capsule and the lentiform nucleus (thus they are described as retrolenticular), and around the inferior horn of the lateral ventricle to end in the visual cortex in the occipital lobe.

- Lesions of this part of the visual pathway depend upon precisely which part of the lateral geniculate body or optic radiation is affected since there is a precise retinotopic arrangement in the optic radiation and visual cortex.
- Revise the connections of the visual pathway with the midbrain (14.11, p. 267) and Figure 14.35 (p. 269) for the pathway of the pupillary light and other reflexes.

Blood supply of visual cortex (Fig. 15.17)

Although the posterior cerebral artery supplies most of the visual cortex, both middle and posterior arteries generally supply the cortex to which the macula of the retina projects. This is one of the explanations given for the phenomenon of macular sparing in which vision at the macula may be preserved even though the surrounding areas of the visual cortex are no longer functional. As with the bilateral cortical innervation of muscles involved in eye movements, there may be an evolutionary basis for this.

Auditory pathways in the brain

The auditory pathways as far back as the cochlear nuclei were considered in Chapter 14 (14.10, p. 261).

Cochlear nuclei, medial geniculate body, auditory cortex

From the cochlear nuclei, neurons pass bilaterally to the inferior colliculi (midbrain, for auditory reflexes) and the medial geniculate bodies (diencephalon). Some neurons pass to other centres (e.g. medial longitudinal fasciculus, reticular formation, spinal cord) for integration with other systems. Axons from medial geniculate bodies project through the internal capsule to the auditory cortex in the upper part of the temporal lobe on the inferior operculum, in the territory of middle cerebral artery.

Note. Visual system: lateral geniculate bodies, superior colliculi; auditory system: medial geniculate bodies, inferior colliculi.

Vestibular pathways in the brain

The vestibular pathways and the cerebellum have been considered above (15.3, p. 291) and in Chapter 14 (14.10, p. 262).

Vestibular nuclei and connections

Most fibres from the vestibular apparatus pass straight to the vestibulocerebellum. Of those that do not, some descend in vestibulospinal tracts to the spinal cord, and others pass to the medial longitudinal fasciculus for integration with eye muscle nuclei. The vestibular system projects to the thalamus and, since we have a conscious awareness of stability in space, impulses may pass to parts of cerebral cortex.

Clinical box

Vertebrobasilar insufficiency
The labyrinthine artery is a branch of the vertebrobasilar system and enters the internal acoustic meatus to supply VII, VIII and the inner ear. Lesions of this artery, or of the vertebrobasilar system, can cause vertigo and unsteadiness. Narrowing of the vertebral arteries by either atherosclerosis or by disease of the cervical spine may lead to these symptoms with neck movements.

Inability to localise sounds in space
A unilateral lesion of the auditory cortex, though not resulting in profound deafness because of bilateral pathways, may lead to difficulty in localising the source of a sound. This is socially awkward and can be dangerous, for example when crossing the road.

Acoustic neuroma
This has been mentioned before. It may compress both VII and VIII causing a nerve deafness, vestibular disorders and, eventually, an ipsilateral facial palsy.

Nystagmus
This also has been mentioned before. Disorders of the vestibular system, the cerebellum, and/or the medial longitudinal fasciculus in the brain stem, may lead to pathological nystagmus with slow eye movements in one direction followed by quick movements in the other. It requires investigation.

15.10 Clinical miscellany

Your attention has already been drawn to clinical conditions illustrating individual points of the anatomy of the head and neck and cranial nerves. The anatomy of the brain is so complex, however, that a single lesion can have profound effects on a combination of different neurological systems and some of these are considered here.

Stroke, cerebrovascular accident (CVA)

- A lesion in the genu of the internal capsule would produce sensory and motor loss in the contralateral side of the head. This may not be complete since there is bilateral cortical innervation of some cranial nerve nuclei. The motor symptoms could produce a pseudobulbar palsy (see p. 298).
- A lesion in the posterior limb of the internal capsule would produce motor and sensory signs in the contralateral side of the body.
- Monoplegia is weakness or paralysis of one limb, possibly arising as a result of a lesion of a specific limb area of one motor cortex.
- Hemiplegia is weakness or paralysis of one side of the body, possibly arising as a result of an internal capsule lesion, or a lesion elsewhere on the corticospinal pathway.
- Quadriplegia is weakness or paralysis of all four limbs, probably arising as a result of injury to the cervical spine which completely sections the spinal cord below the origin of the phrenic nerve (so diaphragmatic breathing is preserved). In these cases, the spinal cord below the lesion is completely cut off from the brain and each spinal cord segment functions only as a component of a segmental reflex. The sphincters innervated by S2–4 would revert to automatic emptying as required as a result of reflex sensory stimulation.

Bilateral upper motor neuron lesions of the lower limbs

Your detective powers may be tried by this until you realise that because of the anatomy of the motor cortex, and the manner in which the body is represented on it, the two motor areas for the lower limbs are actually very close to one another on the medial sides of the two cerebral hemispheres: they are separated only by the falx cerebri. In theory, these symptoms could be produced by occlusion of both anterior cerebral arteries which supply these areas, but, on the ground that one explanation is better than two, the symptoms could be produced by an enlarging tumour of the falx itself which presses on the medial surfaces of both hemispheres. This is a sagittal meningioma.

Pyramidal, extrapyramidal

Paralysis with hyperreflexia and hypertonia probably means a lesion of the corticospinal (pyramidal) tract. These are often called pyramidal symptoms.

Uncontrolled involuntary movements probably means a lesion of the basal ganglia, or tracts descending from them which do not pass deep to the pyramids. These are often called extrapyramidal symptoms.

Medial longitudinal fasciculus

Now that this brief survey of the brain is complete you should revise the medial longitudinal fasciculus and its connections, and nystagmus (14.10, p. 262; 14.11, p. 265).

Multiple sclerosis

Multiple (disseminated) sclerosis is a disease of myelin produced by oligodendrocytes. It can strike anywhere in the central nervous system causing symptoms as a result of defective neurotransmission.

Spinal cord lesions and sensory symptoms

From receptors in one part of the body, some sensory impulses ascend in the contralateral side of the spinal cord, and some in the ipsilateral. To any muscle, most impulses come from the contralateral cortex but descend in the ipsilateral side of the cord. The interpretation of symptoms of spinal cord lesions is therefore not straightforward. For example, if the right half of the spinal cord is damaged at spinal cord segment T6:

- all ipsilateral sensory fibres entering at that level will be affected
- all ipsilateral motor fibres leaving at that level will be affected
- contralateral pain and temperature fibres from the body at all levels below the injury will be interrupted
- ipsilateral dorsal column sensation from the body at all levels below the injury will be interrupted.

It is somewhat less complex with motor symptoms because most motor fibres in the spinal cord pass to the same side of the body.

These detective games are often made more difficult by the fact that there may be other features complicating the clinical picture.

And finally ... **15**

15.11 And finally ...

When you reflect on this brief consideration of the brain, you may be able to perceive a caudal (bottom) to rostral (top) progression in functional terms. Unconscious mechanical functions, such as would be possessed by a primitive vertebrate, seem to be housed in the hindbrain. More sophisticated functions like visual and auditory reflexes, so essential in detecting approaching predators or prey, are prominent in the midbrain. Bodily homeo-

stasis is a function of the diencephalon. The limbic system in the caudal telencephalon deals with urges and emotions and, most rostrally of all, what passes for intellectual function is based in the cortex. You might like to consider whether or not some psychiatric disease is caused by the intellectual activity of the cerebral cortex suppressing the basic urges of the limbic system. If you feel the need to throw this book at someone, and do so, you might be preserving your mental health but you must be prepared to take the consequences.

Self-assessment: questions

Multiple choice questions

1. The following cranial nerves arise as stated:
   a. XII: medulla, lateral to olive.
   b. X: medulla, medial to olive.
   c. VI, VII: cerebellopontine angle.
   d. V: pons.
   e. III: interpeduncular fossa of midbrain.

2. The following are midline structures:
   a. The foramen of Magendie.
   b. The foramen of Monro.
   c. The pineal.
   d. The thalamus.
   e. The pyramid.

3. The following are derivatives of the diencephalon:
   a. The third ventricle.
   b. The substantia nigra.
   c. The retina.
   d. The thalamus.
   e. The neurohypophysis.

4. A voluntary motor impulse from the cerebral cortex to the right biceps brachii muscle:
   a. Passes through the posterior limb of the left internal capsule.
   b. Passes through the left substantia nigra of the midbrain.
   c. Decussates above the pyramids of the medulla.
   d. Descends in the spinal cord in the right lateral corticospinal tract.
   e. Synapses on ventral horn cells in spinal cord segments C5 and C6.

5. Fine touch and vibration sense impulses from the skin over the left patella:
   a. Synapse in the left dorsal root ganglion of L3.
   b. Ascend in the left dorsal column of white matter of the spinal cord.
   c. Decussate in the lower medulla.
   d. Ascend through the brain stem as the right medial lemniscus.
   e. Pass in the midbrain ventral to the substantia nigra.

6. A left pupil that did not respond to the shining of a light into the right eye might result from:
   a. An opaque right cornea and/or lens.
   b. A severed right optic nerve.
   c. Damage to the right lateral geniculate body.
   d. Damage to the right Edinger–Westphal nucleus.
   e. Damage to the left oculomotor nerve.

7. The lateral medullary (Wallenberg's or PICA) syndrome:
   a. May be caused by blockage of the posterior inferior cerebellar artery.
   b. May cause disturbances of facial temperature sensation.
   c. Would impair swallowing and speaking.
   d. May involve the nucleus ambiguus.
   e. Would involve the pyramids.

8. All the following structures are found in the midbrain:
   a. Red nucleus.
   b. Substantia nigra.
   c. Superior colliculus.
   d. Facial colliculus.
   e. Aqueduct of Sylvius.

9. The head and neck area of the motor cortex:
   a. Lies in the postcentral gyrus.
   b. Extends on to the medial surface of the hemisphere.
   c. Is supplied by the anterior cerebral artery.
   d. Is part of the occipital lobe.
   e. Is related to the pterion.

10. In the internal capsule:
    a. The thalamus is related to the anterior and posterior limbs.
    b. The optic radiation occupies the anterior limb.
    c. The anterior limb contains the main motor and sensory tracts.
    d. The caudate nucleus is lateral to the anterior limb.
    e. Blood supply is from branches of the middle cerebral artery.

11. Lower motor neuron lesions are characterised by:
    a. Flaccidity.
    b. Hyporeflexia.
    c. Wasting.
    d. Sensory loss.
    e. Contralateral symptoms with respect to site of lesion.

12. The spinothalamic tracts serve:
   a. Two-point discrimination.
   b. Pain.
   c. Conscious proprioception.
   d. Heat.
   e. Vision.

Matching item questions

Questions 1–12

Match the numbered item to the lettered response. Each lettered response may be used once, more than once, or not at all.
   a. middle cerebral artery or branches
   b. posterior cerebral artery or branches
   c. anterior cerebral artery or branches
   d. vertebrobasilar system
   e. middle meningeal artery or branches
1. motor cortex for upper limb
2. motor cortex for lower limb
3. sensory cortex for head
4. sensory cortex for lower limb
5. motor nucleus for phonation and swallowing
6. most of visual cortex
7. auditory cortex
8. frontal cortex
9. inner ear
10. internal capsule
11. cranial dura
12. diploë

Questions 13–25

Match the numbered item to the lettered response. Each lettered response may be used once, more than once, or not at all.
   a. solitary tract and nucleus
   b. nucleus ambiguus
   c. medial longitudinal fasciculus
   d. spinal nucleus of V
   e. facial nucleus
13. nystagmus
14. speech
15. oral pain
16. chemoreceptor sensation
17. toothache
18. taste sensation from the pharynx
19. earache
20. taste sensation from the tongue
21. facial paralysis
22. muscles of swallowing
23. heat sensation on the tongue
24. hyperacusis
25. facial pain

Questions requiring short answers

1. Trace the course of a motor impulse from the motor cortex to the left masseter muscle. Give details of cell bodies, synapse(s), decussations (if any), and give the blood supply of that part of the pathway within the forebrain.

2. Where is CSF produced, how does it circulate and where is it resorbed? What would happen if its passage through the midbrain were blocked?

3. What and where is the substantia nigra? What is known of its function and its connections?

4. Trace the course of a pain impulse from the left upper incisors. Give details of cell bodies, synapse(s), decussation (if any), and give the blood supply of those parts of the brain to which these impulses are relayed.

5. Describe the connections of the vestibular system. Explain why vestibular disease may give rise to nystagmus.

6. A patient imagines he can detect odours that other people can not. When out walking he is almost knocked down by a car because he did not hear it approaching. After some weeks he begins to notice mood disturbance and personality changes. Can you put this story together with one cause?

7. Following a cerebrovascular accident (stroke), a patient is unable to swallow normally. Trace the course of a motor nerve impulse from the motor cortex to the left pharyngeal musculature. Include details of central pathways, synapses (if any), decussation (if any), and peripheral course. Explain where the lesion might be and add any other notes you wish.

8. Compare and contrast the trigeminal and pterygopalatine ganglia.

Self-assessment: answers

Multiple choice answers

1. a. **False.** XII arises medially, between olive and pyramid.
   b. **False.** It arises lateral to the olive, with IX and XI.
   c. **False.** VI does not, VII does.
   d. **True.**
   e. **True.**

2. a. **True.**
   b. **False.** Each lateral ventricle communicates with the third ventricle through a foramen of Monro, so there are right and left.
   c. **True.**
   d. **False.** There is a right thalamus and a left thalamus.
   e. **False.** There are right and left pyramids.

3. a. **True.**
   b. **False.** The substantia nigra is in the midbrain (mesencephalon).
   c. **True.**
   d. **True.**
   e. **True.**

4. a. **True.**
   b. **False.** It passes anterior to the substantia nigra, not through it.
   c. **False.** It decussates below the pyramids.
   d. **True.**
   e. **True.**

5. a. **False.** Nothing ever synapses in sensory ganglia.
   b. **True.**
   c. **True.**
   d. **True.**
   e. **False.** Sensory tracts are dorsal to the substantia nigra.

6. a. **True.**
   b. **True.**
   c. **False.** Geniculate bodies have nothing to do with the pupillary light reflex.
   d. **False.** The left Edinger–Westphal nucleus would be relevant, but not the right.
   e. **True.**

7. a. **True.**
   b. **True.** The spinal trigeminal nucleus may be affected.
   c. **True.**
   d. **True.**
   e. **False.** The pyramids are medial.

8. a. **True.**
   b. **True.**
   c. **True.**
   d. **False.** It is in the medulla.
   e. **True.**

9. a. **False.** It is in the precentral gyrus.
   b. **False.** The lower limb portion is medial.
   c. **False.** It is supplied by the middle cerebral artery.
   d. **False.** It is part of the frontal lobe.
   e. **True.**

10. a. **True.** It is medial to both.
    b. **False.** The optic radiation is not really part of the internal capsule at all.
    c. **False.** These are in the posterior limb.
    d. **False.** The caudate nucleus is medial to the anterior limb.
    e. **True.**

11. a. **True.**
    b. **True.**
    c. **True.**
    d. **False.** This is a motor lesion.
    e. **False.** Symptoms are ipsilateral with respect to the site of the lesion.

14. a. **False.** This is served by the dorsal columns.
    b. **True.**
    c. **False.** This is served by the dorsal columns.
    d. **True.**
    e. **False.** This is nothing to do with the spinothalamic tracts.

Matching item answers

1. a. This is on the lateral aspect of the cerebrum.
2. c. This is on the medial aspect of the cerebrum.
3. a. This is on the lateral aspect of the cerebrum.
4. c. This is on the medial aspect of the cerebrum.
5. d. The nucleus ambiguus in the medulla supplied by PICA.
6. b.

7. a. The auditory cortex is on the superior surface of the temporal lobe.
8. c.
9. d.
10. a.
11. e.
12. e.
13. c.
14. b.
15. d.
16. a.
17. d.
18. a.
19. d.
20. a.
21. e.
22. b.
23. d.
24. e.
25. d.

Short answers

1. The impulse begins in the right motor cortex deep to pterion (supplied by the middle cerebral artery), and the corticobulbar axon passes through the genu of the internal capsule (supplied by the middle cerebral artery), and the right cerebral peduncle of the midbrain ventral to the substantia nigra. Fibres decussate just before reaching the left trigeminal motor nucleus in the pons, where they synapse on the lower motor neuron cell bodies in the trigeminal nucleus. From there, axons pass in the left trigeminal nerve and branches of the mandibular nerve to the masseter muscle.

2. CSF is produced in the choroid plexus in all ventricles and reabsorbed into the venous system at the arachnoid granulations. Its circulation around the brain and spinal cord is shown in Figure 15.3 (p. 283). If the cerebral aqueduct were blocked, CSF pressure in the lateral and third ventricles would rise.

3. The substantia nigra is an area of pigmented (melanin) grey matter in midbrain, separating the cerebral peduncles from the rest of the midbrain. Depleted dopamine here leads to Parkinson's disease. It is one of the basal ganglia and has connections with the other members of this group (caudate nucleus, putamen, globus pallidus: nigrostriatal) and with the spinal cord (nigrospinal). Unwanted involuntary movements are a feature of basal ganglia (extrapyramidal) disease.

4. Pain impulses pass in palatine branches of the left maxillary nerve (Vb) and then gain the maxillary nerve itself. They then run in Vb through the foramen rotundum to the trigeminal ganglion (cell bodies, no synapse). The trigeminal nerve enters the pons (supplied by the vertebrobasilar system), where pain fibres synapse in the spinal nucleus of V (supplied by the vertebrobasilar system) and axons decussate and ascend to the right thalamus (supplied by the right middle cerebral artery), and on to higher centres including the right sensory cortex (supplied by the right middle cerebral artery).

5. Connections of the vestibular system are:
   • mostly to the cerebellum (flocculonodular node and fastigial nucleus)
   • some to the medial longitudinal fasciculus for coordination of III, IV, VI, etc.
   • some to vomiting and other centres
   • some to trunk muscles for neck movements etc. (e.g. startle reflex).
   Nystagmus results from overstimulation of the medial longitudinal fasciculus as a result of vestibular disease.

6. A temporal lobe tumour is the probable cause. These may present with:
   • olfactory hallucinations: uncus
   • failure to localise the direction of sound: auditory cortex
   • mood changes: components of the limbic system (amygdala, hippocampus).

7. From the right motor cortex, the impulse passes through the genu of the right internal capsule, the right cerebral peduncle, and the right pons, crossing to the left nucleus ambiguus in the medulla. Here it synapses and impulses pass in the left vagus and through pharyngeal branches to pharyngeal muscles. The lesion could be in the left nucleus ambiguus (bulbar palsy), or the corticobulbar tract above it (e.g. right internal capsule).

8. Similarities: both are swellings on nerves, both contain cell bodies. Differences: the trigeminal ganglion is sensory, so has no synapses; the pterygopalatine is parasympathetic, so contains synapses. The trigeminal ganglion is susceptible to anaesthetics; the pterygopalatine is susceptible to neurotransmitter blocking agents.

16 Surface anatomy: revision

Head and neck

Lateral aspect

Position	Significance
Pterion: 4 cm (about) above and anterior to pinna	Anterior division of middle meningeal vessels behind thinnest area of skull, extradural haemorrhages
Pterion: above and behind	Central sulcus of cerebral cortex separating motor cortex (anterior) and sensory cortex (posterior)
2 cm (about) above pinna	Auditory cortex Superficial temporal pulse (often visible)
Between pinna and mandible, extending below angle of mandible	Parotid gland
Anterior to pinna	Parotid nodes
Mastoid process	Mastoid lymph nodes
Temporomandibular joint, below and behind	Terminal branching of external carotid artery

Anterior aspect

Position	Significance
Bridge of the nose, above and behind	Cribriform plate: anterior cranial fossa fractures, anosmia, CSF rhinorrhoea
Supraorbital foramen	Supraorbital nerve (Va) and vessels: fractures
Infraorbital foramen	Infraorbital nerves (Vb) and vessels: fractures
Mental foramen	Mental nerve (Vc) and vessels: fractures

Posterior aspect

Position	Significance
External occipital protuberance, above	Visual cortex
External occipital protuberance	Confluence of sinuses
External occipital protuberance, below	Cerebellum

Neck

Position	Significance	Approx. vertebral level
Hyoid bone, angle of mandible	Tonsillar (jugulo-digastric) node	C2
Ear lobe (roughly) – sternoclavicular joint	Internal jugular vein, deep cervical chain of lymph nodes (deep to sternocleidomastoid)	
Angle of mandible – midpoint of clavicle	External jugular vein	
Lateral to superior border of thyroid cartilage	Bifurcation of common carotid artery, carotid pulse	C3
Behind, and slightly below, thyroid prominence	Vocal cords	C4
Cricothyroid membrane	Laryngotomy site	C5
Cricoid cartilage	Cricopharyngeal sphincter, upper extent of oesophagus, trachea	C6
Sternocleidomastoid, trapezius, clavicle	Boundaries of posterior triangle	
Posterior triangle: one-third of way down posterior border – one-third of way up anterior border	Accessory nerve (XI)	

Thorax

Position	Significance	Approx. vertebral level
Sternoclavicular joint	Formation of brachiocephalic veins (from subclavian, internal jugular)	T2
Suprasternal notch	Trachea	T2
First intercostal space, anteriorly	Formation of superior vena cava	T3
Sternal angle (of Louis)	Bifurcation of trachea, lower limit of arch of aorta	T4
	Hilum of lung	T5/6

Pleural cavities and reflexions

2, 4, 6, 8, 10, 12: 2 cm above clavicle – sternoclavicular joint – second costal cartilage – fourth costal cartilage – sixth costal cartilage (more lateral on the left) – eighth rib, midclavicular line – tenth rib, midaxillary line – twelfth rib (or lower), midscapular line (behind) – side of vertebra L1.

Lungs

These are similar to the pleura except that lung tissue does not extend much below vertebral level T10.

- Oblique fissure (both sides): spine of vertebra T2 or T3 – sixth costal cartilage.
- Horizontal fissure: level of fourth costal cartilage, sternal edge – line of oblique fissure.
- Chest drain: second intercostal space in midclavicular line *or* fourth or fifth space in midaxillary line.

Heart borders

2 × 3 = 6: second intercostal space, left sternal edge – third intercostal space, right sternal edge – sixth intercostal space, right sternal edge – fifth intercostal space, midclavicular line (normal apex) – back to top.

Heart valves

Valve	Position	Best heard
Pulmonary	Retrosternal, level of 3rd rib	2nd space just to left of sternal edge
Aortic	Retrosternal, level of 3rd space	2nd space just to right of sternal edge
Mitral	Retrosternal, level of 4th rib	Apex (5th space, midclavicular line)
Tricuspid	Retrosternal, level of 4th space	Lower sternal edge, side depending upon the condition

Abdomen and pelvis

Anterior abdominal wall

- Nine regions: see Figure 11.1 (p. 100). Of these:
  - epigastrium: stomach, liver, aorta
  - umbilical region: aorta is palpable above the umbilicus
  - hypogastrium or suprapubic region: uterus, bladder
  - right hypochondrium: liver and gall bladder
  - left hypochondrium: enlarged spleen
  - lumbar region: lower poles of the kidneys, colon
  McBurney's point: one–third of the way from the right anterior superior iliac spine to the umbilicus: base of appendix, caecum.
- Quadrants:
  - right upper quadrant (gall bladder, enlarged liver)
  - left upper quadrant (enlarged spleen)
  - right lower quadrant (appendix, caecum, etc.)
  - left lower quadrant (sigmoid colon etc.)

Abdomen, anterior aspect

Position	Significance	Approx. vertebral level
Nipple, fourth intercostal space	Liver, upper limit	T7
Xiphoid process		T10
	Origin of coeliac artery	T12
	Origin of superior mesenteric artery	T12/L1
Tip of 9th costal cartilage	Transpyloric plane: gall bladder, pylorus, duodenojejunal flexure, hilum of kidneys, head of pancreas	L1
Subcostal plane	Origin of gonadal, inferior mesenteric artery (approximate)	L2/3
Umbilicus, just below and to the left	Bifurcation of aorta	L3/4
McBurney's point: one-third of way between right anterior superior iliac spine and umbilicus	Base of appendix, caecum	L4
Anterior superior iliac spine	Lateral cutaneous nerve of thigh, inguinal ligament attachment	L5
Midinguinal point	Femoral pulse	
2 cm above midinguinal point	Deep inguinal ring	
Pubic tubercle, above	Superficial inguinal ring	

Abdomen, posterior aspect

Position	Significance	Approx. vertebral level
Ribs 9, 10, 11	Spleen	T11
Rib 12	Upper pole of kidneys, costodiaphragmatic recess	T12
	Hilum of kidney	L1/2
Line between highest points of iliac crests	Lumbar puncture, extradural anaesthesia	L3/4

Upper limb

Position	Structure, significance
Axilla	Axillary lymph nodes (breast cancer etc.)
Arm: medial to biceps muscle	Brachial pulse
Cubital fossa	Biceps tendon
Cubital fossa: medial to biceps tendon	Brachial pulse
Cubital fossa: medial to brachial pulse	Median nerve
Wrist: radial side of (lateral to) tendon of flexor carpi ulnaris	Radial pulse
Wrist: ulnar side of (medial to) tendon of flexor carpi ulnaris	Ulnar pulse, ulnar nerve
Wrist: midline	Median nerve
Wrist: dorsum/radial side, between tendons of extensors pollicis longus and brevis	Anatomical snuff box, scaphoid (tenderness could signify fractured scaphoid)
Wrist: 2 cm square distal to the distal wrist crease in midline	Flexor retinaculum
Palpable carpal bones	Pisiform, hamate (ulnar side); scaphoid, trapezium (radial side)
Fleshy muscle between thumb and index finger	First dorsal interosseous

Lower limb

Position	Structure, significance	Position	Structure, significance
Gluteal region: midway between posterior superior iliac spine and ischial tuberosity – midway between ischial tuberosity and greater trochanter	Sciatic nerve in gluteal region (to be avoided in injections)	Between biceps femoris, lateral head of gastrocnemius (laterally); semitendinosus, medial head of gastrocnemius (medially)	Popliteal fossa
Inguinal region: midpoint of inguinal ligament	Femoral pulse (arterial blood for blood gases estimations)	Popliteal fossa: upper part, compress artery against popliteal surface of femur	Popliteal pulse (artery here is vulnerable in supracondylar femoral fracture)
Inguinal region: medial to femoral pulse	Femoral vein	Neck of fibula, biceps attachment	Common fibular nerve
Inguinal region: lateral to femoral pulse	Femoral nerve	Ankle: halfway between medial and lateral malleoli	Anterior tibial pulse
Inguinal region: about 2 cm below and lateral to pubic tubercle	Saphenous opening, femoral hernia	Ankle: anterior to medial malleolus Ankle: 2 cm behind medial malleolus	Saphenous vein and nerve at the ankle Posterior tibial pulse, flexor retinaculum
Covering saphenous opening and medial part of inguinal ligament	Inguinal lymph nodes (perineal, lower limb disease)	Foot: between tendons of extensor hallucis longus	Dorsalis pedis pulse
Patella:		and extensor digitorum longus on dorsum of foot	
Extending about 5 cm above upper margin	Suprapatellar bursa	Palpable foot bones	Head of talus, sustentaculum tali, navicular
Anterior Below	Prepatellar bursa Infrapatellar bursa		

Index